D0081458

Physical Therapist Assistant Exam Review

Physical Therapist Assistant Exam Review

Kevin Tenpenny, PTA

Associate Professor

Physical Therapist Assistant, and Massage Therapy Programs

Kaskaskia College

Centralia, Illinois

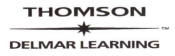

THOMSON

DELMAR LEARNING

Australia　Canada　Mexico　Singapore　Spain　United Kingdom　United States

RM
706
.T467
2004

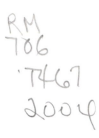

THOMSON
™
DELMAR LEARNING

Physical Therapist Assistant Exam Review
by Kevin Tenpenny

Vice President, Health Care Business Unit:
William Brottmiller

Editorial Director:
Cathy L. Esperti

Developmental Editor:
Maria D'Angelico

Marketing Director:
Jennifer McAvey

Channel Manager:
Tamara Caruso

Marketing Coordinator:
Chris Manion

Acquisitions Editor:
Kalen Conerly

Project Editor:
Jack Pendleton

Technology Coordinator:
Mary Colleen Liburdi

COPYRIGHT © 2004 by Thomson Delmar Learning, a part of The Thomson Corporation. Thomson, the Star logo, and Delmar Learning are trademarks used herein under license.

Printed in the United States of America
1 2 3 4 5 XXX 08 07 06 05 04 03

For more information, contact
Thomson Delmar Learning,
5 Maxwell Drive, Clifton Park, NY 12065
Or find us on the World Wide Web at
http://www.delmarlearning.com

ALL RIGHTS RESERVED. No part of this work covered by the copyright hereon may be reproduced or used in any form or by any means—graphic, electronic, or mechanical, including photocopying, recording, taping, Web distribution or information storage and retrieval systems—without the written permission of the publisher.

For permission to use material from this text or product, contact us by
Tel (800) 730-2214
Fax (800) 730-2215
www.thomsonrights.com

Library of Congress Cataloging-in-Publication Data

Tenpenny, Kevin.
Physical therapist assistant exam review / Kevin Tenpenny.
p. ; cm.
Includes bibliographical references.
ISBN 1-4018-1403-4
1. Physical therapy assistants—Examinations, questions, etc.
[DNLM: 1. Physical Therapy Techniques—Examination Questions. WB 18.2 T312p 2004] I. Title.
RM706.T467 2004
615.8'2'076—dc22

2004041250

NOTICE TO THE READER

Publisher does not warrant or guarantee any of the products described herein or perform any independent analysis in connection with any of the product information contained herein. Publisher does not assume, and expressly disclaims, any obligation to obtain and include information other than that provided to it by the manufacturer.

The reader is expressly warned to consider and adopt all safety precautions that might be indicated by the activities described herein and to avoid all potential hazards. By following the instructions contained herein, the reader willingly assumes all risks in connection with such instructions.

The publisher makes no representations or warranties of any kind, including but not limited to, the warranties of fitness for particular purpose or merchantability, nor are any such representations implied with respect to the material set forth herein, and the publisher takes no responsibility with respect to such material. The publisher shall not be liable for any special, consequential, or exemplary damages resulting, in whole or part, from the reader's use of, or reliance upon, this material.

This book is dedicated to Barb, my partner, friend, and wife,
and to Nathan and Evan, my heroes and sons.
Thank you for your love and endurance.

About the Author

Kevin Tenpenny, PTA, is an Associate Professor at Kaskaskia College in Centralia, Illinois. He is a full-time faculty member for the Physical Therapist Assistant and Massage Therapy programs; he also teaches courses in medical terminology. He began teaching at the community college level in 1995.

Professor Tenpenny earned his Associate of Applied Science Degree while serving in the United States Air Force from 1989 to 1996. He was recognized as the 1994 United States Air Force Outstanding Physical Therapy Specialist of the Year.

He is an active member of the American Physical Therapy Association (APTA) and currently serves as the Secretary/Treasurer for the Southern District of the Illinois Chapter of the APTA. His clinical practice experience is diverse with many years experience in acute, inpatient, skilled care, orthopedics, outpatient, and rehabilitation. He currently practices in neurological, orthopedic, and subacute rehabilitation.

Professor Tenpenny has conducted several professional presentations at the local and state level. His presentations include the areas of kinesiology, therapeutic exercise, physical agents, and educational strategies for developing the affective domain in physical therapy students. His published abstracts include A Model for Learning and Applying Therapeutic Strengthening (AMFLATS), and as co-author for Continuing Clinical Competence Among Community College Faculty. He has created a multitude of innovative learning aids and supplements for physical therapist assistant students.

Contents

Preface

The PTA Exam Review book and CD ROM are essential for preparing to challenge the National Physical Therapist Assistant Examination (NPTAE). It is also a beneficial tool for review by practicing physical therapist assistants. The question often arises, "When should I buy a review book?" Of course, during your education, the first objective is to meet the academic and clinical standards to be eligible to take the licensure exam. However, it is by no means too early to prepare for the NPTAE before graduation. The sooner you begin to improve your multiple-choice testing skills, and improve your clinical reasoning with the exam content, the sooner you can achieve exam competency. This product has been developed based upon the latest content outline and format of the NPTAE. In the near future, the NPTAE will include visual references such as pictures or digital video images.

The first purpose for this book was to provide the greatest number of licensure-related items to cover a broader and deeper content than previous review books. The second purpose was to enhance content-specific review through a diverse set of questions. The items used are based upon input from a variety of academic and clinical professionals. Physical therapist assistant (PTA) students and entry-level and experienced PTAs tested many of the items.

The text is organized into nine chapters. The first section and chapter introduces the process of preparing and taking the NPTAE. This chapter should be completed first to identify common test-taking errors and strategies for success with the practice items and the NPTAE. Chapters 2–9 are divided based upon the major content areas of the NPTAE outline. The objective of each of these chapters is for a content-based review for the user.

Section 2 of the book, which contains Chapters 2 and 3, deals with the critical knowledge and skills related to data collection. Data collection is the smallest content area, addressing 21.3% of the exam or 32 of 150 items on the exam. Chapter 2 covers the first group of tests and measurements for data collection, with 102 items related to measuring muscle strength and length, range of motion, posture, body segments, cognition, reflexes, and sensation. The content area of Chapter 2 addresses 11.3% of the exam or 17 of 150 items on the exam. Chapter 3 covers the second group of tests and measurements for data collection, with 90 items related to the cardiovascular system, pulmonary system, integumentary system, and measuring functional status. The content area of Chapter 3 addresses 10% of the exam or 15 of 150 items on the exam.

Section 3 of the book, which contains Chapters 4–8, deals with knowledge and skills related to nonprocedural and procedural interventions. Intervention is the largest content area as it addresses 60% of the exam or 90 of 150 items on the exam. Chapter 4 covers the nonprocedural interventions with 168 items related to coordination of care, communication, patient/family instructions, and documentation. The content area of Chapter 4 addresses 18.7% of the exam or 28 of 150 items on the exam. Chapter 5 covers the third group of procedural interventions with 96 items related to exercise and manual therapy. The content area of Chapter 5 addresses 10.7% of the exam or 16 of 150 items on the exam.

Chapter 6 covers the second group of procedural interventions with 102 items related to transfers, functional activities, gait training, equipment training, and environment modification. The content area of Chapter 6 addresses 11.3% of the exam or 17 of 150 items on the exam. Chapter 7 covers the third group of procedural interventions with 120 items related to physical agents and modalities. The content area of Chapter 7 addresses 13.3% of the exam or 20 of 150 items on the exam. Chapter 8 covers the fourth group of procedural interventions with 54 items related to airway clearance, wound care, health promotion, wellness, monitoring patient responses, and modifying interventions. The content area of Chapter 8 addresses 18.7% of the exam or 28 of 150 items on the exam.

The fourth and last section of the book covers critical knowledge and skills related to standards of care. The content area addresses 18.7% of the exam or 28 of 150 items on the exam. Chapter 9 has 168 items that deal with patient confidentiality, professional issues, legal and ethical issues, body mechanics, positioning, safety, first aid, cardiopulmonary resuscitation, sterile technique, universal precautions, and equipment preparation.

In addition of these 950 items in Chapters 2–9, the CD ROM includes three full-length (150 item) practice exams. Each of these exams is constructed with the ratio of content areas outlined in the current version of the NPTAE. The CD ROM practice exams are timed to facilitate the appropriate pacing through the electronic version of the exam.

Acknowledgments

I wish to thank Ronald DeVera Barredo, PT, EdD, GCS, CMT, for his contributions to Chapter 1 and for introducing me to this project. I also thank the reviewers for their meticulous and valuable critique of the manuscript. Thanks to my students and colleagues for their patience and their willingness to "try it out." I especially thank my wife Barb, who provided unwavering support and detailed critique when I would listen to no one else. I would also like to give a special thanks to Maria D'Angelico and Chris Manion at Thomson Delmar Learning for their encouragement, foresight, and timeliness. They made a first publishing experience survivable.

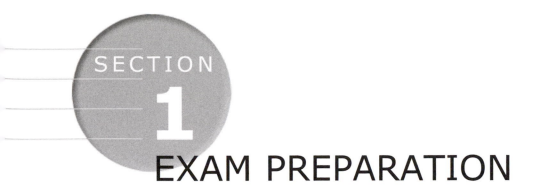

SECTION 1

EXAM PREPARATION

An Introduction to the Physical Therapist Assistant Examination

INTRODUCTION

"To pass or not to pass," that is the question. This is perhaps one of the most important questions an exam candidate has to contend with when faced with the reality of professional practice. For one, the licensing exam is the prospective practitioner's passport to gainful employment and a professional career. In addition, successful passage of the licensing exam demonstrates to the public that the licensee possesses the entry-level competence to practice in the profession.

The purpose of this text is to provide you, the exam candidate, an opportunity not only to understand the context of the Physical Therapist Assistant (PTA) licensing examination but also to develop strategies in preparation for and during the exam. Chapters 2–9 include 950 questions in the same ratio of standardized content areas used in the current exam. This format allows you to identify specific content areas for improvement. In addition, a CD ROM is included with the text containing three full-length simulations (150 questions each) of the computer-based delivery of the exam. The strengths of this text are the 1,400 unduplicated practice questions. In addition, the answer key provides a rationale for each question and published references for further study. Recommended readings are also included in the text.

FIRST THINGS FIRST

There are basically two fundamental reasons why exam candidates fail the licensing exam. The first is related to dealing with the exam format. Challenges related to exam format may include the following:

- Inexperience with multiple-choice exams, especially for applicants who are used to other methods of testing such as essays and identification questions.

- Unfamiliarity with the medium used to deliver the exam, that is, the use of computers especially for applicants who are technologically challenged.

The second reason for failure has to do with the exam content areas. Content-related problems may include the following:

- Applicants possessing a weak body of knowledge and skills related to the standards of the profession.

- Applicants possessing the required competencies, but lacking problem solving and critical thinking skills required to select the correct response to exam questions.

The key to addressing problems associated with format begins with familiarizing yourself with the testing medium and practicing with multiple-choice exam formats. Doing so will allow you the opportunity to sharpen your test taking skills and identify errors in multiple-choice selections. Therefore, the utilization of licensing exam review books especially those with access to computer-based testing formats is ideal.

Problems associated with content require a systematic approach. Applicants need to identify weak content areas relative to entry-level competencies and professional expectations, and develop a plan of remediation to address these content deficiencies. Sometimes, taking one version of the exam helps to identify content areas for improvement. After working on these content areas, taking another version of the exam may be helpful in evaluating the effectiveness of the review. Areas of weakness are also determined through the content-specific questions and answers given in Chapters 2–9.

A CLOSER LOOK AT THE LICENSING EXAM

Exam Content

Through its website, the Federation of State Boards of Physical Therapy (FSBPT) provides a breakdown of exam content for the licensing exam (go to www.fsbpt.org). The exam has three general content areas: Data Collection, Interventions, and Standards of Care. These areas are covered through 150 multiple-choice questions.[1] Distribution of items for each content area is as follows:

- *Data Collection*—21.30% of the exam, or 32 items

- *Interventions*—60.00% of the exam, or 90 items

- *Standards of Care*—18.70% of the exam, or 28 items

This book is organized into sections and chapters similar to the outline used by the FSBPT for the PTA examination. When reading the content outline do not focus much on how many questions will come from each area; rather, emphasis should be placed on asking yourself whether or not the content outline matches your skills and knowledge.

Exam Items

Candidates for the PTA licensing examination currently have $3\frac{1}{2}$ h to answer 175 items. An item poses a question (or stem) for making choices. Each item has four choices, and one of these items is the BEST choice.

The other choices that are less correct are called distracters. Currently, the items are intended to provide four good choices for an item and require the PTA to reason out the BEST response. These items are written by qualified volunteer item writers and further refined in collaboration with and by approval from the higher levels of the examination construction process. The item writers come from diverse backgrounds, clinical experiences, and levels of education. A particular item may be more difficult for you based upon the published references and choices used by the individual writer. The FSBPT makes an effort to approve items and choices that are considered more common. Avoid trying to read every published physical therapy text. You will not be informed as to which items you have answered correctly or incorrectly.

Twenty-five of the 175 items are not included in the calculation of your exam score. These items are being field-tested to determine if they are appropriate. Therefore, only 150 items are used to test the examinees. You will not be informed which 25 items are being excluded from your exam score. Therefore, you need to treat all 175 items as though they are part of the exam. In addition, the exam score is based on the number of items correctly answered; it would be to your benefit to answer every item, even if you are unsure of the correct choice. There is no penalty for guessing at answers. Items not answered are considered incorrect.

The licensing exam items are multiple-choice in format and computer-based in delivery. An introductory tutorial is offered prior to the actual administration of the exam to acquaint you with the process of selecting the best item and moving from one question to the next. You are also given the ability to "mark" questions so that you may move onto another item and return later to answer the marked items. The time utilized during the tutorial does not count against the $3\frac{1}{2}$ h for the test itself. You have approximately 1 min 12 s per exam item, pace yourself for comprehension and clarity.

STUDY SKILLS AND STRATEGIES

Planning for the Exam

Assess Areas of Strength and Weakness

The best way to assess areas of strength and weakness is to take a sample exam without studying, and score the exam accordingly, or perhaps studying only your notes and texts from PTA school. Based on the items answered correctly and incorrectly, you can determine your content areas of strength and weakness. Once the self-assessment is complete, your study time and study strategy can begin.

Develop and Maintain a Realistic and Systematic Study Schedule

Most exam candidates have more usable study time than they would acknowledge. In the event that there appears to be little time for review, then make efficient use of your time! You need to know which content to study for which duration of time. For example, the schedule may be *linear*, with only a single pass of a long block of time for each content area until the arrival of the exam date. The linear approach to studying is more appropriate for the exam candidates who typically study in this manner, and those who tend to manage their time well. On the other hand, the schedule may be cyclical, with several passes of shorter blocks of time for each content area until the arrival of the exam date. The *cyclical* approach is more appropriate for the "less organized" exam candidates, or those who need to improve several areas of content knowledge. Also, try short breaks during the day to review content areas, or practice 10–20 questions.

Sample Study Schedule

Linear Approach

Week One:
1. Review content area: Tests and Measurements Groups I and II (see Table of Contents)
2. Take Chapters 2 and 3 practice questions
3. Review areas for improvement

Week Two:
1. Review content area: Nonprocedural Interventions (see Table of Contents)
2. Take Chapter 4 practice questions
3. Review areas for improvement

Week Three:
1. Review content area: Procedural Interventions Group I (see Table of Contents)
2. Take Chapter 5 practice questions
3. Review areas for improvement

Week Four:
1. Review content area: Procedural Interventions Group II (see Table of Contents)
2. Take Chapter 6 practice questions
3. Review areas for improvement

Week Five:
1. Review content area: Procedural Interventions Groups III and IV (see Table of Contents)
2. Take Chapters 7 and 8 practice questions
3. Review areas for improvement

Week Six:
1. Review content area: Standards of Care (see Table of Contents)
2. Take Chapter 9 practice questions
3. Review areas for improvement

Week Seven:
1. Take practice exams on CD ROM
2. Review areas for improvement

Week Eight: Pass the Exam!

Cyclical Approach

Week One: Take Practice Exam One

Week Two: Review Chapters 2–5 content areas for improvement

Week Three: Review Chapters 6–9 content areas for improvement

Week Four: Take Practice Exam Two

Week Five: Review Chapters 2–9 content areas for improvement

Week Six: Take Practice Exam Three

Week Seven: Review Chapters 2–9 content areas for improvement

Week Eight: Pass the Exam!

The Eve of the Big Day

Eat, Sleep, Relax, and Enjoy

When eating meals, make sure that the meals are not out of your common diet to minimize the effects of stomach indigestion or bladder/bowel irritation. The use of some caffeine may provide some increase in mental alertness. However, for some people this may do more to increase nervousness and impair focus. You should develop and abide by a study schedule that allows you to complete your review two days before the exam date. In doing so, you can use the day before the exam to relax and enjoy. If the exam center is more than 90 min from your residence, consider staying at a nearby hotel the night before. The importance of getting enough productive sleep the night before the exam cannot be emphasized enough.

Know the location and travel time to the exam center. Take a practice trip to the exam center and, if allowed, view the facility and procedures for checking in on your scheduled day. Allow plenty of time to arrive early, and prepare some quiet activity to occupy your time if you arrive far in advance of your scheduled time. By the way, we do not recommend cram time. You will typically need a photo identification or other documents to validate your identity as the exam candidate.

Hygiene and Attire

Although you do not get points for being clean and dressing comfortably, a good rule of thumb to follow is that feeling fresh may help with your attitude. Taking a stimulating shower can enhance mental and physical alertness. Dressing comfortably, but smart may do a lot to boost your morale. Of course, it does not hurt to wear your lucky socks, too. Avoid wearing tight or restrictive clothing during the exam. If you are not sure about the testing environment, wear layered clothing so that you may adjust your temperature to comfort. Remember, you may need to sit comfortably for up to $3\frac{1}{2}$ h.

Exam Day Cometh

Success

Why do most people fail objective structured exams? Studies show that the *ability of the person to reason* with what he or she knows *is more important* than what he or she really knows.[2]

Example: A person with a spinal cord injury underwent surgical fusion of the fifth to seventh cervical vertebrae four weeks ago. Now, they are beginning to regain function at the sixth cervical neurological level. The physical therapist sets a goal for compensatory grasp utilizing tenodesis. Which of the following interventions would NOT be appropriate?

    ——— a. keep interphalangeal joints flexed during upper extremity weight bearing

    ——— b. stretch into wrist and finger flexion, hold for 30 s or more

    ——— c. provide passive range of motion into finger flexion, abduction, and extension to neutral

    ——— d. stretch into wrist extension and finger extension, hold for 30 s or more

Correct answer: (d)

Rationale: If a stretch is applied to the long finger flexors concurrently across the wrist and finger joints, the flexor tendons may lose the required tendon tension for a tenodesis grasp.

Reference: Somers, M. (2001). *Spinal cord injury: Functional rehabilitation* (2nd ed., p. 178). New Jersey: Prentice Hall.

In this case, the concept of tenodesis may be familiar, but you are required to apply this using clinical reasoning to choices that are unfamiliar.

When unsure, use a deductive reasoning approach to questions. Begin with what you know about the topic. Avoid false logic. Two true statements may be linked by a word that makes them false.

Example: "The rectus femoris is indicated for therapeutic strengthening *because* of a positive result on the Thomas test."

The question may indicate the intervention of therapeutic strengthening, but the Thomas test is not used to determine strength.

Over- and Underreading

Also known as rationalization, overreading exam items may cause you to read more into the question than what the question is actually asking. Rationalization is usually the result of adding unreliable details or previous personal experiences that are not included in the item. On the other hand, underreading is rooted in the applicants failing to comprehend key words or phrases in the context of the question. As a result, they totally miss the meaning of the question and consequently choose the incorrect answer. In order to avoid over- and underreading, the best solution is to read and understand the question at face value.

Dealing with Multiple-Choice Questions

The following are ten suggested tips that may be helpful when dealing with multiple-choice exams in general and the licensing exam in particular.

1. Read the entire item, including the stem and all of the choices, regardless of whether or not you think that you have already identified the correct answer. One of the most common reasons for answering a multiple-choice question incorrectly is not understanding what is being asked.

   Example: A person, who recently underwent open reduction with internal fixation of the left femur and right tibia, has orders to ambulate bilateral partial weight bearing. The physical therapist evaluates the patient and sets a short-term goal for the patient to be accurate and safe with a four-point alternating gait pattern. Which of the following ambulation aids would be MOST appropriate to begin instruction?

   _____ a. bilateral large base quad canes
   _____ b. parallel bars
   _____ c. reciprocal walker
   _____ d. Lofstrand crutches

   Correct answer: (b)

   In this example, it is easy to be distracted by the four-point gait pattern. The specific question is which ambulation aid is MOST appropriate to begin instruction. Take your time to comprehend what the item is asking.

2. Select the best answer of the four choices provided. Remember that each of the choices given in the licensing exam is a feasible option.

3. Eliminate the obvious. The obviously wrong choices are eliminated first, leaving a greater probability of choosing the correct item. Eliminate a choice once you have a clear reason that it is not the best or most appropriate.

4. Avoid selecting or eliminating choices because of vague terms used in the wording of the item. Translate the contextual meaning of the items if possible.

5. Look for the choice that has been most carefully constructed. Oftentimes, the correct answer may be the one that has been most carefully constructed in order to be the most correct.[3, 4]

6. When exam items and choices are read carefully, first thoughts and selections are usually the correct answers. If you have no clue, mark the item, conserve time to return to the item later, reconsider, and make a choice.

7. Be aware of key words, otherwise known as indicators. The following are classifications of the most frequently used indicators in multiple-choice questions:

   - Frequency indicators include, but are not limited to, words such as always, never, often, sometimes, usually, and typically.
   - Inclusion and exclusion indicators include, but are not limited to, words such as all, some, none, most, except, and not.
   - Sequencing and preference indicators include, but are not limited to, words such as first, best, and most.

- These indicators provide the context to make the correct choice for the item. Just because the wording of an item seems familiar and the choice that was correct on some previous test is available, does not necessarily mean that it is appropriate for the current item.

8. Use the "Left-Hand Method." Read the question accurately without looking at the choices. If you are right-handed, cover the choices with your left hand. Decide what you believe is the correct answer before reading the choices. Reread the question and then look at the choices provided. Is your choice available? If so, that is most likely the answer. If your answer is not among the choices, two things may be true. First, you may have misread the question. Second, the test item may provide a correct and acceptable alternative answer that is the best among the given choices.

9. Do not be afraid to skip exam items for which you do not have immediate answers. It is not imperative for you to answer the exam sequentially. You can skip items and go back to them as long as there is time available to do so. Sometimes, other exam items may provide the trigger for you to answer the previous items you have skipped. In addition, the positive momentum of answering several questions comfortably does a lot to boost your confidence and positive attitude.

10. As a last resort, just guess. Do not leave any unanswered questions. Unanswered questions are scored as wrong answers. In addition, since guesses that turn out to be correct are not penalized, it is to the advantage of the exam taker to answer all the questions.

In summary, remember that the exam is intended to determine if you can choose the safest, most ethical, and best standard of practice. So look for these choices on the exam, and we wish you success!

REFERENCES

[1]Federation of State Boards of Physical Therapy (2002, July 29). *Physical Therapist Assistant Examination Content Outline* [On-line]. Available: http://www.fsbpt.org/pdf/PTA_Content_Outline_2002.pdf

[2]Carman, R., & Adams, W. (1984). *Study skills: A student's guide for survival* (2nd ed.). New York: Wiley.

[3]Coman, M., & Heavers, K. (1994). *How to improve your study skills.* Lincolnwood, IL: VGM Career Horizons.

[4]Fry, R. (1994). *Ace any test* (2nd ed.). Hawthorne, NJ: Career Press.

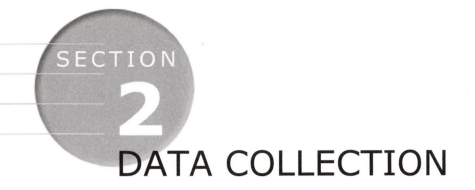

DATA COLLECTION

2

Tests and Measurements Group I: Body Segments, Girth, Posture, Range of Motion, Muscle Length, Strength, Cognition, Reflexes, and Sensation

OVERVIEW

This chapter includes questions covering clinical tests and measurements included in the exam. There are 102 questions in this chapter that deal with measuring muscle strength and length, range of motion, posture, body segments, cognition, reflexes, and sensation.

KEY POINTS FOR REVIEW

Girth Measurement and Body Segment

- Inch-centimeter conversion
- Anatomical reference points
- Segmental lengths and ratios

Posture

- Normal spinal curves
- Spine, girdle, and extremity deviations
- Muscle imbalances
- Plumb line

Range of Motion and Muscle Length

- Positioning
- Landmarks
- Muscle attachments
- Normal values
- Passive insufficiency

Manual Muscle Testing

- Positioning
- Grading
- Direction of pressure
- Transverse and vertical planes
- Muscle actions
- Active insufficiency

Cognition

- Alertness
- Orientation
- Glasgow Coma Scale
- Terminology

Reflexes and Muscle Tone

- Myotomes
- Deep tendon and reflex testing
- Terminology
- Upper versus lower motor neurons

Sensory Integrity

- Dermatomes
- Proprioception, discrimination, and kinesthesia testing
- Terminology

ANTHROPOMETRICS, GIRTH, AND LENGTH

Seven Items

1. You are performing the forward reach test to observe the length of a person's hamstrings. During which of the following age ranges would you expect to observe a person's inability to reach their toes due to a longer limb to trunk ratio?

   _____ a. 3–7 years of age

   _____ b. 11–14 years of age

_____ c. 40–44 years of age

_____ d. 68–72 years of age

2. Which of the following anatomical landmarks is typically the MOST difficult to locate on a person with moderate ankle swelling due to its size and location?

_____ a. medial malleolus

_____ b. lateral malleolus

_____ c. tibial tuberosity

_____ d. fibular head

3. You are asked by the physical therapist to measure and record segmental length of a person's right lower extremity. Which of the following anatomical landmarks are both located on a person's femur?

_____ a. greater trochanter to anterior superior iliac spine

_____ b. anterior-superior iliac spine to the superior medial pole

_____ c. greater trochanter to the lateral epicondyle

_____ d. anterior-superior iliac spine to the lateral tubercle

4. A person stands with equilateral postures of the foot and knee, but an apparent leg length discrepancy. Which of the following observations is necessary to determine if a person has a true leg length discrepancy?

_____ a. radiologic view of lengths from the anterior-superior iliac spine to the ipsilateral tibial tuberosities, comparing the involved and uninvolved limbs

_____ b. position the person in supine, and measure angle of the anterior-superior iliac spine to the midpatellar to the tibial tubersities, and compare bilaterally

_____ c. position the person in prone, measure and compare the lengths of the involved and uninvolved femurs and tibias

_____ d. position the person in supine, measure and compare the lengths of the involved and uninvolved limbs from the anterior-superior iliac spine to the medial malleolus

5. After applying edema reduction interventions to a person's left upper extremity, you take several girth measurements. When recording these measurements in the patient's physical therapy record, you realize that you incorrectly wrote one of the measurements in inches. What is the correct conversion of inches to centimeters?

_____ a. 25″ equals 63.5 cm

_____ b. 11″ equals 29.8 cm

_____ c. 10″ equals 26.4 cm

_____ d. 10″ equals 28.4 cm

6. Which of the following girth measurements reflect the effectiveness of an edema intervention?

_____ a. measurement after a treatment session

_____ b. measurement before a treatment session

_____ c. measurements before and after a treatment session

_____ d. measurements prior to previous treatment session and after today's treatment session

7. Girth measurements MUST be taken at which of the following locations?

    _____ a. at the location of greatest girth

    _____ b. at a location distal to the greatest girth

    _____ c. at a location proximal to the greatest girth

    _____ d. at the same location on the uninvolved limb

POSTURE OBSERVATIONS

Eighteen Items

1. The presence of postural scoliosis is BEST observed by which of the following?

    _____ a. palpate the spine in ipsilateral sidebending

    _____ b. palpate the spine in forward bending

    _____ c. palpate the spine in contralateral sidebending

    _____ d. palpate the spine in static standing

2. A young person is participating in interventions to address a 28° left thoracic scoliosis due to cerebral palsy. Which of the following classifications of scoliosis does this person's condition describe?

    _____ a. congenital scoliosis

    _____ b. neuromuscular scoliosis

    _____ c. nonstructural scoliosis

    _____ d. structural scoliosis

3. A person's radiologic report notes a curvature of the spine in the sagittal plane, with a convexity directed posteriorly. This would be consistent with which of the following postures?

    _____ a. kyphosis

    _____ b. lordosis

    _____ c. scoliosis

    _____ d. posterior pelvic tilt

4. A person with paralysis associated with a spinal cord injury sits with their head and shoulders slouched forward, and they appear to be in an anterior pelvic tilt. This position will MOST likely produce which of the following thoracic spine postures?

    _____ a. flat low back posture

    _____ b. swayback posture

    _____ c. lordosis posture

    _____ d kyphosis–lordosis posture

5. A person is strength-tested and found to have poor plus strength of their lower abdominals. Weakness of the lower abdominal muscles is MOST often associated with which of the following postures?

_____ a. flat low back

_____ b. swayback

_____ c. anterior pelvic tilt

_____ d. lordosis

6. A person stands with a lordotic curve in their lumbar spine. Based upon this clinical observation, the person has which of the following?

_____ a. weak erector spinae, weak lower abdominals, and short iliopsoas

_____ b. short abdominals, weak iliopsoas, short gluteus maximus, and weak rectus femoris

_____ c. short lumbar paraspinals, weak gluteus maximus, short rectus femoris, and weak lower abdominals

_____ d. normal alignment of the spine

7. A person with an anterior pelvic tilt will often have which of the following sets of muscle imbalances?

_____ a. erector spinae shortened, rectus abdominus lengthened, iliopsoas shortened, and hamstrings lengthened

_____ b. iliopsoas shortened, sternocleidomastoid lengthened, and sartorius lengthened

_____ c. erector spinae lengthened, rectus abdominus shortened, ilipsoas lengthened, and hamstrings shortened

_____ d. iliopsoas lengthened, sternocleidomastoid shortened, and sartorius shortened

8. A person sits with a posterior pelvic tilt; upon standing, they assume an anterior pelvic tilt. Which of the following sets of muscle imbalances accounts for these clinical observations?

_____ a. short paraspinals and weak rectus femoris

_____ b. short rectus femoris and weak lower abdominals

_____ c. short rectus femoris and weak lumbar paraspinals

_____ d. short paraspinals and weak lower abdominals

9. A person is standing without shoes on a thinly carpeted floor in a physical therapy setting. Upon palpation you find that the person's pubis symphysis aligns anterior to the anterior superior iliac spines. Which of the following postures does this observation suggest?

_____ a. anterior pelvic tilt

_____ b. posterior pelvic tilt

_____ c. swayback

_____ d. flat low back

10. A person stands with a leg length discrepancy. Which of the following femoral deformities is the MOST likely explanation for ipsilateral shortness with this discrepancy?

_____ a. coxa varus

_____ b. coxa valgus

_____ c. femoral anteversion

_____ d. femoral retroversion

11. A physical therapist evaluated a person and documented that the person has an increased Q angle. What are the biomechanical effects of an increased Q angle?
    _____ a. increased lateral force by the quads on the patella
    _____ b. decreased medial force by the quads on the patella
    _____ c. decreased superior pull by the iliotibial band on the patella
    _____ d. increased inferior pull by the tensor fascia latae via the iliotibial band on the patella

12. A person with genu varus is MOST likely to have which of the following skeletal alignments?
    _____ a. coxa varus
    _____ b. pes cavus
    _____ c. anterior pelvic tilt
    _____ d. femoral retroversion

13. Upon observation, you find that a person has a posteriorly tilted pelvis in standing. In addition, their knees are hyperextended, and they demonstrate a forward head and a flat low-back posture. Which of the following postures would MOST accurately classify these findings?
    _____ a. scoliotic posture
    _____ b. typical adult male posture
    _____ c. swayback posture
    _____ d. kyphotic–lordotic posture

14. A person with coxa valgus is more susceptible to which of the following?
    _____ a. hip fractures
    _____ b. hip dislocations
    _____ c. pes cavus
    _____ d. decreased apparent leg length

15. Which of the following is MOST likely to occur with a person who has genu recurvatum?
    _____ a. increased laxity of the posterior cruciate ligament
    _____ b. increased laxity of the anterior cruciate ligament
    _____ c. decreased laxity of the medial collateral ligament
    _____ d. increased laxity of the lateral retinaculum

16. A person is standing in a pain-free and flat-footed posture bilaterally. Which of the following MOST likely contributed to this person's pronated posture?
    _____ a. swayback posture
    _____ b. anterior pelvic tilt
    _____ c. flat low-back posture
    _____ d. prolonged overstretching of the Achilles tendon

17. When observing a person in standing their head appears forward, their scapulae are each 2″ from their spinous processes, their olecranon processes are directed posterior-laterally, and their anterior-

superior iliac spine are in the same frontal plane as the pubis symphysis. Based upon these observations and palpations, which of the following is a valid deduction?

_____ a. the person has bilateral shortness of humeral internal rotators

_____ b. the person has bilateral weakness of sternocleidomastoids

_____ c. the person has bilateral shortness of rectus femoris

_____ d. the person has bilateral weakness of middle trapezius

18. A person stands with a forward shoulder posture, flat low back, and a posterior pelvic tilt. Which of the following therapeutic exercise interventions is most appropriate to address this person's posture?

_____ a. middle trapezius strength test

_____ b. rectus femoris length test

_____ c. lower abdominal strength test

_____ d. rhomboid strength test

RANGE OF MOTION AND MUSCLE LENGTH

Sixteen Items

1. You are observing a physical therapist perform the Thomas test with a person's left lower extremity. When the person's knee is flexed, the leg lowers to 40° of hip flexion. When the person's knee is extended, their extremity lowers to 30° of hip flexion. Which of the following is MOST likely present with these results?

_____ a. short psoas major

_____ b. short rectus femoris

_____ c. short tensor fascia latae

_____ d. short rectus femoris and ilopsoas

2. A person who extends their elbow to 2°, and extends their shoulder to 10°, is demonstrating which of the following:

_____ a. passive insufficiency of the biceps brachii

_____ b. active insufficiency of the biceps brachii

_____ c. normal range of motion in the humeral-ulnar and glenohumeral joints

_____ d. none of these

3. You observe a patient in supine, with their right hip positioned at 90° and their right knee at 22° when passively extended. From this you would determine that the patient

_____ a. has 2+/5 strength of rectus femoris

_____ b. has passively insufficient hamstrings

_____ c. has 2+/5 strength of hamstrings

_____ d. has an actively insufficient rectus femoris

4. When attempting to goniometrically measure a person's shoulder flexion in hooklying, with their lumbar spine flat on the table, you find that they are unable to fully flex their shoulder unless allowed to internally rotate their humerus or arch their back. Which of the following is a logical explanation for this observation?

   _____ a. shortness of subscapularis

   _____ b. shortness of pectoralis major

   _____ c. shortness of latissimus dorsi

   _____ d. shortness of levator scapula

5. When taking goniometric measurement of a person's right knee extension in supine, the result is 12°. In short-sitting, their right knee reaches 20°. Which of the following is the most logical explanation?

   _____ a. weakness of the quadriceps femoris

   _____ b. shortness of the gastrocnemius

   _____ c. shortness of the hamstrings

   _____ d. shortness of the rectus femoris

6. After taking a person's left lower extremity passively through knee flexion to 142°, which of the following indicates weakness of the hamstrings muscle group?

   _____ a. active tibiofemoral flexion to 128°

   _____ b. passive tibiofemoral flexion to 136°

   _____ c. active tibiofemoral flexion to 150°

   _____ d. active tibiofemoral extension to 22°

7. To accurately perform the modified Ober's test, which of the following sequences of steps are taken to effectively position the patient?

   _____ a. extend the hip, abduct the hip, and externally rotate the hip

   _____ b. extend the hip, externally rotate the hip, and abduct the hip

   _____ c. externally rotate the hip, abduct the hip, and extend the hip

   _____ d. abduct the hip, avoid rotating the hip, and extend the hip

8. A person is placed in sidelying and found to have a positive Ober's test. Which of the following would represent a positive Ober's test?

   _____ a. 45° of passive hip abduction

   _____ b. 0° of passive hip adduction

   _____ c. 10° of passive hip adduction

   _____ d. 125° of passive hip flexion

9. Which of the following is MOST true about the parts of a universal goniometer?

   _____ a. the scale is located on the stationary arm of the goniometer

   _____ b. the scale is typically divided into increments of five

   _____ c. the scale is located on the moving arm of the goniometer

   _____ d. the moving arm is typically aligned with the proximal anatomical landmark of the patient

10. A person is being treated with interventions to address hamstring shortness. Today their progress is going to be documented based upon several clinical measurements. Which of the following pieces of equipment is necessary to accurately and reliably determine a person's hamstring length using the forward reach test?

    _____ a. goniometer

    _____ b. padded table

    _____ c. flexible tape measure

    _____ d. dynamometer

11. Two physical therapist assistants measured active left knee flexion for a person who recently underwent anterior cruciate ligament reconstruction. The first PTA documented that the patient had 84° of active left knee flexion in the morning. That afternoon, the second PTA documented that the patient had 104° of active left knee flexion. Based on measurement standards, which of the following describes this variation?

    _____ a. satisfactory intertester reliability

    _____ b. poor intratester reliability

    _____ c. satisfactory intratester reliability

    _____ d. poor intertester reliability

12. Which of the following is the BEST example of good intratester reliability?

    _____ a. one tester observes passive radiocarpal extension to 58°, 56°, and 58°

    _____ b. one tester observes a positive Ober's test, the next tester observes a positive Ober's test, and a third tester observes a positive Ober's test

    _____ c. one tester observes 70° glenohumeral internal rotation, and then observes 90° glenohumeral lateral rotation

    _____ d. one tester observes tibiofemoral hyperextension during the midstance phase of gait repeatedly, and another tester observes tibiofemoral hyperextension during the midstance phase of gait repeatedly

13. Which of the following is the BEST example of test validity?

    _____ a. the measurement of a person's internal rotation was obtained by four different testers and compared

    _____ b. the measurement of a person's hamstring length is a predictor of posture

    _____ c. the measurement of a person's hamstring length was repeated by the tester and compared

    _____ d. the measurement of a person's internal rotation is compared with the uninvolved limb

14. Today, you are to update a person's progress towards their short-term goal of increasing glenohumeral range of motion by 8°. What is the preferred position for measuring glenohumeral internal rotation?

_____ a. supine with the humerus adducted to 90°

_____ b. supine with the humerus abducted to 0°

_____ c. supine with the humerus abducted to 90°

_____ d. sitting with the humerus abducted to 90°

15. A person had a right total knee arthroplasty three days ago. Which of the following positions is MOST effective when measuring a person's full available tibiofemoral extension?

_____ a. sidelying

_____ b. prone with a support under the distal anterior femur

_____ c. supine with a support under the calcaneus

_____ d. sitting on the edge of an adjustable mat table

16. Which of the following sequences is accurate for performing the two-joint hip flexor length test? The subject begins seated at end of table, and is cradled onto their back placing their sacrum flat onto the table.

_____ a. lower extended leg onto table, if it fails to reach the table it is due to shortness of the iliopsoas

_____ b. lower extended leg onto table, if it fails to reach the table, reattempt with flexed knee, if it fails to reach the table it is due to shortness of the iliopsoas

_____ c. lower flexed knee onto table, if it fails to reach the table it is due to shortness of the rectus femoris

_____ d. lower flexed knee onto table, if it fails to reach the table, reattempt with extended knee, if it fails to reach the table it is due to shortness of the rectus femoris

MUSCLE PERFORMANCE — MANUAL MUSCLE TESTING

Sixteen Items

1. According to the manual muscle testing strength grades, which of the following is MOST accurate?

_____ a. a person with fair strength must be tested in the horizontal plane

_____ b. a person with trace muscle strength will only complete partial range in the horizontal plane

_____ c. the fair strength grade may be detected in any position

_____ d. the trace strength grade may be detected in any position

2. A patient has been scheduled for therapeutic exercise three times a week, for two weeks to address biceps weakness. The physical therapist evaluated her strength as 3/5 for the biceps. In which position was the patient tested? Which position would BEST challenge the patient's strength?

_____ a. standing/sitting

_____ b. prone/prone

_____ c. sitting/prone or sitting

_____ d. sitting/sitting or standing

3. During an initial evaluation with the physical therapist, it is determined that a patient has 2−/5 strength in their left iliopsoas. In which position is the person placed in during the manual muscle test?

    _____ a. hooklying, leg supported by unaffected extremity

    _____ b. seated, left femur supported

    _____ c. supine, left femur supported

    _____ d. sidelying

4. To accurately and effectively test the strength of someone with weakness of the middle trapezius, you would position them in prone with the humerus in which of the following positions?

    _____ a. abducted, internally rotated, and horizontally abducted

    _____ b. abducted, externally rotated, and horizontally abducted

    _____ c. adducted and internally rotated

    _____ d. abducted and externally rotated

5. Which of the following antigravity manual muscle tests are NOT typically performed in supine?

    _____ a. ankle dorsiflexion

    _____ b. biceps brachii

    _____ c. peroneals

    _____ d. ankle plantarflexion

6. The physical therapist states in a SOAP note that a patient has 4+/5 strength in their left wrist extensors. In which position was the patient placed in during the manual muscle test?

    _____ a. standing, forearm supported by unaffected extremity

    _____ b. seated, forearm supported

    _____ c. supine, humerus supported

    _____ d. sidelying, radial-ulnar joint supported

7. When observing length and strength of muscles, it is important to know whether they act upon single or multiple joints. Which of the following muscle acts upon more than one joint?

    _____ a. anterior deltoid

    _____ b. gastrocnemius

    _____ c. posterior deltoid

    _____ d. soleus

8. A physical therapist has documented that a patient tested positive for hip flexor shortness, specifically the tensor fascia latae. Which of the following is NOT true about the tensor fascia latae?

    _____ a. the tensor fascia latae attaches to the iliotibial band

    _____ b. the tensor fascia latae attaches indirectly to the knee

    _____ c. the tensor fascia latae performs iliofemoral internal rotation

    _____ d. the tensor fascia latae performs volitional knee extension

9. A person who was gross strength tested at 5/5 for knee flexion in sitting is next placed prone, with their knee flexed to 65°. In this position, their hamstring strength is manually tested and found to be

4−/5. Most likely the person was substituting during the gross strength test by the following:

_____ a. dorsiflexing the ankle

_____ b. externally rotating the hip

_____ c. plantarflexing the ankle

_____ d. pronating the hind foot

10. Based on the principles of Kendall's manual muscle testing, which of the following are accurate?

_____ a. one-joint muscles are tested at overall midrange

_____ b. one-joint muscles are tested at completion of range, two-joint muscles are tested at their overall midlength

_____ c. two-joint muscles are tested simultaneously with one-joint muscles

_____ d. two-joint muscles must be tested first in antigravity, one-joint muscles can be tested either in antigravity or against manual resistance

11. Which of the following MOST accurately represents the strength test position of the supraspinatus muscle?

_____ a. in sitting, with the shoulder flexed, abducted, and externally rotated

_____ b. humerus at the side, initiating abduction

_____ c. humerus at 90° abduction

_____ d. humerus in the scapular plane, externally rotating

12. A therapist initially documented that a person with bilateral anterior-medial pain has left hamstring strength of 4−/5. Which position would be MOST accurate for comparing strength of the medial versus lateral hamstrings?

_____ a. flex their knee to 70°, internally rotate the femur, to detect the strength of the biceps femoris

_____ b. flex their knee to 70°, externally rotate the femur, to detect the strength of the biceps femoris

_____ c. flex their knee to 70°, internally rotate the tibia, to detect the strength of the biceps femoris

_____ d. flex their knee to 70°, externally rotate the tibia, to detect the strength of the biceps femoris

13. During manual muscle testing of the wrist extensors, you observe the person's wrist deviate laterally during extension. After repeated verbal and tactile cueing, it is still unresolved. Weakness of which of the following muscles could explain this substitution?

_____ a. extensor carpi radialis

_____ b. extensor carpi ulnaris

_____ c. flexor carpi radialis

_____ d. flexor carpi ulnaris

14. A person with a weak left gluteus medius would MOST likely demonstrate which of the following deviations in single limb standing on their left leg?

   ____ a. ipsilateral increase in adduction

   ____ b. ipsilateral increase in abduction

   ____ c. contralateral increase in abduction

   ____ d. contralateral increase in adduction

15. Which of the following is a functional example of active insufficiency?

   ____ a. grip strength is increased with slight wrist extension

   ____ b. glenohumeral flexion is more difficult with the elbow flexed

   ____ c. prone hip extension with the knee extended allows participation of the hamstrings

   ____ d. extension of the knee is more difficult with the hip in flexion

16. Which manual muscle testing strength grades have the highest level of reliability?

   ____ a. fair and fair plus

   ____ b. poor and fair minus

   ____ c. good and normal

   ____ d. poor minus and fair minus

AROUSAL, ATTENTION, AND CHECKING COGNITION

Eleven Items

1. A person who is oriented to person, place, and time is documented with which of the following entries?

   ____ a. oriented $\times$ 3

   ____ b. oriented $\times$ 2

   ____ c. fully alert

   ____ d. alert $\times$ 3 and oriented

2. A person who has difficulty comprehending spoken words has which of the following neurological conditions?

   ____ a. expressive aphasia

   ____ b. receptive aphasia

   ____ c. global aphagia

   ____ d. receptive aphagia

3. A person with a brain injury was scored as a seven on the Glasgow Coma Scale. Which of the following is a category used in the Glasgow Coma Scale?

   ____ a. opening of the eyes

   ____ b. autonomic function

   ____ c. response to humor

   ____ d. manual muscle strength in hands

4. A person recently suffered a closed head injury as an unrestrained passenger in a motorized vehicle. The person is rated as a Rancho Los Amigos Grade I, which is most consistent with which of the following descriptions?

    _____ a. responds to touch

    _____ b. does not respond to stimulus

    _____ c. follows one step commands

    _____ d. is dead

5. When a person is stuck on a task or word, it is often described as which of the following terms?

    _____ a. perseveration

    _____ b. expressive apraxia

    _____ c. aphasia

    _____ d. dementia

6. Upon visiting a patient bedside, you introduce yourself and wish to determine if the person is oriented to person, place, and time. Which of the following questions would detect a person's orientation to place?

    _____ a. What is the name of the building you are in?

    _____ b. What is today's date?

    _____ c. Where were you born?

    _____ d. Where does the President of the United States live?

7. Before beginning a treatment with a person beside, you ask the person, "Do you know where you are at this time?" Which of the following elements of orientation have you not addressed?

    _____ a. orientation to person

    _____ b. orientation to place and person

    _____ c. orientation to time and person

    _____ d. orientation to time and place

8. Upon entering a person's room in a hospital setting, you check to see if they are alert and oriented. The person is sitting in a recliner with their eyes open and facing towards the television show they are watching. You introduce yourself and use the person's name. You follow with the question—"Do you know where you are?" If the person does not respond you can accurately determine which of the following?

    _____ a. they lack orientation to place

    _____ b. they lack orientation to time

    _____ c. they lack orientation to person

    _____ d. they may have heard you and repeat your introduction

9. When working with a person, you are unsure of their cognitive ability. Prior to proceeding with multi-step instructions or other potentially difficult teaching techniques, you attempt to determine their current cognitive status. Which of the following questions is MOST appropriate to determine a person's

general cognitive status?

_____ a. What did you have for breakfast this morning?

_____ b. What season is it today?

_____ c. Which is longer, a yard or two feet?

_____ d. Do you remember what my name is?

10. A person has been diagnosed with recurrent transient ischemia attacks. What is the primary difference between transient ischmia attacks and cerebral vascular accidents?

_____ a. focal effects

_____ b. duration of effects

_____ c. intensity of symptoms

_____ d. lobe affected

11. Which of the following is LEAST likely to occur with a mild cerebral vascular accident?

_____ a. bladder infection

_____ b. loss of consciousness

_____ c. hypotonicity

_____ d. death

CHECKING REFLEXES AND MUSCLE TONE

Nineteen Items

1. When checking a person's muscle tone in their left lower extremity you find no response to reflex or voluntary action. Which of the following terms is BEST used to document these observations?

_____ a. fasciculation

_____ b. spasticity

_____ c. clonus

_____ d. flaccidity

2. A person recently suffered a spinal cord injury in the cervical region. What is the primary concern for the person with injury affecting the fourth cervical neurological level?

_____ a. grip function

_____ b. diaphragm function

_____ c. bladder function

_____ d. cardiac function

3. Which of the following manual muscle testing procedures would reflect the function of the eleventh cranial nerve?

_____ a. instruct the person to clinch their teeth

_____ b. instruct the person to look medially and inferiorly

_____ c. instruct the person to track an object visually

_____ d. instruct the person to shrug their shoulders

4. Which of the following clinical observations is used to check reflex activity at the sixth cervical neurological level?

    _____ a. tapping the deltoid, when the humerus is abducted to 90°

    _____ b. place the elbow in 90° flexion, and manually push into extension against the person's flexion effort

    _____ c. tapping the brachioradialis, when the forearm is supported at 90° elbow flexion

    _____ d. tapping the biceps, with the forearm supinated, and supported at 90° elbow flexion

5. Which of the following nerve roots would be indicated by a decrease or absent patellar tendon reflex?

    _____ a. C8

    _____ b. T10

    _____ c. L2

    _____ d. L4

6. The anterior tibialis is innervated primarily from which nerve roots?

    _____ a. L2-L3

    _____ b. L3-L4

    _____ c. L4-L5

    _____ d. all of these

7. A person is having recurrent low back pain, with sciatic consistent symptoms. Which of the following is the reflex test for the fifth lumbar neurological level?

    _____ a. Achilles tendon reflex

    _____ b. there is no reflex for the fifth lumbar level

    _____ c. anal sphincter reflex

    _____ d. patellar reflex

8. A person who has an injury to their spinal cord has the benefit of sacral sparing. Which of the following myotomes is MOST consistent with the first sacral nerve distribution?

    _____ a. anal sphincter

    _____ b. soleus muscle

    _____ c. anterior tibialis

    _____ d. tensor fascia latae

9. A person in an intensive care setting is unresponsive, and currently being treated bedside. In their evaluation the physical therapist noted that they have a positive Babinski sign. The Babinski sign is tested by which of the following?

    _____ a. stroking the lateral-plantar aspect of the foot

    _____ b. stroking the anterior-plantar aspect of the foot

_____ c. stroking the medial-plantar aspect of the foot

_____ d. tapping the plantar aspect of the foot, while the person's eyes are closed

10. Which of the following is MOST accurate about the reflex arc?

_____ a. specific sensations are transmitted to the anterior horn of the spinal cord, and immediately exit through the anterior horn of the spinal cord for a motor response

_____ b. specific sensations are transmitted to the posterior horn of the spinal cord, and immediately exit out the anterior horn of the spinal cord for a motor response

_____ c. specific sensations are transmitted to the posterior horn of the spinal cord, and simultaneously send ascending signals to the brain, and out the anterior horn of the spinal cord for a motor response

_____ d. specific sensations are transmitted to the anterior horn of the spinal cord, and simultaneously send ascending signals to the brain, and out the posterior horn of the spinal cord for a motor response

11. A lesion involving the median nerve would MOST likely result in impaired function with which of the following functional activities?

_____ a. bending the elbow

_____ b. reaching overhead

_____ c. shrugging of the shoulders

_____ d. grasp

12. With an isolated injury to the radial nerve, which set of muscles would MOST likely be affected?

_____ a. triceps, supinator, and biceps

_____ b. brachioradialis, triceps, and extensor carpi radialis

_____ c. supinator, pronator, and biceps

_____ d. extensor carpi radialis, triceps, and biceps

13. A person experienced a crushing injury to their low back, and has neurological impairment to both of their lower extremities. Which of the following methods is BEST for detecting which myotomes remain intact?

_____ a. lightly brush the skin in various locations of their lower extremities

_____ b. use a two-point discrimination tool to compare sensation in various locations of their lower extremities

_____ c. perform manual muscle testing of their lower extremities

_____ d. all of the above

14. Neurological lesions affecting the anterior horn of the spinal cord will LEAST likely result in which of the following impairments?

_____ a. weakness

_____ b. hypotonicity

_____ c. flaccidity

_____ d. spasticity

15. Which of the following terms is accurately described as a peripheral nerve injury, often a result of transient ischemia, or temporary compression, without autonomic compromise? There is also typically a decrease in strength and loss of sensation, which may spontaneously be recovered in less than three months.

_____ a. axonotmesis

_____ b. neurotmesis

_____ c. neuropraxia

_____ d. axonitis

16. After a head injury, a person demonstrates a primitive reflex of upper extremity extension towards the direction their head is facing, and withdrawal of the contralateral upper extremity. This sign describes which primitive reflex?

_____ a. asymmetrical tonic neck reflex

_____ b. symmetrical tonic neck reflex

_____ c. Landau reflex

_____ d. rooting

17. While a person is sitting, you passively dorsiflex their ankle. This stimulates a cyclical tonic resistance. Which of the following neurological signs does this demonstrate?

_____ a. fasciculation

_____ b. spasticity

_____ c. clonus

_____ d. flaccidity

18. A person with a peripheral nerve injury is MOST likely to experience which of the following clinical signs?

_____ a. spasticity

_____ b. muscle fasciculations

_____ c. paresis

_____ d. hypertonicity

19. A person is being treated with neuromuscular reeducation interventions to address flaccidity. Which of the following neurological conditions would LEAST likely result in flaccidity?

_____ a. diffuse upper motor neuron injury

_____ b. peripheral nerve compression injury

_____ c. spinal cord compression injury

_____ d. acute cerebral vascular accident

SENSORY INTEGRITY: SENSATION, PROPRIOCEPTION, AND KINESTHESIA

Fifteen Items

1. A person's sensory impairment can be anatomically mapped based generally agreed upon innervations. What are the anatomical divisions of skin sensation referred to as?

   _____ a. dermatomes

   _____ b. myotomes

   _____ c. neurotomes

   _____ d. axonatomes

2. A person who has an injury to their spinal cord, classified on the American Spinal Injury Association Impairment Scale as C5-A, would still have normal sensation at which of the following dermatomes?

   _____ a. skin over their superior-medial scapular angle

   _____ b. skin over their throat

   _____ c. skin over their nipple line

   _____ d. skin over their navel region

3. A person with a Brown–Sequard syndrome lesion of the spinal cord is MOST likely to experience which of the following?

   _____ a. ipsilateral weakness, impairment of position sense, and vibration below the level of the lesion, and contralateral impairment of temperature sensation

   _____ b. impairment of upper extremity function, with preservation of lower extremity function

   _____ c. lower extremity motor and sensory impairment, with preservation of perianal sensation, and active toe flexion

   _____ d. impairment of motor function, pain, and temperature sensation (below the level of the lesion), with preservation of light touch and position sense below the level of lesion

4. A person diagnosed with discogenic impingement upon the sixth cervical nerve root is MOST likely to experience sensory impairment at which of the following locations?

   _____ a. the skin over the deltoid

   _____ b. the skin over the medial humerus

   _____ c. the skin over the thumb

   _____ d. the skin over the inferior scapular angles

5. A person is asked to visually observe the placement of their right foot by the physical therapist assistant. After that, the assistant instructs the person to close their eyes and describe the direction and magnitude of joint motion. During which of the following sensory tests is the patient asked to identify the direction and magnitude of joint motion?

_____ a. kinesthesia

_____ b. proprioception

_____ c. graphesthesia

_____ d. stereognosis

6. A person is describing the pain they have in their right lower extremity. Pain sensation from the lower extremities is transmitted along which of the following spinal tracts?

_____ a. lateral spinothalamic

_____ b. ventral trigeminothalamic

_____ c. rubrospinal

_____ d. lateral corticospinal

7. A person whose referring diagnosis is lower back pain, primarily complains of increasing burning and numbness in the anterior distal aspect of their left thigh. Which of the following dermatomes is affected by these symptoms?

_____ a. L5

_____ b. L4

_____ c. L3

_____ d. L1

8. Sensations at the nipple line are anatomically consistent with which of the following dermatomes?

_____ a. C3

_____ b. T4

_____ c. T10

_____ d. T8

9. A physical therapist assistant instructs a person to close their eyes. The assistant then places their foot in a 20° plantarflexed position, and then releases the foot and requests the person to place their foot back into the same position. Based upon these instructions, the assistant is MOST likely testing which of the following sensations?

_____ a. kinesthesia

_____ b. proprioception

_____ c. graphesthesia

_____ d. stereognosis

10. A person with a peripheral nerve injury reports altered sensation in the skin over the medial, fourth, and lateral fifth finger. This subjective information is MOST consistent with distribution of which peripheral nerve?

_____ a. radial nerve

_____ b. median nerve

_____ c. medial antebrachial nerve

_____ d. ulnar nerve

11. When checking a person's motor-sensory status, a common test is the Semmes–Weinstein monofilament test. Which of the following diameters should the patient be able to detect in order to indicate protective sensation?

    _____ a. 6.84 mm

    _____ b. 8.92 mm

    _____ c. 5.07 mm

    _____ d. 1.28 mm

12. The tenth thoracic neurological level primarily innervates the skin over which of the following anatomical locations?

    _____ a. deltoid

    _____ b. naval line

    _____ c. nipple line

    _____ d. gluteals

13. Which syndrome of spinal cord injury results in loss of proprioception and paralysis on one half of the body, with impairment of somatic pain and temperature sensation on the other side?

    _____ a. anterior cord syndrome

    _____ b. lateral cord syndrome

    _____ c. posterior cord syndrome

    _____ d. central cord syndrome

14. A person who is experiencing difficulty performing rapidly alternating movements with two limbs may be referred to as having which of the following?

    _____ a. bilateral dystonia

    _____ b. agnosia

    _____ c. chorea

    _____ d. dysdiadochokinesia

15. Which of the following statements is MOST accurate regarding spinal cord injuries?

    _____ a. most persons recover from spinal cord injuries with little or no spasticity within five years

    _____ b. most spinal cord injuries result in complete impairment of the corresponding cord level

    _____ c. persons with spinal cord injuries do not typically recover any function, and must gain skills to maximize daily function

    _____ d. persons who recover from spinal cord injury may regain motor and sensation after function but may still have abnormal reflex activity

ANSWERS AND RATIONALE

ANTHROPOMETRICS, GIRTH, AND LENGTH

Seven Items

1. Correct answer: (b)

   Rationale: At this age the limbs typically grow at a faster rate than the trunk. It is not necessary to reach the toes during the forward reach test. The inability of other age ranges to touch their toes may occur, but not due to trunk to extremity ratio.

   Reference: Kendall, F., et al. (1993). *Muscles: Testing and function* (4th ed., p. 48). Baltimore: Williams & Wilkins.

2. Correct answer: (a)

   Rationale: The medial malleolus is smaller and more difficult to locate than the lateral malleolus. Both landmarks may be nonpalpable with severe swelling.

   Reference: Hoppenfeld, S. (1976). *Physical examination of the spine and extremities* (p. 205). Norwalk, CT: Appleton & Lange.

3. Correct answer: (c)

   Rationale: The anterior-superior iliac spine is a landmark on the pelvis. The superior-medial pole is a landmark on the proximal patella. The lateral tubercle is a landmark on the proximal tibia.

   Reference: Hoppenfeld, S. (1976). *Physical examination of the spine and extremities* (p. 145, 176). Norwalk, CT: Appleton & Lange.

4. Correct answer: (d)

   Rationale: The first and third choices are invalid. The second choice determines the Q angle, the last choice is the correct position and alignment for clinically determining true leg length.

   Reference: Hoppenfeld, S. (1976). *Physical examination of the spine and extremities* (p. 165). Norwalk, CT: Appleton & Lange.

5. Correct answer: (a)

   Rationale: One inch equals 2.54 cm. Be prepared to perform some calculations by hand.

   Reference: Rothstein, J., et al. (1998). *The rehabilitation specialist's handbook* (2nd ed.). Philadelphia: FA Davis (back cover).

6. Correct answer: (c)

   Rationale: This choice allows a comparison of girth prior to, and after the application of, the intervention.

   Reference: Kisner, C., & Colby, L. (2002). *Therapeutic exercise: Foundations and techniques* (4th ed., p. 720). Philadelphia: FA Davis.

7. Correct answer: (a)

    Rationale: Each of these measurements is necessary to represent the girth and contour of the body part. However, the measurement that must be recorded is the location of the greatest girth.

    Reference: Pierson, F. (2002). *Principles and techniques of patient care* (3rd ed., p. 312). Philadelphia: WB Saunders.

POSTURE OBSERVATIONS

Eighteen Items

1. Correct answer: (b)

    Rationale: In flexion, the curvature becomes more prominent. The convex side in the thoracic region designates the name to the scoliotic curve.

    Reference: Magee, D. J. (2002). *Orthopedic physical assessment* (4th ed., p. 882). Philadelphia: WB Saunders.

2. Correct answer: (b)

    Rationale: Congenital scoliosis occurs with malformation, neuromuscular is a deficiency of support to the spine, and nonstructural and structural are apparent discrepancies and fixed skeletal conditions, respectively.

    Reference: Seymour, R. (2002). *Prosthetics and orthotics: Lower limb and spinal* (p. 431). Philadelphia: Lippincott Williams & Wilkins.

3. Correct answer: (a)

    Rationale: Kyphosis is a posterior convexity of the thoracic spine.

    Reference: Sahrmann, S. (2002). *Diagnosis and treatment of movement impairment syndromes* (p. 199). St. Louis: Mosby.

4. Correct answer: (d)

    Rationale: Kyphosis–lordosis is the only choice related to the thoracic region, and is consistently seen with the given alignments.

    Reference: Kendall, F., et al. (1993). *Muscles: Testing and function* (4th ed., p. 84). Baltimore: Williams & Wilkins.

5. Correct answer: (c)

    Rationale: Weakness of the lower abdominal muscles is associated with an anterior pelvic tilt.

    Reference: Kendall, F., et al. (1993). *Muscles: Testing and function* (4th ed., p. 150). Baltimore: Williams & Wilkins.

6. Correct answer: (d)

    Rationale: A lordotic curve is an ideal spinal postural alignment. Excessive lordosis may suggest muscular imbalance, but not a normal lordosis. The term lordosis means the condition of bending, and is misused to describe an excessive curve of the lumbar region.

Reference: Kendall, F., et al. (1993). *Muscles: Testing and function* (4th ed., p. 83). Baltimore: Williams & Wilkins.

7. Correct answer: (a)

Rationale: The superior-anterior muscles of the pelvis lengthen, while the superior-posterior muscles shorten. The inferior-anterior muscles of the pelvis shorten, while the inferior-posterior muscles lengthen.

Reference: Kendall, F., et al. (1993). *Muscles: Testing and function* (4th ed., p. 350). Baltimore: Williams & Wilkins.

8. Correct answer: (c)

Rationale: A short rectus femoris will produce an anterior pelvic tilt in standing. In sitting, the rectus femoris is slack proximally and allows the pelvis to tilt posteriorly, exacerbated by weak lumbar paraspinals.

Reference: Kendall, F., et al. (1993). *Muscles: Testing and function* (4th ed., p. 213). Baltimore: Williams & Wilkins.

9. Correct answer: (b)

Rationale: The anterior-superior iliac spines should be in the same plane as the pubic symphysis. In this scenario, these are posterior of the symphysis (stated differently), and therefore describe a posterior pelvic tilt.

Reference: Kendall, F., et al. (1993). *Muscles: Testing and function* (4th ed., p. 83). Baltimore: Williams & Wilkins.

10. Correct answer: (a)

Rationale: Coxa varus is a decrease in femoral neck angle, which results in an increase in ipsilateral femoral length.

Reference: Smith, L., et al. (1996). *Brunnstrom's clinical kinesiology* (5th ed., p. 269). Philadelphia: FA Davis.

11. Correct answer: (a)

Rationale: The Q angle is the angle of pull on the patella by the quadriceps. Normally a 15°–20° lateral pull is acceptable, any increase in that angle results in excessive lateral forces during knee excursion.

Reference: Smith, L., et al. (1996). *Brunnstrom's clinical kinesiology* (5th ed., p. 311). Philadelphia: FA Davis.

12. Correct answer: (d)

Rationale: Femoral retroversion often results in genu varum and pes planus.

Reference: Kisner, C., & Colby, L. (2002). *Therapeutic exercise: Foundations and techniques* (4th ed., p. 388). Philadelphia: FA Davis.

13. Correct answer: (c)

Rationale: This posture is also known as resting on their ligaments, secondary to the posterior displacement of the upper trunk.

Reference: Kendall, F., et al. (1993). *Muscles: Testing and function* (4th ed., p. 85). Baltimore: Williams & Wilkins.

14. Correct answer: (b)

Rationale: A person with coxa valgus has a femoral neck angle greater than 120°, and is therefore less susceptible to fracture, but more susceptible to iliofemoral dislocation.

Reference: Norkin, C., & Levangie, P. (1992). *Joint structure and function: A comprehensive analysis* (2nd ed., p. 333). Philadelphia: FA Davis.

15. Correct answer: (b)

Rationale: The anterior cruciate ligament prevents forward displacement of the tibia when moving on the femur. Genu recurvatum is excessive extension of the knee, during which the tibia is displaced abnormally forward upon the femur. Recurrence of this hyperextension leads to laxity (over stretching) of the anterior cruciate ligament.

Reference: Sahrmann, S. (2002). *Diagnosis and treatment of movement impairment syndromes* (p. 43). St. Louis: Mosby.

16. Correct answer: (b)

Rationale: An anterior pelvic tilt may result in genu valgus, lateral tibial torsion, pes planus, and hallux valgus.

Reference: Kisner, C., & Colby, L. (2002). *Therapeutic exercise: Foundations and techniques* (4th ed., p. 391). Philadelphia: FA Davis.

17. Correct answer: (a)

Rationale: The olecranon reflects an internally rotated position of the humerus, most likely due to short humeral internal rotators. Forward head is more likely due to sternocleidomastoid shortness. The anterior-superior iliac spine is supposed to be in the same frontal plane at the pubis symphysis. Scapula positioned within 2" of the spinous processes would be considered an ideal alignment.

Reference: Sahrmann, S. (2002). *Diagnosis and treatment of movement impairment syndromes* (p. 198). St. Louis: Mosby.

18. Correct answer: (a)

Rationale: Forward shoulder posture is often a result of weak middle trapezius and short pectoral muscles. Persons with posterior pelvic tilt and flat low back often have short hamstrings, or gluteus maximus.

Reference: Kendall, F., et al. (1993). *Muscles: Testing and function* (4th ed., p. 287). Baltimore: Williams & Wilkins.

RANGE OF MOTION AND MUSCLE LENGTH

Sixteen Items

1. Correct answer: (d)

   Rationale: When the knee is flexed and the hip taken towards extension, it is limited by the length of the rectus femoris. When the knee is extended and the hip taken towards extension, it is limited only by the iliopsoas. Since the femur failed to reach neutral with either position of the knee, then both hip flexors are indicted as short.

   Reference: Kendall, F., et al. (1993). *Muscles: Testing and function* (4th ed., p. 34). Baltimore: Williams & Wilkins.

2. Correct answer: (a)

   Rationale: Passive insufficiency means that a muscle could lengthen no further. The posture in this item is the lengthening positions of the biceps muscle.

   Reference: Lippert, L. (2000). *Clinical kinesiology for physical therapist assistants* (3rd ed., p. 39). Philadelphia: FA Davis.

3. Correct answer: (b)

   Rationale: Passive insufficiency means that a muscle could lengthen no further. The normal length for the hamstrings in sitting is to allow full knee flexion.

   Reference: Lippert, L. (2000). *Clinical kinesiology for physical therapist assistants* (3rd ed., p. 39). Philadelphia: FA Davis.

4. Correct answer: (c)

   Rationale: The latissimus dorsi attaches to the medial humerus and the lumbar spine. In hooklying and shoulder flexion, the fibers must lengthen to allow full shoulder flexion. Substitutions for short latissimus dorsi include medial rotation of the humerus or lumbar extension.

   Reference: Kendall, F., et al. (1993). *Muscles: Testing and function* (4th ed., p. 63). Baltimore: Williams & Wilkins.

5. Correct answer: (c)

   Rationale: In short-sitting, the hamstrings are lengthened proximally due to the flexed position of the hip. In supine, the hip is closer to neutral and allows the knee to extend further.

   Reference: Kendall, F., et al. (1993). *Muscles: Testing and function* (4th ed., p. 210). Baltimore: Williams & Wilkins.

6. Correct answer: (a)

   Rationale: Active range of motion is typically equal to or slightly less than available range of motion. Active range of motion reflects the volitional recruitment of muscles. The first choice shows significantly deficient active excursion through the available range of motion. Passive range of motion reflects muscle length or joint available range.

Reference: Kendall, F., et al. (1993). *Muscles: Testing and function* (4th ed., p. 210). Baltimore: Williams & Wilkins.

7. Correct answer: (d)

   Rationale: The hip is abducted prior to extension in order to place the iliotibial band over the greater trochanter. Avoid rotation of the femur.

   Reference: Kendall, F., et al. (1993). *Muscles: Testing and function* (4th ed., p. 57). Baltimore: Williams & Wilkins.

8. Correct answer: (b)

   Rationale: Normal length during the Ober's test will result in 10° of hip adduction. Less than that is positive for iliotibial band shortness.

   Reference: Kendall, F., et al. (1993). *Muscles: Testing and function* (4th ed., p. 57). Baltimore: Williams & Wilkins.

9. Correct answer: (a)

   Rationale: The scale of a universal goniometer is located on the stationary arm, in increments of 1°.

   Reference: Norkin, C., & White, D. (1995). *Measurement of joint motion: A guide to goniometry* (2nd ed., p. 18). Philadelphia: FA Davis.

10. Correct answer: (c)

    Rationale: Measurements should occur on an unpadded surface, with use of a goniometer. A tape measure is not needed for the forward reach test. Dynamometers are used for strength testing.

    Reference: Kendall, F., et al. (1993). *Muscles: Testing and function* (4th ed., p. 33). Baltimore: Williams & Wilkins.

11. Correct answer: (d)

    Rationale: Measurement of the same motion taken by two or more different persons is a comparison of intertester reliability. Goniometric measurements should have a reliability of 3° within and among testers.

    Reference: Norkin, C., & White, D. (1995). *Measurement of joint motion: A guide to goniometry* (2nd ed., p. 37). Philadelphia: FA Davis.

12. Correct answer: (a)

    Rationale: Intratester reliability is a comparison of results obtained by a single tester, repeatedly. Goniometry measurement should vary by no more than 3°–5°.

    Reference: Norkin, C., & White, D. (1995). *Measurement of joint motion: A guide to goniometry* (2nd ed., p. 41). Philadelphia: FA Davis.

13. Correct answer: (b)

    Rationale: The first and third choices are examples of intertester and intratester reliability, respectively. Validity relates to how accurately a measurement represents what it intends.

    Reference: Norkin, C., & White, D. (1995). *Measurement of joint motion: A guide to goniometry* (2nd ed., p. 35). Philadelphia: FA Davis.

14. Correct answer: (c)

Rationale: Sitting is an acceptable alternative position, but supine provides more stabilization to the trunk, and decreases substitutions.

Reference: Norkin, C., & White, D. (1995). *Measurement of joint motion: A guide to goniometry* (2nd ed., p. 62). Philadelphia: FA Davis.

15. Correct answer: (c)

Rationale: Many times a person with total knee replacements is measured in sitting on the edge of a mat table. However, the question in this item is not about these persons. The preferred position is supine with gravity assisting.

Reference: Norkin, C., & White, D. (1995). *Measurement of joint motion: A guide to goniometry* (2nd ed., p. 143). Philadelphia: FA Davis.

16. Correct answer: (d)

Rationale: The leg is first tested with the knee flexed, if shortness is suspected, the knee is extended to eliminate passive insufficiency of the rectus femoris.

Reference: Kendall, F., et al. (1993). *Muscles: Testing and function* (4th ed., p. 35). Baltimore: Williams & Wilkins.

MUSCLE PERFORMANCE—MANUAL MUSCLE TESTING

Sixteen Items

1. Correct answer: (d)

Rationale: The fair strength grade must be tested against gravity. A trace strength grade is an absence of volitional range, and given only in the presence of a visible or palpable muscle contraction.

Reference: Hislop, H., & Montgomery, J. (2002). *Daniels and Worthingham's muscle testing techniques of manual examination* (7th ed., p. 7). Philadelphia: WB Saunders.

2. Correct answer: (d)

Rationale: These are the antigravity positions for testing and strengthening the biceps muscle.

Reference: Hislop, H., & Montgomery, J. (2002). *Daniels and Worthingham's muscle testing techniques of manual examination* (7th ed., p. 116). Philadelphia: WB Saunders.

3. Correct answer: (d)

Rationale: Sidelying achieves the horizontal plane necessary to detect poor minus strength.

Reference: Kendall, F., et al. (1993). *Muscles: Testing and function* (4th ed., p. 187). Baltimore: Williams & Wilkins.

4. Correct answer: (d)

Rationale: Prone is used to achieve the antigravity position. External rotation of the humerus elimates contributions from the rhomboid muscles.

Reference: Kendall, F., et al. (1993). *Muscles: Testing and function* (4th ed., p. 284). Baltimore: Williams & Wilkins.

5. Correct answer: (d)

   Rationale: The gastrocnemius and soleus are typically tested in prone or standing.

   Reference: Kendall, F., et al. (1993): *Muscles: Testing and function* (4th ed., pp. 204–206). Baltimore: Williams & Wilkins.

6. Correct answer: (b)

   Rationale: This is the antigravity position required to detect a good plus strength grade.

   Reference: Kendall, F., et al. (1993). *Muscles: Testing and function* (4th ed., pp. 260–261). Baltimore: Williams & Wilkins.

7. Correct answer: (b)

   Rationale: The gastrocnemius also crosses the knee joint posteriorly, and can be a contributor to knee flexion when the ankle is dorsiflexed.

   Reference: Hislop, H., & Montgomery, J. (2002). *Daniels and Worthingham's muscle testing techniques of manual examination* (7th ed., p. 2). Philadelphia: WB Saunders.

8. Correct answer: (d)

   Rationale: Each of these statements are true.

   Reference: Kendall, F., et al. (1993). *Muscles: Testing and function* (4th ed., p. 216). Baltimore: Williams & Wilkins.

9. Correct answer: (a)

   Rationale: Dorsiflexing the foot allows the gastrocnemius to assist with knee flexion.

   Reference: Kendall, F., et al. (1993). *Muscles: Testing and function* (4th ed., p. 210). Baltimore: Williams & Wilkins.

10. Correct answer: (b)

    Rationale: This is one of the primary principles to manual muscle testing with the methods given in the reference below.

    Reference: Kendall, F., et al. (1993). *Muscles: Testing and function* (4th ed., pp. 182–183). Baltimore: Williams & Wilkins.

11. Correct answer: (b)

    Rationale: The supraspinatus initiates shoulder abduction.

    Reference: Kendall, F., et al. (1993). *Muscles: Testing and function* (4th ed., p. 272). Baltimore: Williams & Wilkins.

12. Correct answer: (d)

    Rationale: The differentiation in action and strength between the medial and lateral group is ipsilateral rotation.

    Reference: Kendall, F., et al. (1993). *Muscles: Testing and function* (4th ed., pp. 208–209). Baltimore: Williams & Wilkins.

13. Correct answer: (b)

    Rationale: Both wrist extensors are required to have pure wrist extension. Activation of the extensor carpi radialis without activation of the extensor carpi ulnaris will cause lateral tracking towards the radius.

    Reference: Hislop, H., & Montgomery, J. (2002). *Daniels and Worthingham's muscle testing techniques of manual examination* (7th ed., p. 140). Philadelphia: WB Saunders.

14. Correct answer: (a)

    Rationale: This compensation occurs to avoid isometric tension in a weak gluteus medius muscle.

    Reference: Kendall, F., et al. (1993). *Muscles: Testing and function* (4th ed., p. 222). Baltimore: Williams & Wilkins.

15. Correct answer: (b)

    Rationale: When flexing the shoulder with the elbow, the biceps is shortening across the elbow and shoulder, and becomes actively insufficient; "a" is an example of good length-tension ratio, "c" is not an example of length-tension insufficiency, and "d" is an example of passive insufficiency of the hamstrings.

    Reference: Lippert, L. (2000). *Clinical kinesiology for physical therapist assistants* (3rd ed., pp. 38–39). Philadelphia: FA Davis.

16. Correct answer: (a)

    Rationale: There is less reliability with the descriptors used to assign strength grades for the "good" grades and the partial active range of motion grades. Fair and fair plus are more reliable.

    Reference: Hislop, H., & Montgomery, J. (2002). *Daniels and Worthingham's muscle testing techniques of manual examination* (7th ed., p. 5). Philadelphia: WB Saunders.

AROUSAL, ATTENTION, AND CHECKING COGNITION

Eleven Items

1. Correct answer: (a)

    Rationale: This entry represents that a person is oriented to person, place, and time.

    Reference: O'Sullivan. *Physical rehabilitation assessment and treatment* (4th ed., p. 135). Philadelphia: FA Davis.

2. Correct answer: (b)

    Rationale: Receptive aphasia refers to comprehension of language, expressive is speaking language. Aphagia is the inability to swallow.

    Reference: Berryman Reese, N. (1999). *Muscle and sensory testing* (p. 452). Philadelphia: WB Saunders.

3. Correct answer: (a)

   Rationale: The three categories of the Glasgow Coma Scale are opening eyes, motor response, and verbal response.

   Reference: Anemaet, W., et al. (2000). *Home rehabilitation: Guide to clinical practice* (p. 368). St. Louis: Mosby.

4. Correct answer: (b)

   Rationale: Grade I is classified as unresponsive to any stimulus.

   Reference: Anemaet, W., et al. (2000). *Home rehabilitation: Guide to clinical practice* (p. 369). St. Louis: Mosby.

5. Correct answer: (a)

   Rationale: This is the neurological condition that can occur with injury to the brain.

   Reference: O'Sullivan. (2001). *Physical rehabilitation assessment and treatment* (4th ed., p. 375). Philadelphia: FA Davis.

6. Correct answer: (a)

   Rationale: When checking a person's orientation to place, it is in reference to their current location. Applications can include building, street, city, state, country, etc.

   Reference: Berryman Reese, N. (1999). *Muscle and sensory testing* (p. 451). Philadelphia: WB Saunders.

7. Correct answer: (c)

   Rationale: This question addressed only orientation to place.

   Reference: O'Sullivan. (2001). *Physical rehabilitation assessment and treatment* (4th ed., p. 135). Philadelphia: FA Davis.

8. Correct answer: (d)

   Rationale: A person with hearing deficits may not respond to verbal questions. Care should be taken to confirm the ability to hear prior to assessing alertness and orientation. A person without deficits may be distracted by a television.

   Reference: O'Sullivan. (2001). *Physical rehabilitation assessment and treatment* (4th ed., p. 136). Philadelphia: FA Davis.

9. Correct answer: (c)

   Rationale: This is the only cognitively directed question. The first two choices are directed towards orientation, and the last choice towards memory.

   Reference: O'Sullivan. (2001). *Physical rehabilitation assessment and treatment* (4th ed., p. 136). Philadelphia: FA Davis.

10. Correct answer: (b)

    Rationale: A transient attack is short in duration. The effects may be intense or mild, and affect one or several areas of the brain.

    Reference: O'Sullivan. (2001). *Physical rehabilitation assessment and treatment* (4th ed., p. 523). Philadelphia: FA Davis.

11. Correct answer: (d)

    Rationale: A mild stroke would not cause death.

    Reference: O'Sullivan. (2001). *Physical rehabilitation assessment and treatment* (4th ed., p. 523). Philadelphia: FA Davis.

CHECKING REFLEXES AND MUSCLE TONE

Nineteen Items

1. Correct answer: (d)

   Rationale: Flaccidity is the absence of muscular tone or volitional recruitment.

   Reference: O'Sullivan. (2001). *Physical rehabilitation assessment and treatment* (4th ed., p. 184). Philadelphia: FA Davis.

2. Correct answer: (b)

   Rationale: The third to fifth cervical nerve roots innervate the diaphragm.

   Reference: Nixon, V., & Schneider, F. (1985). *Spinal cord injury: A guide to functional outcomes in physical therapy management* (p. 48). Maryland: Aspen.

3. Correct answer: (d)

   Rationale: The upper trapezius and sternocleidomastoid receive innervation from the spinal accessory nerve, and the third and fourth cervical nerves. The other choices are the fifth, fourth, and third cranial nerves, respectively.

   Reference: Cipriano, J. (2003). *Photographic manual of regional orthopedic and neurologic tests* (4th ed., pp. 443–446). Philadelphia: Lippincott Williams & Wilkins.

4. Correct answer: (c)

   Rationale: The brachioradialis reflex is innervated primarily at the C6 neurological level. The second choice is a strength test, not a reflex. The deltoid is innervated primarily by C5.

   Reference: Hoppenfeld, S. (1976). *Physical examination of the spine and extremities* (p. 121). Norwalk, CT: Appleton & Lange.

5. Correct answer: (d)

   Rationale: The contributions to this reflex arise from the second to fourth lumbar nerve roots, but primarily from the fourth.

   Reference: Hoppenfeld, S. (1976). *Physical examination of the spine and extremities* (p. 250). Norwalk, CT: Appleton & Lange.

6. Correct answer: (c)

   Rationale: This muscle is the L4-L5 myotome.

   Reference: Hoppenfeld, S. (1976). *Physical examination of the spine and extremities* (p. 250). Norwalk, CT: Appleton & Lange.

7. Correct answer: (b)

   Rationale: There is no reflex test for the fifth lumbar neurological level.

   Reference: Hoppenfeld, S. (1976). *Physical examination of the spine and extremities* (p. 252). Norwalk, CT: Appleton & Lange.

8. Correct answer: (b)

   Rationale: The spinal cord terminates at the first or second lumbar level. The first two sacral nerves innervate the soleus muscle.

   Reference: Hoppenfeld, S. (1976). *Physical examination of the spine and extremities* (p. 253). Norwalk, CT: Appleton & Lange.

9. Correct answer: (a)

   Rationale: The other choices are similar, but not the correct method for the Babinski. A positive sign occurs with extension and abduction of the toes during the test.

   Reference: O'Sullivan. (2001). *Physical rehabilitation assessment and treatment* (4th ed., p. 183). Philadelphia: FA Davis.

10. Correct answer: (c)

    Rationale: Posterior = sensory, anterior = motor. Sensory signals enter the posterior cord, and do exit immediately through the anterior horn, but they also continue to the brain. In many events, there is a motor response before sensory interpretation by the brain.

    Reference: Somers, M. (2001). *Spinal cord injury: Functional rehabilitation* (2nd ed., p. 26). New Jersey: Prentice Hall.

11. Correct answer: (d)

    Rationale: Muscles of the thenar eminence and opposition muscles are innervated by the median nerve.

    Reference: Rothstein, J., et al. (1998). *The rehabilitation specialist's handbook* (2nd ed., p. 323). Philadelphia: FA Davis.

12. Correct answer: (b)

    Rationale: The radial nerve supplies the triceps, anconeus, brachioradialis, supinator, and distal extensor muscles.

    Reference: Lippert, L. (2000). *Clinical kinesiology for physical therapist assistants* (3rd ed., p. 75). Philadelphia: FA Davis.

13. Correct answer: (c)

    Rationale: Myotomes are the anatomical reference points to the spinal nerve roots used to map muscle function and impairment.

    Reference: Cipriano, J. (2003). *Photographic manual of regional orthopedic and neurologic tests* (4th ed., p. 93). Philadelphia: Lippincott Williams & Wilkins.

14. Correct answer: (d)

    Rationale: The first three choices are signs that are consistent with lower motor neuron injuries. The anterior horn of the spinal cord is where motor tracts exit the spinal cord. Impairment of these would result in a decrease in tone and volition. Spasticity is consistent with an upper motor neuron injury.

Reference: Lippert, L. (2000). *Clinical kinesiology for physical therapist assistants* (3rd ed., p. 67). Philadelphia: FA Davis.

15. Correct answer: (c)

Rationale: This is the definition of neuropraxia.

Reference: O'Sullivan. (2001). *Physical rehabilitation assessment and treatment* (4th ed., p. 233). Philadelphia: FA Davis.

16. Correct answer: (a)

Rationale: The ATNR reflex is a similar posture to shooting an arrow or aiming a rifle.

Reference: O'Sullivan. (2001). *Physical rehabilitation assessment and treatment* (4th ed., p. 532). Philadelphia: FA Davis.

17. Correct answer: (c)

Rationale: Clonus is an undesired cyclical and spasmodic response to stretching.

Reference: O'Sullivan. (2001). *Physical rehabilitation assessment and treatment* (4th ed., p. 183). Philadelphia: FA Davis.

18. Correct answer: (c)

Rationale: Paresis is a weakness, commonly associated with impairment of lower motor neurons. Each of the other choices are clinical signs of upper motor neuron lesions.

Reference: Lippert, L. (2000). *Clinical kinesiology for physical therapist assistants* (3rd ed., p. 67). Philadelphia: FA Davis.

19. Correct answer: (a)

Rationale: Upper motor neuron injuries typically result in hypertonicity. Injuries to the spinal cord may also involve upper motor neurons. The initial response of cerebral vascular accidents is flaccidity and hypotonia.

Reference: Lippert, L. (2000). *Clinical kinesiology for physical therapist assistants* (3rd ed., p. 67). Philadelphia: FA Davis.

SENSORY INTEGRITY: SENSATION, PROPRIOCEPTION, AND KINESTHESIA

Fifteen Items

1. Correct answer: (a)

Rationale: "Derma" means skin, "tome" means division.

Reference: Lippert, L. (2000). *Clinical kinesiology for physical therapist assistants* (3rd ed., p. 71). Philadelphia: FA Davis.

2. Correct answer: (a)

Rationale: The throat is located in the C3 dermatome. An injury at C5 would compromise sensation at the nipple line (T4) and navel (T10).

Reference: Lippert, L. (2000). *Clinical kinesiology for physical therapist assistants* (3rd ed., p. 71). Philadelphia: FA Davis.

3. Correct answer: (a)

Rationale: The second choice describes central cord syndrome, the third, sacral sparing. The last choice is invalid.

Reference: Somers, M. (2001). *Spinal cord injury: Functional rehabilitation* (2nd ed., p. 28) New Jersey: Prentice Hall.

4. Correct answer: (c)

Rationale: The other choices are the C5, T2, and T6 dermatomes, respectively.

Reference: O'Sullivan. (2001). *Physical rehabilitation assessment and treatment* (4th ed., p. 143). Philadelphia: FA Davis.

5. Correct answer: (a)

Rationale: Kinesthesia is the awareness motion, both in direction and magnitude.

Reference: O'Sullivan. (2001). *Physical rehabilitation assessment and treatment* (4th ed., p. 145). Philadelphia: FA Davis.

6. Correct answer: (a)

Rationale: The lateral spinothalamic tract carries sensory signals from the trunk and extremities, and the ventral trigeminothalamic from the face. The rubrospinal carries efferent impulses to the upper extremities, and the lateral corticospinal carries efferent impulses to the distal limbs.

Reference: Berryman Reese, N. (1999). *Muscle and sensory testing* (p. 426). Philadelphia: WB Saunders.

7. Correct answer: (c)

Rationale: This is the general dermatome for the third lumbar nerve root.

Reference: Somers, M. (2001). *Spinal cord injury: Functional rehabilitation* (2nd ed., p. 26). New Jersey: Prentice Hall.

8. Correct answer: (b)

Rationale: This is the universal dermatome for the fourth thoracic nerve root, used in mapping sensory function.

Reference: O'Sullivan. (2001). *Physical rehabilitation assessment and treatment* (4th ed., p. 143). Philadelphia: FA Davis.

9. Correct answer: (b)

Rationale: Proprioception is the sensation of joint position.

Reference: O'Sullivan. (2001). *Physical rehabilitation assessment and treatment* (4th ed., p. 145). Philadelphia: FA Davis.

10. Correct answer: (d)

    Rationale: This is within the cutaneous distribution of the ulnar nerve.

    Reference: Berryman Reese, N. (1999). *Muscle and sensory testing* (p. 425). Philadelphia: WB Saunders.

11. Correct answer: (c)

    Rationale: This is the standard for the Semmes–Weinstein monofilament test.

    Reference: O'Sullivan. (2001). *Physical rehabilitation assessment and treatment* (4th ed., p. 591). Philadelphia: FA Davis.

12. Correct answer: (b)

    Rationale: This is the standard dermatome mapping for T10.

    Reference: Somers, M. (2001). *Spinal cord injury: Functional rehabilitation* (2nd ed., p. 26) New Jersey: Prentice Hall.

13. Correct answer: (b)

    Rationale: Lateral cord syndrome is also known as Brown–Sequard sydrome. Anterior cord syndrome primarily results in motor impairment, posterior cord in fine discrimination and proprioception, and central cord syndrome results more upper extremity impairment than lower.

    Reference: Somers, M. (2001). *Spinal cord injury: Functional rehabilitation* (2nd ed., p. 28). New Jersey: Prentice Hall.

14. Correct answer: (d)

    Rationale: This is the definition of dysdiadochokinesia.

    Reference: O'Sullivan. (2001). *Physical rehabilitation assessment and treatment* (4th ed., p. 160). Philadelphia: FA Davis.

15. Correct answer: (d)

    Rationale: None of the other statements are completely true. Individuals, who even regain the skill of walking, may experience abnormal reflexes.

    Reference: Somers, M. (2001). *Spinal cord injury: Functional rehabilitation* (2nd ed., pp. 24–28). New Jersey: Prentice Hall.

Test and Measures Group II: Cardiovascular System, Pulmonary System, Integumentary System, and Measuring Functional Status

OVERVIEW

This chapter includes questions covering clinical tests and measurements included in the exam. There are 90 questions in this chapter that deal with the cardiovascular system, pulmonary system, integumentary system, and measuring functional status.

KEY POINTS FOR REVIEW

Aerobic Capacity and Endurance

- Cardiac limitations
- Perceived level of exertion
- Metabolic equivalence tables
- Terminology

Circulation and Vital Signs

- Edema grades
- Autonomic nervous system
- Pulse and blood pressure

Ventilation and Respiration

- Respiration rate
- Dyspnea index
- Terminology
- Oxygen saturation

Integumentary System

- Skin grafts
- Rule of nines
- Staging and grading of wounds
- Skin anatomy
- Terminology

Measurement and Selection of Assistive and Adaptive Devices

- Wheelchair fitting
- Ambulation and adaptive devices

Gait, Locomotion, and Balance

- Phases and events of normal gait
- Balance tests and grading
- Balance strategies
- Terminology

Checking Pain

- Pain scales
- Terminology

Ergonomics and Body Mechanics

- Ideal postures
- Normal anatomy
- Observations for body mechanics
- Terminology

AEROBIC CAPACITY AND ENDURANCE

Twelve Items

1. Which of the following treatment sequences would be MOST appropriate for a person participating in an ambulation-based cardiac rehabilitation?

    _____ a. perform active range of motion, check vital signs, ambulate, check vital signs, perform active range of motion, and check perceived level of exertion

_____ b. check vital signs, perform active range of motion, check vital signs, ambulate, check perceived level of exertion, and check vital signs

_____ c. check vital signs, perform active range of motion, check vital signs, ambulate, check perceived level of exertion, check vital signs, perform active range of motion, and check vital signs

_____ d. ask perceived level of exertion, check vital signs, perform active range of motion, ambulate, and check vital signs

2. When monitoring the cardiovascular exertion of a child 10 years of age, which of the following is considered a normal value for heart rate?

_____ a. 100 beats per minute

_____ b. 50 beats per minute

_____ c. 150 beats per minute

_____ d. 200 beats per minute

3. You are ambulating with a person who is having difficulty with energy conservation. After educating the patient on energy conserving strategies, which of the following is LEAST necessary to monitor energy expenditure?

_____ a. perceived level of exertion

_____ b. monitor heart rate

_____ c. cardiac telemetry

_____ d. treadmill testing

4. Some individuals, who have spent a prolonged time in bed, experience orthostatic hypotension. Which of the following activities is MOST appropriate to reduce the effects of orthostatic hypotension during the first or second treatment day?

_____ a. have the person perform active range of motion in the bed

_____ b. have the person sit upright several times during the day

_____ c. have the person sit upright and perform active range of motion several times during the day

_____ d. have the person perform sit-to-stand several times during the day

5. The physical therapist has evaluated a person and designed a cardiac rehabilitation program in an inpatient setting. Today they have requested that you perform endurance training with the person at a 3–4 MET level. Which of the following activities is MOST appropriate to meet the plan of care?

_____ a. ambulate with the person in the hallway for 8–10 minutes, as tolerated

_____ b. ambulate with the person up and down one flight of stairs using at least one handrail, as tolerated

_____ c. have the person sit bedside in a recliner for at least 25 minutes, as tolerated

_____ d. have the person perform closed-chain, low-exertion activities in standing, as tolerated

6. Which of the following exercise interventions are LEAST appropriate for addressing endurance?

_____ a. an endurance training program at moderate intensity to significantly reverse a loss of cardiovascular capacity in an older adult

_____ b. aerobic exercise to reduce the risk of developing type I diabetes mellitus in an older adult

_____ c. endurance exercise to accelerate the synthesis of growth hormones from the pituitary gland

_____ d. aerobic activity to improve endurance, performed three days a week, for more than 10 minutes

7. A person is participating in endurance interventions in an inpatient setting. Which of the following signs or symptoms is MOST appropriate following endurance exercise?

_____ a. dyspnea

_____ b. claudication

_____ c. insomnia

_____ d. fatigue

8. A person with multiple sclerosis is experiencing recurrent fatigue and poor tolerance to endurance activities. Which of the following strategies is MOST appropriate based upon this information?

_____ a. have the person decrease the duration of endurance activities

_____ b. utilize therapeutic heating source to decrease muscle soreness and increase vasodilatation to muscles

_____ c. discuss with the person how to pace their daily activities

_____ d. avoid strenuous activities during remission of their disease

9. Which of the following clinical observations is LEAST critical when a person is participating in endurance training?

_____ a. rate of perceived exertion

_____ b. duration of activity

_____ c. respiration rate

_____ d. blood pressure

10. Which of the following observations is the MOST appropriate physiological response for a person performing endurance exercise?

_____ a. an increase in heart rate less than 25 beats per minute during exertion

_____ b. a decrease in resting heart rate and resting respiratory rate immediately following the endurance activity

_____ c. an increase in heart rate less than 10 beats per minute, when taking beta-blockers

_____ d. an increase in resting respiratory rate during exertion

11. Which of the following clinical tests MOST closely approximates peak oxygen consumption during endurance activities?

_____ a. ambulation with or without an assistive device, using the total distance divided by the elapsed time

_____ b. the Borg scale

_____ c. the 6 minute walk test

_____ d. the Tinetti assessment tool

12. Which of the following is MOST appropriate to address the goal of improving muscular endurance?

_____ a. patient to perform stationary bike for 10 minutes

_____ b. patient to perform leg press with 5 pounds for 40 repetitions

_____ c. patient to perform five sets of ten repetitions with a medium resistance elastic band

_____ d. patient to perform treadmill at 15% grade for 20 minutes

CIRCULATION AND VITAL SIGNS

Eleven Items

1. The physical therapist delegates to you interventions for a woman, 42 years of age, who just had removal of lymphatic nodes from the left axillary region secondary to cancer. The therapist instructs you to address postsurgical edema through measurement and application of a compression garment and massage. Which of the following will give the BEST results?

_____ a. perform compression pump therapy first, then apply the compression garment

_____ b. massage the proximal lymphatic nodes first, then the rest of the extremity

_____ c. massage the distal lymphatic nodes first, then the rest of the extremity

_____ d. apply the compression garment first, then perform the massage

2. A soft area of movable edema, which leaves an imprint after pressure is removed, is described as which of the following?

_____ a. brawning edema

_____ b. chronic edema

_____ c. pitting edema

_____ d. disputary edema

3. The autonomic nervous system regulates the rate of myocardial contraction. Sympathetic impulses cause the heart rate to do which of the following?

_____ a. increase

_____ b. decrease

_____ c. sustain

_____ d. fluctuate

4. After a warm-up on the stationary bike, you check your patient's heart rate and find that it is tachycardic; this means that his heart rate is which of the following?

_____ a. less than 90 beats per minute

_____ b. greater than 90 beats per minute

_____ c. less than 100 beats per minute

_____ d. greater than 100 beats per minute

5. Prior to beginning a treatment session with a person who is being treated in an inpatient setting, it is important to check their vital signs. Which of the following blood pressure readings would you find while taking blood pressure that MOST qualifies a person as hypertensive?

    ____ a. 140/92

    ____ b. 140/80

    ____ c. 130/66

    ____ d. 120/84

6. When documenting girth measurements for a person with an acute ankle sprain, which of the following would be the MOST appropriate statement in your SOAP note?

    ____ a. left ankle 17″ in girth

    ____ b. pretreatment left ankle girth was 17″ across medial and lateral malleoli, 14″ at 4″ proximal to malleoli, and 15″ at 2″ distal

    ____ c. posttreatment left ankle girth was 17″, 14″, and 15″, (at malleoli, 8 centimeters proximal, and 5 centimeters distal)

    ____ d. girth not measured this date secondary to edema

7. Vascularization of the brain can remain intact, even in the event of occlusion, because of which anatomical structure?

    ____ a. Brown-Sequard

    ____ b. circle of Williams

    ____ c. anterior communicating artery

    ____ d. circle of Willis

8. A physical therapist assistant is measuring capillary refill time for a person with compromised circulation. What is the normal capillary refill time?

    ____ a. less than 3 seconds

    ____ b. 3–5 seconds

    ____ c. 5–7 seconds

    ____ d. greater in the upper extremities than the lower

9. A person has lymphedema affecting their left upper extremity. Girth measurements reveal generally a 4 centimeter difference between the left and right upper extremities. Which lymphedema classification MOST accurately describes these observations?

    ____ a. negligible

    ____ b. mild

    ____ c. moderate

    ____ d. severe

10. A physical therapist assistant is performing peripheral pulse assessment of a person's extremity. The assistant palpates the pulse and determines it is easy to palpate, but not bounding. Which pulse grade SHOULD be recorded in the objective portion of their documentation?

_____ a. 0

_____ b. 1+

_____ c. 2+

_____ d. 3+

11. In which position SHOULD peripheral pulses be assessed?

    _____ a. supine

    _____ b. an elevated position of the affected limb

    _____ c. sitting

    _____ d. a dependent position of the affected limb

VENTILATION AND RESPIRATION

Eight Items

1. You observe that a person whom you are treating with endurance interventions is to be monitored by pulse oximetry during exertion. At which vascular structure does air exchange occur in the lungs?

    _____ a. pulmonary arteries

    _____ b. pulmonary veins

    _____ c. aorta

    _____ d. alveoli

2. A person is about to participate in an endurance activity. Which of the following observations is the MOST acceptable for an adult?

    _____ a. oxygen saturation greater than 84%

    _____ b. a resting rate greater than 20 respirations per minute

    _____ c. a duration ratio of 1:2, inspiration to expiration

    _____ d. dyspnea and use of accessory muscles for ventilation

3. A person who is recovering from surgery performed yesterday is MOST likely to suffer respiratory problems due to which of the following reasons?

    _____ a. pain medications may stimulate normal ciliary action of the tracheobronchial tree

    _____ b. pain medications may stimulate the cough reflex

    _____ c. pain medications may stimulate hyperventilation

    _____ d. pain medications may depress respiratory activity

4. A person with respiratory impairment is participating in therapeutic interventions to improve endurance. The person complains of shortness of breath during activity. Using the dyspnea index to assess shortness of breath, the person inhales, then counts out loud and slowly to fifteen. The person counts to six, takes a breath, counts to eleven, takes a breath, and then finishes the count to fifteen. Which of the following scores represents the dyspnea index for this person?

_____ a. six

_____ b. eleven

_____ c. forty-five

_____ d. two

5. A person is ambulating with a wheeled walker and minimal contact assistance. Presently the person begins to complain of shortness of breath. During periods of increased dyspnea, which of the following postures would assist the person in recovering their breathing?

_____ a. sitting, with their upper extremities unsupported

_____ b. semirecumbent, leaning back against a wall

_____ c. standing, leaning forward onto the assistive device

_____ d. standing, with their upper extremities unsupported

6. When observing a person's breathing pattern, you detect a rapid rate, shallow depth, regular rhythm, and accessory muscle contribution. Based upon these observations, which of the following breathing patterns is being exhibited?

_____ a. dyspnea

_____ b. orthopnea

_____ c. hyperpnea

_____ d. eupnea

7. Which of the following clinical observations reflects the amount of oxygen perfusion into the extremities during periods of rest and exertion?

_____ a. respiration rate

_____ b. inspirometer

_____ c. pulse oximetry

_____ d. blood pressure

8. When observing a person's ventilation efficiency, you generally observe their skeletal posture. Which of the following skeletal postures functionally limits vital capacity of the lungs?

_____ a. lordosis

_____ b. s-curve scoliosis

_____ c. professorial posture

_____ d. posterior pelvic tilt

INTEGUMENTARY SYSTEM

Fifteen Items

1. After whirlpool and debridement interventions, it is determined that a patient needs an autograft. What does this mean?

_____ a. the skin graft will be donated from another human donor

_____ b. human skin from an anonymous donor will be used

_____ c. lamb skin will be applied to automatically facilitate healing

_____ d. the skin will be transplanted from another part of the body

2. An adult receiving whirlpool intervention for burns on the head, neck, and full trunk would be classified at what percent of the affected body surface?

_____ a. 45%

_____ b. 9%

_____ c. 36%

_____ d. 18%

3. A burn that includes damage to the epidermis and dermis, which is very painful and has some bleeding present, is classified as which of the following?

_____ a. full thickness

_____ b. superficial

_____ c. partial thickness

_____ d. stage IV

4. An adult person with burn injuries covering their bilateral upper extremities would be classified by the rule of nines as having burnt what percentage of their body?

_____ a. 9%

_____ b. 18%

_____ c. 36%

_____ d. 27%

5. Upon admission to a medical facility, a person's risk for developing pressure sores is assessed using the Braden scale. This assessment tool is repeated a few days later, with a resulting score of fourteen. Which of the following levels of risk is consistent with this score?

_____ a. negligible risk level

_____ b. mild risk

_____ c. moderate risk level

_____ d. high risk level

6. Which of the following conditions is MOST consistent with a lower extremity that is excessively cool to touch?

_____ a. arterial insufficiency

_____ b. diabetes

_____ c. venous insufficiency

_____ d. Raynaud's phenomenon

7. A person experiences a burn injury over the distal half of the anterior lower leg. Using the rule of nines, this person would most likely be classified as having which of the following percentages of

total body surface injury?

_____ a. 2.2%

_____ b. 4.5%

_____ c. 9%

_____ d. 13.5 %

8. A person has a pressure ulcer, which exposes destruction of underlying muscle and bone tissue. Which of the following pressure ulcer classifications would be MOST accurate when describing this person's wound?

_____ a. stage I

_____ b. stage II

_____ c. stage III

_____ d. stage IV

9. A person suffers an injury to the skin, resulting in loss of perception of pressure and vibration. Which of the following is MOST accurate about this person's injury?

_____ a. the person has suffered a superficial partial-thickness injury

_____ b. the person has suffered a deep partial-thickness injury

_____ c. the person has suffered a deep thickness injury

_____ d. the person has suffered a superficial thickness injury

10. Which of the following wound measurement techniques facilitates consistency between clinicians when referring to wound descriptions?

_____ a. document the location of variations in the surface of the skin using north, south, east, or west

_____ b. document the location of wounds, describing any variations as in the direction of a clock, using 12:00 in reference to the nearest bony anatomical landmark

_____ c. document the location of tunnels by referencing them to soft tissue anatomical landmarks

_____ d. document the location of tunnels by referencing them as clocks, with 12:00 being referenced cephalically

11. A person received an injury while getting into a wheelchair. When describing the injury to the skin in an incident report, which of the following terms is MOST consistent with a scraping lesion to the skin?

_____ a. incision injury

_____ b. laceration injury

_____ c. abrasion injury

_____ d. excoriation injury

12. A person has an open wound with moderate exudate. When describing wound drainage that is thin, watery, pale red, or pink, which of the following terms can be used for documentation?

_____ a. purulent

_____ b. serous

_____ c. serosanguineous

_____ d. sanguineous

13. A person's right distal lower extremity has a skin ulceration that appears cool, dry, and with dermal atrophy. Which type of skin ulcer is typically being described?

_____ a. arterial ulcer

_____ b. diabetic ulcer

_____ c. venous ulcer

_____ d. intrinsic ulcer

14. A person with nonblanchable, warm, erythematous skin, who does not have any open areas, would have that location of their skin graded at which classification of skin pressure ulceration?

_____ a. stage I

_____ b. stage II

_____ c. stage III

_____ d. stage IV

15. A child who stepped into an open receptacle suffered a steam burn injury throughout nearly all of their left lower extremity. Based upon this information, which of the following percentages of their body surface is injured?

_____ a. 5.5%

_____ b. 18%

_____ c. 9%

_____ d. 26%

MEASURE AND SELECT ASSISTIVE AND ADAPTIVE DEVICES

Sixteen Items

1. You are preparing to instruct a person in the use of Lofstrand crutches. Which of the following is NOT one of the advantages of using Lofstrand crutches?

_____ a. Lofstrand crutches reduce the likelihood of axillary region compression

_____ b. Lofstrand crutches provide less stability than a standard cane

_____ c. Lofstrand crutches are more functional on stairs than a small-base quad cane

_____ d. Lofstrand crutches provide less stability than a standard walker

2. A person unable to perform safe locomotion without maximal assistance is given a standard manual wheelchair with a sling seat. Which of the following postures are facilitated with the use of a sling seat?

_____ a. anterior pelvic tilt

_____ b. femoral adduction

_____ c. femoral external rotation

_____ d. postural symmetry

3. Adjusting the armrests of a wheelchair to the appropriate height is necessary for upper body support. Which of the following is the appropriate reference point for adjusting the armrests on a motorized wheelchair?

_____ a. the distance from the seat cushion to the olecranon process when the elbow is at 90°

_____ b. the distance from the seat cushion to the olecranon process minus 1"

_____ c. the distance from the seat cushion to the olecranon process plus 1"

_____ d. the distance from the seat cushion to the ulnar styloid when the elbow is at 90°

4. A person was recently fitted with a manual wheelchair. Which of the following is NOT the correct angle of alignment for a manual wheelchair?

_____ a. elbow at 120° angle maximum when propelling from superior surface of wheel

_____ b. knees at 105° angle when placed upon legrests

_____ c. ankles at 70° angle when placed upon footrests

_____ d. hips at 100° angle when seated on cushion

5. Which of the following measurement observations for adjusting a person's standard cane is accurate?

_____ a. the cane should be adjusted to the height of the iliac crests

_____ b. the cane should be adjusted to the height of the greater trochanter

_____ c. the cane should be adjusted to within 6" of their olecranon

_____ d. the cane should be adjusted to the height that allows 20°–25° of elbow flexion

6. A person with significant neurogenic muscle weakness in all four extremities is being fitted for a dailyuse wheelchair. Which of the following wheelchair options will BEST address the need to provide regular pressure relief?

_____ a. elevating legrests

_____ b. proportional drive

_____ c. tilt in space

_____ d. motorized frame

7. A person is preparing to ambulate, with their left lower extremity weight bearing as tolerated using a cane in their right hand. Which of the following parameters SHOULD be used to adjust the height of a standard cane?

_____ a. greater trochanter

_____ b. dorsal crease of radiocarpal joint

_____ c. elbow at 20°–30° flexion

_____ d. 4" inferior to the iliac crest

8. Which of the following is an error in adjusting axillary crutches that could lead to the devices being too short?

_____ a. the person elevates their shoulders during the height check

_____ b. the person stands in a tripod position during the height check

_____ c. the person is not wearing shoes during the initial fit

_____ d. the person is standing on an uneven surface

9. A standard wheelchair is MOST appropriate for individuals with which of the following clinical considerations?

_____ a. a person with decreased mobility function, who weighs 260 pounds

_____ b. a person with bilateral distal femoral amputations

_____ c. a person, 74 years of age, with weakness due to central cord syndrome

_____ d. a person with recent bilateral total knee arthroplasty

10. When standing, for a person to adjust forearm crutches for first time use, how is the device positioned on the floor to establish the correct support and check dimensions?

_____ a. 4″ from their toes at a 45° angle

_____ b. 6″ from their toes at a 45° angle

_____ c. 4″–6″ from their toes at 30° angle

_____ d. 2″ lateral and 2″ anterior to the toes

11. A person is initially unable to tolerate standing. The physical therapist has requested that you see the person bedside and let the person attempt standing with axillary crutches. Which of the following parameters can be used to establish an initial estimate of the correct crutch height?

_____ a. 77% of the person's height

_____ b. the length of the person's upper extremity minus 2″–4″

_____ c. 85% of the person's height

_____ d. the length of the lower extremity plus 58% of the length of the lower extremity

12. You are adjusting a manual wheelchair for a person in a hospital setting. Which of the following parameters are required to allow smooth propulsion of the wheelchair over uneven surfaces and turns?

_____ a. place a leg strap across the anterior lower extremities and wrap around the legrests

_____ b. place padded armrests facing the person

_____ c. select removable legrests

_____ d. position footrests at least 2″ from the floor

13. A person is seated in a wheelchair with the brakes locked and lower extremities on the elevated legrests. Which of the following landmarks is the anatomical reference point for checking back height?

_____ a. olecranon process

_____ b. vertebra prominens

_____ c. inferior angle of scapula

_____ d. acromion process

14. When training a person to stand for the first time, using a wheeled walker, which of the following observations is necessary for observing a good fit of the assistive device?

_____ a. the elbow should be flexed to 25°

_____ b. the handgrip of the device should be at the level of the greater trochanter

_____ c. the device should be placed 4"–6" anterior to the toes

_____ d. the device should be placed 2"–4" laterally

15. You are selecting and adjusting a manual wheelchair for a person who recently underwent a posterior approach left hip arthroplasty. Which of the following manual wheelchair options is LEAST important for this person?

_____ a. reclining seat back for positioning

_____ b. removable armrests for transfers

_____ c. large wheels for propulsion

_____ d. long handled brakes

16. A person with pulmonary dysfunction and recurrent lower extremity edema is using a standard wheelchair. Which of the following features of a standard wheelchair is MOST important for this person to use?

_____ a. reclining seat back

_____ b. elevating legrests with calf supports

_____ c. removable armrests

_____ d. raising footplate

GAIT, LOCOMOTION, AND BALANCE

Fourteen Items

1. A person who has a decreased recruitment of their gluteus medius is more likely to demonstrate weakness of the muscle during ambulation. Gluteus medius activity is greatest at which of the following phases of gait?

_____ a. midswing

_____ b. loading response

_____ c. midstance

_____ d. initial swing

2. Iliopsoas activity is greatest at which of the following phases of gait?

_____ a. initial swing

_____ b. initial contact

_____ c. terminal swing

_____ d. midstance

3. A person who recently had a rupture of the quadriceps tendon is currently under precautions for quad activity. Quadriceps activity is greatest at which of the following phases of gait?

_____ a. terminal stance

_____ b. initial swing

_____ c. loading response

_____ d. midswing

4. Which of the following pregait activities would BEST challenge a person for stability?

_____ a. short-sitting balance with perturbations

_____ b. quadruped reaching for colored cones

_____ c. ambulation in parallel bars

_____ d. standing frame

5. A person who experiences exacerbation of vertigo with their eyes closed would MOST likely exhibit signs during which of the following tests?

_____ a. timed up and go

_____ b. Romberg test

_____ c. Tinetti assessment tool

_____ d. Berg test

6. A person who lacks the ability to reach 6″ in the modified reach balance test, would MOST likely be described as which of the following?

_____ a. without impairment

_____ b. with minimal impairment

_____ c. at a high risk for falls

_____ d. at a low risk for falls

7. Relatively small perturbations in a person's base of support SHOULD be compensated for by which balance strategy?

_____ a. ankle strategy

_____ b. parachute strategy

_____ c. stepping strategy

_____ d. hip strategy

8. You are observing a person ambulating two weeks after a right total knee arthroplasty. You notice that the person lacks knee flexion during preswing and midswing. What is the normal range of motion in the knee on level surfaces during these phases of gait?

_____ a. 20°–40° of knee flexion

_____ b. 40°–60° of knee flexion

_____ c. 10°–30° of knee flexion

_____ d. 60°–80° of knee flexion

9. When observing a person ambulate, you mark and measure the distances between the initial contacts of their left heel and right heel. Which of the following gait analysis parameters have you observed?

_____ a. step length

_____ b. gait cycle

_____ c. step pattern

_____ d. stride length

10. Which of the following iliofemoral muscles is the primary agonist during midstance to heel off?

_____ a. tensor fascia latae and iliopsoas

_____ b. gluteus maximus and biceps femoris long head

_____ c. gluteus medius

_____ d. no hip muscle activity occurs during late midstance

11. When performing observational gait analysis, the pelvis is observed to drop during contralateral stance periods. In which plane SHOULD this pelvic transition occur?

_____ a. midsagittal

_____ b. sagittal

_____ c. transverse

_____ d. coronal

12. During which of the following phases of gait do you expect the axial skeleton to be at its highest elevation from the walking surface?

_____ a. early terminal swing

_____ b. late midswing

_____ c. early midstance

_____ d. early midswing

13. Which of the following plantar flexor muscles produces the greatest amount of torque upon the ankle joint during the normal gait cycle?

_____ a. gastrocnemius

_____ b. tibialis posterior

_____ c. soleus

_____ d. flexor hallucis longus

14. A person is able to maintain standing balance without support, but is unable to sufficiently respond to any external challenges to their stability. Which of the following functional balance grades is described by these observations?

_____ a. normal

_____ b. good

_____ c. fair

_____ d. poor

CHECKING PAIN

Eight Items

1. Tenderness over the tibial tuberosity epiphysis, common in male athletes and juveniles, is referred to as which of the following conditions?

_____ a. Frenkel's sign

_____ b. Osgood–Schlatter's disease

_____ c. Parkinson–Guillian disease

_____ d. Thomas' sign

2. A male who is 48 years of age is referred to physical therapy with the chief complaint of a dull ache located over the medial epicondyle. Using this information, which of the following conditions would MOST likely be suspected?

_____ a. tennis elbow

_____ b. little league's elbow

_____ c. nursemaid's elbow

_____ d. golfer's elbow

3. A person is asked to rate their symptoms using a visual analog pain scale. Which of the following is MOST accurate about the visual analog pain scale?

_____ a. it uses a horizontal or semicircular line

_____ b. it uses a line 10 centimeters in length

_____ c. it uses a line 100 millimeters in length, with 10 millimeters increments

_____ d. it uses a line 100 millimeters in length, with pain descriptors every 20 millimeters

4. Which of the following is MOST appropriate in regards to checking a person's pain?

_____ a. pain reported at the end of a treatment session may be sequentially recorded in either the subjective or plan section of a SOAP note

_____ b. acute inflammatory pain should be assessed using only open-ended questions

_____ c. assess chronic recurrent pain through the use of specified closed-ended questions

_____ d. reports of pain initiated by the patient do not require further questioning

5. Which of the following observations is MOST useful in recording a person's complaints of extremity numbness?

_____ a. ask the person to rate degree of numbness

_____ b. comparison of subjective description between involved and uninvolved limbs

_____ c. description of response to touch

_____ d. comparison of previous normal and current abnormal sensations

6. Which of the following methods of rating a person's symptoms would use a line without increments, and a request for them to indicate their level of symptoms?

_____ a. ten scale

_____ b. McGill questionnaire

_____ c. visual analog

_____ d. pain thermometer

7. A person is complaining of intermittent causalgia and numbness in their left posterior thigh. Which of the following spinal tracts transmit information about pain and temperature?

_____ a. corticospinal

_____ b. rubrospinal

_____ c. spinothalamic

_____ d. lemniscal

8. You are documenting a person's specific symptoms, including activities that exacerbate and relieve the discomfort. Which of the following ranges are MOST consistent within the painful arc of the glenohumeral joint?

_____ a. $60°-130°$

_____ b. $30°-60°$

_____ c. $120°-160°$

_____ d. initial motion up to $30°$

ERGONOMICS AND BODY MECHANICS

Six Items

1. A person who stands in genu valgus will have an increase in stress in which structures, and is MOST likely to be associated with which of the following foot postures?

_____ a. lateral collateral ligaments; supination

_____ b. medial collateral ligaments; pronation

_____ c. medial collateral ligaments; supination

_____ d. lateral collateral ligaments; pronation

2. Which of the following MOST accurately describes the purpose of the posterior longitudinal ligament?

_____ a. compress the lumbar vertebrae and protect the spinal cord

_____ b. limit vertebral extension

_____ c. limit vertebral flexion

_____ d. limit vertebral lateral flexion and rotation

3. During a treatment visit to a person's home, a physical therapist assistant observed the person ascend and descend their stairs. The preferred height of a stair step is which of the following?

_____ a. height less than 6", depth less than 11"

_____ b. height less than 7", depth greater than 11"

_____ c. height less than 8″, depth less than 14″

_____ d. height greater than 4″, depth greater than 8″

4. Which of the following activities is the LEAST useful indicator of a person's body mechanics during activities of daily living?

_____ a. squatting

_____ b. forward bending

_____ c. plumb line

_____ d. lifting and carrying

5. Which of the following techniques should be avoided MOST with effective body mechanics?

_____ a. using larger muscles of the extremities and trunk

_____ b. positioning your center of gravity over your base of support

_____ c. lifting immediately after prolonged inactivity

_____ d. using the momentum of simultaneous trunk flexion and rotation

6. Which of the following is an application of effective body mechanics related to the principle of using translatory motion versus lifting?

_____ a. keeping your head aligned directly over your feet during a stand-pivot transfer

_____ b. lifting a person to standing position, and repositioning your feet prior to pivoting the person to the mat table, when they are dependent in mobility

_____ c. performing a sliding board transfer with a person who is dependent in mobility

_____ d. placing your feet in an offset position prior to performing a stand-pivot transfer

ANSWERS AND RATIONALE

AEROBIC CAPACITY AND ENDURANCE

Twelve Items

1. Correct answer: (c)

   Rationale: It is important to check vital signs at the beginning, during, and after treatment session. It is also important with cardiac rehabilitation to perform an active warm-up and cool-down period, and to check perceived level of exertion.

   Reference: O'Sullivan. (2001). *Physical rehabilitation assessment and treatment* (4th ed., p. 498). Philadelphia: FA Davis.

2. Correct answer: (a)

   Rationale: The normal range for an infant is 100–130 beats per minute, and for children 1–7 years old it is 80–120 beats per minute. For a child 10 years of age, 100 beats per minute is the best of these choices.

Reference: Pierson, F. (2002). *Principles and techniques of patient care* (3rd ed., p. 52). Philadelphia: Saunders.

3. Correct answer: (d)

    Rationale: Heart rate provides an acceptable estimate of energy expenditure. The perceived level of exertion is a subjective indicator of a person's tolerance to an activity.

    Reference: O'Sullivan. (2001). *Physical rehabilitation assessment and treatment* (4th ed., p. 292). Philadelphia: FA Davis.

4. Correct answer: (b)

    Rationale: Upright posture produces enough challenges to orthostatic hypotension in early treatment sessions. Active range of motion may be excessively challenging.

    Reference: O'Sullivan. (2001). *Physical rehabilitation assessment and treatment* (4th ed., p. 498). Philadelphia: FA Davis.

5. Correct answer: (a)

    Rationale: This is considered within 3–4 METs, the other choices are 4–5 and 1.5–2 for the last two choices.

    Reference: O'Sullivan. (2001). *Physical rehabilitation assessment and treatment* (4th ed., p. 499). Philadelphia: FA Davis.

6. Correct answer: (b)

    Rationale: Each of the statements is true with the correction to type II diabetes.

    Reference: Goodman, C., & Snyder, T. (2000). *Differential diagnosis in physical therapy* (3rd ed., p. 825). Philadelphia: WB Saunders.

7. Correct answer: (d)

    Rationale: Each of the other signs and symptoms are indications of excessive activity levels.

    Reference: O'Sullivan. (2001). *Physical rehabilitation assessment and treatment* (4th ed., p. 497). Philadelphia: FA Davis.

8. Correct answer: (c)

    Rationale: Heat will typically magnify fatigue the person experiences, and strenuous activities should be avoided during exacerbation of their disease. The most appropriate strategy is discussing energy conservation strategies such as pacing.

    Reference: O'Sullivan. (2001). *Physical rehabilitation assessment and treatment* (4th ed., p. 729). Philadelphia: FA Davis.

9. Correct answer: (b)

    Rationale: Each of the first three choices, including pulse rate, are critical to gauge response to endurance training.

    Reference: O'Sullivan. (2001). *Physical rehabilitation assessment and treatment* (4th ed., p. 496). Philadelphia: FA Davis.

10. Correct answer: (c)

    Rationale: Beta-blockers are used to limit increases in heart rate. A heart rate increase of up to twenty (not twenty-five) beats is also appropriate. A decrease in their resting respiratory rate does not occur immediately after exercise.

    Reference: O'Sullivan. (2001). *Physical rehabilitation assessment and treatment* (4th ed., p. 498). Philadelphia: FA Davis.

11. Correct answer: (c)

    Rationale: The 6 minute walk test is considered a positive predictor when the person completes at LEAST 300 meters during the exam.

    Reference: Prentice, W., & Voight, M. (2001). *Techniques in musculoskeletal rehabilitation* (p. 128). New York: McGraw-Hill.

12. Correct answer: (a)

    Rationale: Low resistance and high duration activities to address muscular endurance. The stationary bike is more appropriate, given the duration of activity. The treadmill is less appropriate and gives the increased effort with a 15% grade.

    Reference: Prentice, W., & Voight, M. (2001). *Techniques in musculoskeletal rehabilitation* (p. 69). New York: McGraw-Hill.

CIRCULATION AND VITAL SIGNS

Eleven Items

1. Correct answer: (b)

   Rationale: Massage for edema should begin with clearing the proximal first, then removal of fluid from the involved tissue.

   Reference: Goodman, C., & Snyder, T. (2000). *Differential diagnosis in physical therapy* (3rd ed., p. 497). Philadelphia: WB Saunders.

2. Correct answer: (c)

   Rationale: Pitting edema is a sign of moderate to severe edema.

   Reference: O'Sullivan. (2001). *Physical rehabilitation assessment and treatment* (4th ed., p. 111). Philadelphia: FA Davis.

3. Correct answer: (a)

   Rationale: The sympathetic nervous systems stimulate the release of norepinephrine which excites the contraction of myocardial tissue.

   Reference: Goodman, C., & Snyder, T. (2000). *Differential diagnosis in physical therapy* (3rd ed., p. 383). Philadelphia: WB Saunders.

4. Correct answer: (d)

   Rationale: "Tachy" means fast, "cardia" means pertaining to the heart. Resting heart rates greater than 100 are considered tachycardiac for an adult.

   Reference: Pierson, F. (2002). *Principles and techniques of patient care* (3rd ed., p. 54). Philadelphia: WB Saunders.

5. Correct answer: (a)

   Rationale: The resting systolic pressure is the standard to determine hypertension.

   Reference: Pierson, F. (2002). *Principles and techniques of patient care* (3rd ed., p. 56). Philadelphia: WB Saunders.

6. Correct answer: (b)

   Rationale: The use of multiple reference points and distance from anatomical landmarks provide an effective representation of extremity girth.

   Reference: Lukan, M. (2001). *Documentation for physical therapist assistants* (2nd ed., p. 77). Philadelphia: FA Davis.

7. Correct answer: (d)

   Rationale: The brain requires constant and immediate vascular support. This is achieved largely by the supply from the circle of Willis.

   Reference: O'Sullivan. (2001). *Physical rehabilitation assessment and treatment* (4th ed., p. 523). Philadelphia: FA Davis.

8. Correct answer: (a)

   Rationale: Normal capillary refill should take less than 3 seconds.

   Reference: Myers, B. (2004). *Wound management, principles and practice* (p. 57). Upper Saddle River, NJ: Prentice Hall.

9. Correct answer: (c)

   Rationale: Two to five centimeters difference between the extremities is classified as moderate edema.

   Reference: Myers, B. (2004). *Wound management, principles and practice* (p. 364). Upper Saddle River, NJ: Prentice Hall.

10. Correct answer: (c)

    Rationale: Zero is given for an absent pulse, 1+ for a diminished pulse, 2+ for a normal pulse, and 3+ for a bounding pulse.

    Reference: Myers, B. (2004). *Wound management, principles and practice* (p. 57). Upper Saddle River, NJ: Prentice Hall.

11. Correct answer: (a)

    Rationale: Peripheral pulses are palpated in supine with the person resting.

    Reference: Myers, B. (2004). *Wound management, principles and practice* (p. 57). Upper Saddle River, NJ: Prentice Hall.

VENTILATION AND RESPIRATION

Eight Items

1. Correct answer: (d)

   Rationale: The alveoli are the locations for oxygen to enter the vascular system, and wastes to be dispersed.

   Reference: Hillegass, E., & Sadowsky, H. (2001). *Essentials of cardiopulmonary physical therapy* (2nd ed., p. 25). Philadelphia: WB Saunders.

2. Correct answer: (c)

   Rationale: This is the normal ration for inspiration to expiration. Oxygen saturation should be at least 90%. Resting respiration rate should normally not be greater than 20 per minute.

   Reference: Hillegass, E., & Sadowsky, H. (2001) *Essentials of cardiopulmonary physical therapy* (2nd ed., p. 621). Philadelphia: WB Saunders.

3. Correct answer: (d)

   Rationale: Pain medications typically decrease respiratory function, cough reflex, and ciliary action.

   Reference: Kisner, C., & Colby, L. (2002). *Therapeutic exercise: Foundations and techniques* (4th ed., p. 702). Phildelphia: FA Davis.

4. Correct answer: (d)

   Rationale: The dyspnea index is the number of breaths required to count to fifteen aloud.

   Reference: Hillegass, E., & Sadowsky, H. (2001). *Essentials of cardiopulmonary physical therapy* (2nd ed., p. 666). Philadelphia: WB Saunders.

5. Correct answer: (c)

   Rationale: Sitting with the upper extremities supported, or standing and leaning against a wall are also positions that allow improved contribution by the diaphragm and accessory muscles.

   Reference: Hillegass, E., & Sadowsky, H. (2001). *Essentials of cardiopulmonary physical therapy* (2nd ed., p. 658, 659). Philadelphia: WB Saunders.

6. Correct answer: (a)

   Rationale: Dyspnea means difficult breathing. Orthopnea is difficult breathing in other than full erect postures. Hyperpnea is normal rate, but increased depth of respiration. Eupnea means normal breathing.

   Reference: Hillegass, E., & Sadowsky, H. (2001). *Essentials of cardiopulmonary physical therapy* (2nd ed., p. 622). Philadelphia: WB Saunders.

7. Correct answer: (c)

   Rationale: The pulse oximeter detects the capillary perfusion of oxygen into the peripheral tissues such as the fingers or toes.

Reference: Hillegass, E., & Sadowsky, H. (2001). *Essentials of cardiopulmonary physical therapy* (2nd ed., p. 639, 640). Philadelphia: WB Saunders.

8. Correct answer: (b)

Rationale: The curvature of the spine can compress the lung sections and reduce potential ventilation space.

Reference: Hillegass, E., & Sadowsky, H. (2001). *Essentials of cardiopulmonary physical therapy* (2nd ed., p. 617). Philadelphia: WB Saunders.

INTEGUMENTARY SYSTEM

Fifteen Items

1. Correct answer: (d)

Rationale: An autograft is the use of a person's own body parts, transplanting them to another function or location.

Reference: O'Sullivan. (2001). *Physical rehabilitation assessment and treatment* (4th ed., p. 858). Philadelphia: FA Davis.

2. Correct answer: (a)

Rationale: Using the rule of nines, the head and neck constitute 9%, and the trunk anterior plus posterior make up 36% of the total surface area of the body.

Reference: O'Sullivan. (2001). *Physical rehabilitation assessment and treatment* (4th ed., p. 853). Philadelphia: FA Davis.

3. Correct answer: (c)

Rationale: This describes a superficial to deep partial-thickness burn.

Reference: O'Sullivan. (2001). *Physical rehabilitation assessment and treatment* (4th ed., p. 848). Philadelphia: FA Davis.

4. Correct answer: (b)

Rationale: The anterior surface of each upper extremity constitutes 4.5% of the body surface. The same quantity is attributed for the each posterior upper extremity.

Reference: O'Sullivan. (2001). *Physical rehabilitation assessment and treatment* (4th ed., p. 853). Philadelphia: FA Davis.

5. Correct answer: (c)

Rationale: The Braden scale for predicting sore risk uses a scale of 6–23. A person is considered at mild risk with a score of 16–17, at moderate risk with a score of 13–15, and at high risk with a score of 12 or less.

Reference: Myers, B. (2004). *Wound management, principles and practice* (p. 267). Upper Saddle River, NJ: Prentice Hall.

6. Correct answer: (a)

   Rationale: A lack of warm temperature is an indication of decreased arterial supply which brings warmed blood from the body's core.

   Reference: Anemaet, W., et al. (2000). *Home rehabilitation: Guide to clinical practice* (p. 477). St. Louis: Mosby.

7. Correct answer: (b)

   Rationale: The entire anterior surface of the lower leg would be classified as 9%. Since only the anterior surface was affected, the percentage is 4.5%.

   Reference: Anemaet, W., et al. (2000). *Home rehabilitation: Guide to clinical practice* (p. 469). St. Louis: Mosby.

8. Correct answer: (c)

   Rationale: Stage IV ulcers have full-thickness loss of skin, with damage to muscle, bones, tendons, and joint capsules.

   Reference: Anemaet, W., et al. (2000). *Home rehabilitation: Guide to clinical practice* (p. 474). St. Louis: Mosby.

9. Correct answer: (b)

   Rationale: The injury has compromised sensory receptors that are contained in the deep or reticular dermis.

   Reference: O'Sullivan. (2001). *Physical rehabilitation assessment and treatment* (4th ed., p. 850). Philadelphia: FA Davis.

10. Correct answer: (d)

    Rationale: The superior direction of the person's body is the 12:00 reference point to describe direction and variation of the wound.

    Reference: Anemaet, W., et al. (2000). *Home rehabilitation: Guide to clinical practice* (p. 850). St. Louis: Mosby.

11. Correct answer: (c)

    Rationale: An abrasion is a scrape.

    Reference: Anemaet, W., et al. (2000). *Home rehabilitation: Guide to clinical practice* (p. 476). St. Louis: Mosby.

12. Correct answer: (c)

    Rationale: This term is used to describe the drainage of serous and blood fluids.

    Reference: Anemaet, W., et al. (2000). *Home rehabilitation: Guide to clinical practice* (p. 467). St. Louis: Mosby.

13. Correct answer: (a)

    Rationale: These descriptions are consistent with those of an arterial skin ulcer. The person may also have extremity hair loss and sharp, burning pain.

Reference: Anemaet, W., et al. (2000). *Home rehabilitation: Guide to clinical practice* (p. 477). St. Louis: Mosby.

14. Correct answer: (a)

Rationale: This is an early description of a pressure ulceration.

Reference: Anemaet, W., et al. (2000). *Home rehabilitation: Guide to clinical practice* (p. 460). St. Louis: Mosby.

15. Correct answer: (d)

Rationale: The skin over the anterior and posterior thigh is 4% each, the anterior and posterior lower leg is 5.5% each, and the foot is 3.5% each side.

Reference: Frazier, M., et al. (2000). *Essentials of human disease and conditions* (2nd ed., p. 464). Philadelphia: WB Saunders.

MEASURE AND SELECT ASSISTIVE AND ADAPTIVE DEVICES

Sixteen Items

1. Correct answer: (d)

Rationale: It is true that Lofstrand crutches provide less stability than a standard walker, but this is not an advantage.

Reference: Pierson, F. (2002). *Principles and techniques of patient care* (3rd ed., p. 218). Philadelphia: WB Saunders.

2. Correct answer: (b)

Rationale: A sling seat produces a posterior pelvic tilt, femoral adduction with internal rotation, and postural asymmetry.

Reference: O'Sullivan. (2001). *Physical rehabilitation assessment and treatment* (4th ed., p. 1067). Philadelphia: FA Davis.

3. Correct answer: (c)

Rationale: The extra inch is added to unweight the shoulder girdle and stabilize the trunk by allowing upper extremity weight-bearing.

Reference: Pierson, F. (2002). *Principles and techniques of patient care* (3rd ed., p. 168). Philadelphia: WB Saunders.

4. Correct answer: (c)

Rationale: The ankle should be at a 90° angle when placed upon the footrests.

Reference: Anemaet, W., et al. (2000). *Home rehabilitation: Guide to clinical practice* (p. 341). St. Louis: Mosby.

5. Correct answer: (d)

   Rationale: Although the greater trochanter can be used as a landmark, it is necessary for adjusting the size of an assistive device.

   Reference: Pierson, F. (2002). *Principles and techniques of patient care* (3rd ed., p. 219). Philadelphia: WB Saunders.

6. Correct answer: (c)

   Rationale: The tilt in space option for either the manual or motorized wheelchair provides significant pressure relief positions.

   Reference: O'Sullivan. (2001). *Physical rehabilitation assessment and treatment* (4th ed., p. 1084). Philadelphia: FA Davis.

7. Correct answer: (c)

   Rationale: Although the greater trochanter and dorsal wrist crease are common anatomical reference points for the height of a cane, the fit must accomplish the 20°–30° of elbow flexion.

   Reference: Minor, M., & Minor, S. (1999). *Patient care skills*.

8. Correct answer: (c)

   Rationale: The first choice would most likely result in the axillary crutches being too long. The second choice is the appropriate posture for initially adjusting axillary crutches.

   Reference: Pierson, F. (2002). *Principles and techniques of patient care* (3rd ed., p. 221). Philadelphia: WB Saunders.

9. Correct answer: (d)

   Rationale: A standard wheelchair is designed for persons up to 200 pounds. Persons with amputations are fitted in chairs with the axle shifted 2″ posteriorly to compensate for their altered center of gravity. A person with central cord syndrome would have upper extremity motor impairment and may require power assistance for propulsion.

   Reference: Pierson, F. (2002). *Principles and techniques of patient care* (3rd ed., p. 168). Philadelphia: WB Saunders.

10. Correct answer: (b)

    Rationale: This is the correct placement to achieve the correct base of support.

    Reference: Minor, M., & Minor, S. (1999). *Patient care skills*.

11. Correct answer: (a)

    Rationale: Generally, 77% of a person's height is just below the axilla.

    Reference: Pierson, F. (2002). *Principles and techniques of patient care* (3rd ed., p. 220). Philadelphia: WB Saunders.

12. Correct answer: (d)

    Rationale: Two inches of floor clearance is required to accommodate for minimal elevation changes and turns.

Reference: O'Sullivan. (2001). *Physical rehabilitation assessment and treatment* (4th ed., p. 169). Philadelphia: FA Davis.

13. Correct answer: (c)

   Rationale: The back of the seat should be at the level of the inferior angle of the scapula.

   Reference: Minor, M., & Minor, S. (1999). *Patient care skills.*

14. Correct answer: (a)

   Rationale: The second and third choices refer to the fitting of axillary crutches.

   Reference: Pierson, F. (2002). *Principles and techniques of patient care* (3rd ed., p. 222). Philadelphia: WB Saunders.

15. Correct answer: (b)

   Rationale: A person who recently had a posterior approach total hip replacement needs to avoid excessive hip flexion through low transfers that require removable armrests. Reaching forward to propel the wheelchair, apply the brakes, or standing and sitting from a standard seat back exacerbates hip flexion posture.

   Reference: Pierson, F. (2002). *Principles and techniques of patient care* (3rd ed., p. 175). Philadelphia: WB Saunders.

16. Correct answer: (b)

   Rationale: Elevating legrests reduces the effects of the dependent positioning of the lower extremities in sitting.

   Reference: Minor, M., & Minor, S. (1999). *Patient care skills.*

GAIT, LOCOMOTION, AND BALANCE

Fourteen Items

1. Correct answer: (b)

   Rationale: Loading response is the peak activity phase for the majority of lower extremity muscles.

   Reference: Perry, J. (1992). *Gait analysis: Normal and pathological function* (p. 152). Thorofare, NJ: Slack.

2. Correct answer: (a)

   Rationale: The peak phase of gait for the iliopsoas is during initial swing.

   Reference: Perry, J. (1992). *Gait analysis: Normal and pathological function* (p. 164). Thorofare, NJ: Slack.

3. Correct answer: (c)

   Rationale: The weight of the body is loaded onto the forward foot during loading response, causing a flexor moment, which is addressed with quadriceps activity.

   Reference: Perry, J. (1992). *Gait analysis: Normal and pathological function* (p. 160). Thorofare, NJ: Slack.

4. Correct answer: (a)

Rationale: Stability activities are directed towards maintaining a posture against gravity.

Reference: O'Sullivan. (2001). *Physical rehabilitation assessment and treatment* (4th ed., p. 412). Philadelphia: FA Davis.

5. Correct answer: (b)

Rationale: The Romberg test compares balance with the eyes open versus the eyes closed.

Reference: O'Sullivan. (2001). *Physical rehabilitation assessment and treatment* (4th ed., p. 195). Philadelphia: FA Davis.

6. Correct answer: (c)

Rationale: The inability to reach 6″ makes a person four times more likely to fall.

Reference: Anemaet, W., et al. (2000). *Home rehabilitation: Guide to clinical practice* (p. 316). St. Louis: Mosby.

7. Correct answer: (a)

Rationale: The ankle strategy is the appropriate reaction to small perturbations. The hip accommodates larger disturbances, and stepping reestablishes a new base of support.

Reference: O'Sullivan. (2001). *Physical rehabilitation assessment and treatment* (4th ed., p. 194). Philadelphia: FA Davis.

8. Correct answer: (b)

Rationale: A person who utilizes less than $40°-60°$ of knee flexion during preswing to midswing will typically compensate with increased hip flexion, or circumduction.

Reference: O'Sullivan. (2001). *Physical rehabilitation assessment and treatment* (4th ed., p. 262). Philadelphia: FA Davis.

9. Correct answer: (a)

Rationale: The distance between contralateral initial contacts is the step length.

Reference: O'Sullivan. (2001). *Physical rehabilitation assessment and treatment* (4th ed., p. 259). Philadelphia: FA Davis.

10. Correct answer: (d)

Rationale: From midstance to heel off, there is an extension moment acting upon the hip joint, without any required muscle activity at the hip.

Reference: O'Sullivan. (2001). *Physical rehabilitation assessment and treatment* (4th ed., p. 263). Philadelphia: FA Davis.

11. Correct answer: (d)

Rationale: This osteokinematic motion is the closed chain effect of hip adduction, which occurs in the coronal plane.

Reference: Perry, J. (1992). *Gait analysis: Normal and pathological function* (p. 267). Thorofare, NJ: Slack.

12. Correct answer: (a)

    Rationale: During early terminal swing the axial segments are highest elevated from the floor.

    Reference: Perry, J. (1992). *Gait analysis: Normal and pathological function* (p. 139). Thorofare, NJ: Slack.

13. Correct answer: (c)

    Rationale: The gastrocnemius, tibialis posterior, and flexor hallicus longus produce only 68%, 1.8%, and 1.8%, respectively of the total torque produced by the soleus muscle.

    Reference: Perry, J. (1992). *Gait analysis: Normal and pathological function* (p. 58). Thorofare, NJ: Slack.

14. Correct answer: (b)

    Rationale: Good balance is the ability to maintain static standing posture.

    Reference: O'Sullivan. (2001). *Physical rehabilitation assessment and treatment* (4th ed., p. 196). Philadelphia: FA Davis.

CHECKING PAIN

Eight Items

1. Correct answer: (b)

   Rationale: Osgood–Schlatter's results from repeated trauma upon the tibial tuberosity by tension from the patellar tendon during periods of physical activity and long bone growth.

   Reference: Prentice, W., & Voight, M. (2001). *Techniques in musculoskeletal rehabilitation* (p. 564). New York: McGraw-Hill.

2. Correct answer: (d)

   Rationale: Golfer's elbow is medial epicondylitis, or inflammation of the wrist flexors or pronator teres.

   Reference: Kisner, C., & Colby, L. (2002). *Therapeutic exercise: Foundations and techniques* (4th ed., p. 404). Philadelphia: FA Davis.

3. Correct answer: (b)

   Rationale: The visual analog scale for pain is a 10 centimeter line, vertical or horizontal, without increments, and has the words "no pain" and "worst pain" at the ends of the line.

   Reference: Rothstein, J., et al. (1998). *The rehabilitation specialist's handbook* (2nd ed., p. 773). Philadelphia: FA Davis.

4. Correct answer: (a)

   Rationale: Information gained at the end of a treatment session can be recorded in the subjective or plan section when using the SOAP format. Both open-ended and close-ended questions are useful in assessing a person's pain or other symptoms. Further questions are always appropriate when a person reports a new symptom.

Reference: Goodman, C., & Snyder, T. (2000). *Differential diagnosis in physical therapy* (3rd ed., p. 38). Philadelphia: WB Saunders.

5. Correct answer: (c)

   Rationale: Response to touch descriptions can better qualify the type of afferent neuron impairment.

   Reference: O'Sullivan. (2001). *Physical rehabilitation assessment and treatment* (4th ed., p. 145). Philadelphia: FA Davis.

6. Correct answer: (c)

   Rationale: Of the choices, this is the only choice without increments of symptoms provided in the tool.

   Reference: Rothstein, J., et al. (1998). *The rehabilitation specialist's handbook* (2nd ed., p. 773). Philadelphia: FA Davis.

7. Correct answer: (c)

   Rationale: The spinothalamic tract is the ascending tract in the spinal that transmits pain and temperature impulses towards the brain.

   Reference: O'Sullivan. (2001). *Physical rehabilitation assessment and treatment* (4th ed., p. 137). Philadelphia: FA Davis.

8. Correct answer: (a)

   Rationale: The painful arc usually occurs within 50°–130° of glenohumeral motion.

   Reference: Saidoff, D., & McDonough, A. (2002). *Critical pathways in therapeutic intervention, extremities and spine* (p. 111). St. Louis: Mosby.

ERGONOMICS AND BODY MECHANICS

Six Items

1. Correct answer: (b)

   Rationale: The medial collateral ligament attaches at the medial knee, and is intended to resist medial articular surface separation. Genu valgus is a medial vector at the knee, resulting in a pronated foot posture.

   Reference: Hoppenfeld, S. (1976). *Physical examination of the spine and extremities* (p. 172). Norwalk, CT: Appleton & Lange.

2. Correct answer: (c)

   Rationale: The posterior longitudinal ligament attaches to the posterior vertebral bodies and prevents excessive spinal flexion.

   Reference: Lippert, L. (2000). *Clinical kinesiology for physical therapist assistants* (3rd ed., p. 272). Phildelphia: FA Davis.

3. Correct answer: (b)

   Rationale: The preferred height of a stair step should be up to 7″, with a depth of at LEAST 11″.

   Reference: O'Sullivan. (2001). *Physical rehabilitation assessment and treatment* (4th ed., p. 337). Philadelphia: FA Davis.

4. Correct answer: (c)

   Rationale: The plumb line is not a dynamic activity where many of the body's imbalances are revealed.

   Reference: Kisner, C., & Colby, L. (2002). *Therapeutic exercise: Foundations and techniques* (4th ed., p. 778). Philadelphia: FA Davis.

5. Correct answer: (d)

   Rationale: Simultaneous trunk flexion and rotation should be avoided.

   Reference: Pierson, F. (2002). *Principles and techniques of patient care* (3rd ed., p. 69). Philadelphia: WB Saunders.

6. Correct answer: (c)

   Rationale: Push, pull, or slide heavy objects versus lifting when possible.

   Reference: Pierson, F. (2002). *Principles and techniques of patient care* (3rd ed., p. 69). Philadelphia : WB Saunders.

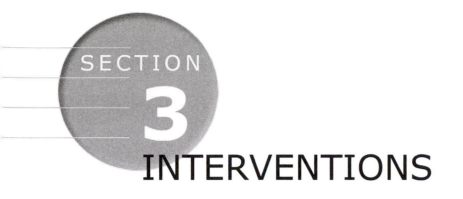

SECTION 3

INTERVENTIONS

Nonprocedural Interventions— Coordination of Care, Interpersonal Communication, Documentation, Terminology, and Providing Education and Instruction

OVERVIEW

This chapter includes questions covering nonprocedural interventions included in the exam. There are 168 questions in this chapter that deal with the coordination of care, interpersonal communication, documentation, terminology, and providing education and instruction.

KEY POINTS FOR REVIEW

Coordination of Care

- Communication with the physical therapist
- Progressing treatment within plan of care
- Directing tasks to support personnel

Interpersonal Communication

- Communicating with patients, families, and caregivers
- Communicating with the physical therapist and health care providers

- Communicating the roles of the physical therapist and physical therapist assistant

Documentation

- Reviewing medical charts

- Objectively documenting measurements, interventions, responses, progress, and outcomes

Terminology

- Medical and physical therapy terminology

Patient Instruction

- Demonstrating and explaining treatment procedures

- Written instructions

- Determining effectives of instruction

- Modified instruction as needed

- Selecting an effective teaching environment

- Providing instruction based upon educational theories

- Considering the developmental level, cultural background, social history, home situation, and geographic barriers of others

COORDINATION OF CARE—COMMUNICATION WITH THE PHYSICAL THERAPIST

Twelve Items

1. Which of the following recommendations is MOST appropriate for an entry-level physical therapist assistant to make to the physical therapist?
   _____ a. recommend that the patient does not require evaluation by the therapist, based on their recent history of treatment
   _____ b. recommend changes and additions of long-term goals
   _____ c. recommend proper size and form of wheelchair cushions
   _____ d. recommend a change of weight-bearing status

2. A physical therapist assistant has completed a treatment session with a person in an inpatient setting. Which of the following is LEAST necessary after treating a person in an inpatient setting?
   _____ a. the treatment should be documented clearly and accurately in the person's medical record
   _____ b. each progress note should be cosigned by the supervisory physical therapist

_____ c. the appropriate and valid charges should be recorded for the physical therapy department

_____ d. the physical therapist should be notified of any changes in the patient's status or response to treatment

3. At which times SHOULD the physical therapist assistant consult with the physical therapist?

_____ a. at least monthly, to update the therapist on the current plan of care

_____ b. every twelve visits, regardless of time since the patient's last evaluation

_____ c. prior to minor modification of the plan of care

_____ d. prior to the planned date of discharge

4. Which of the following is LEAST appropriate for an entry-level physical therapist assistant to recommend to the physical therapist?

_____ a. recommendations regarding an assistive device

_____ b. recommendations regarding an adaptive device

_____ c. recommendations regarding an orthotic device

_____ d. recommendations regarding dynamic splints

5. Which type of information is MOST important for the physical therapist assistant to discuss with the physical therapist?

_____ a. increases in available range of motion

_____ b. increases in ambulation distance

_____ c. increases in idiopathic crepitus

_____ d. increases in weighted pulley exercise repetitions

6. A physical therapist assistant is treating a patient after surgical repair of their right rotator cuff. During today's treatment session, the patient complains of right shoulder pain. Which of the following actions is MOST appropriate?

_____ a. taking goniometric measurements and discussing with the supervisory physical therapist after the treatment session

_____ b. performing Hawkin's special test and discussing the results to the supervisory physical therapist after the treatment session

_____ c. asking the patient for more specific information and discussing with the supervisory physical therapist after the treatment session

_____ d. performing a manual muscle test of the supraspinatus and discussing the results to the supervisory physical therapist after the treatment session

7. Which of the following skills is considered beyond the scope of the entry-level physical therapist assistant?

_____ a. recommendations to a patient to apply protective taping after an ankle sprain

_____ b. recommendations to a patient to apply an additional ply of covering over a residual limb before donning a prosthesis

_____ c. recommendations to the supervisory physical therapist for a static splint to prevent a patient's range of motion loss

_____ d. recommendations to the supervisory physical therapist that a person may not be safe to return home alone

8. The supervisory physical therapist is communicating with a physical therapist assistant regarding the status of a current patient. Which of the following communication strategies is LEAST appropriate during this type of communication?

_____ a. positioning near each other to reduce the invasion of privacy for the patient

_____ b. positioning near each other to improve communication between the individuals

_____ c. positioning near each other to allow physical contact during the discussion

_____ d. positioning near each other to increase attention from both individuals

9. A person is participating in physical therapy after having a total knee replacement. Which of the following observations about this patient is MOST important to report to the physical therapist?

_____ a. the physical assistance the person requires to perform a straight leg raise

_____ b. the initial adjustments to the height of the person's assistive device

_____ c. the level of assistance required for the person when performing a supine to sit transfer

_____ d. the ongoing lack of available range of motion

10. Which of the following is LEAST appropriate for an entry-level physical therapist assistant?

_____ a. progress the assistive device a person is using

_____ b. advise the person regarding use of the assistive device for entrance into the home

_____ c. alter the person's gait from a step-to to a step-through pattern

_____ d. advise the person when the person may return to driving

11. Physical therapy standards regarding the need for the supervisory physical therapist to examine the patient do NOT include which of the following?

_____ a. monthly, or at a higher frequency if indicated

_____ b. every twelve visits, regardless of time since the patient's last evaluation

_____ c. prior to major modifications to the plan of care

_____ d. prior to the planned date of discharge

12. A person is working with a physical therapist assistant two weeks after a Bankart repair. Which of the following occurrences SHOULD immediately be reported to the patient's physical therapist?

_____ a. pain in the lower extremity

_____ b. myalgia in the involved extremity

_____ c. myogenic symptoms in the involved extremity

_____ d. neurogenic symptoms in the upper extremity

COORDINATION OF CARE—PROGRESSING TREATMENT WITHIN THE PLAN OF CARE

Ten Items

1. Which of the following patient documentation formats can appropriately be recorded in pencil for frequent updates in progress by many health care disciplines?

   _____ a. individualized educational program

   _____ b. SOAP note

   _____ c. interim note

   _____ d. cardex

2. A person is participating in gait training with a physical therapist assistant. The person is safe with ambulation on level surfaces, and now needs to practice for the 7″ stair steps to enter their home. Which of the following tasks provides the BEST progression towards this activity?

   _____ a. initially using incremental height training steps

   _____ b. initially using 8″ steps to provide sufficient confidence in the task

   _____ c. initially using a stairwell in the facility with both handrails

   _____ d. initially using a wheeled walker during the activity

3. A physical therapist assistant is working with a person to address their current short-term goals. These include improving relaxation and breathing techniques, energy conservation, and physical endurance, towards specific parameters and a given timeline. Which of the interventions will typically require the greatest amount of time to accomplish?

   _____ a. breathing techniques

   _____ b. energy conservation

   _____ c. physical endurance

   _____ d. relaxation skills

4. Which of the following interventions is MOST appropriate to address the short-term goal of increasing ambulation endurance?

   _____ a. using mat exercises and increase repetitions

   _____ b. using an assistive device initially, then reducing reliance on the device

   _____ c. having the person increase distance by 10′ in each session

   _____ d. having the person walk as far as possible without a device

5. A person has had a prolonged hospitalization, and is currently working on standing tasks in the parallel bars. Which of the following preambulation tasks MOST immediately precedes initiating gait training?

   _____ a. weight shifting

   _____ b. hip hiking

_____ c. stepping forward

_____ d. side stepping

6. What is the purpose of an individualized educational program in a public school setting?

_____ a. to provide a weekly update in the plan of care for a child in a public school setting

_____ b. to provide the physical therapist assistant a standardized record of educational goals and objectives

_____ c. to maintain a law-mandated record of meetings between professional services and parents of the child

_____ d. to provide a format for planning physical therapy, occupational therapy, speech therapy, and psychological services, in an educational setting

7. A physical therapist assistant has been performing peripheral joint mobilization with a person who has capsular restriction of the glenohumeral joint. The patient is now experiencing pain with gliding towards the restricted range. Which of the following actions is MOST appropriate?

_____ a. applying a grade II traction force in the direction of restriction

_____ b. applying a glide in the pain-free direction

_____ c. applying a traction force in the pain-free direction

_____ d. applying a grade III glide in the direction of restriction

8. A person currently ambulates without an assistive device, but appears unsteady and experiences an occasional lack of balance. The physical therapist evaluated the patient and determined that the person required full-time use of an assistive device. Which pregait activity is the MOST basic one for addressing initial gait training?

_____ a. side stepping in the parallel bars

_____ b. lateral weight shifting in the parallel bars

_____ c. braiding in the parallel bars

_____ d. stepping up and down from a small step in the parallel bars

9. Which of the following interventions is MOST appropriate to address the short-term goal of increasing a person's available range of motion after an ankle sprain?

_____ a. passive inversion and plantar flexion

_____ b. active inversion and eversion

_____ c. passive dorsiflexion and plantar flexion

_____ d. resistive eversion and dosiflexion

10. A person is being discharged from a subacute physical therapy setting to an outpatient physical therapy setting. Which activity is LEAST appropriate for coordinating care between these two physical therapy settings?

_____ a. faxing a copy of the physical therapy record

_____ b. refusing to disclose any information regarding the person's care in the subacute setting

_____ c. mailing a referral letter

_____ d. telephone conferencing between the current and future supervisory physical therapist

COORDINATION OF CARE—DIRECTING TASKS TO SUPPORT PERSONNEL

Ten Items

1. Which of the following activities is MOST appropriate for delegating to support personnel by the physical therapist?

   _____ a. any activity determined to be within the scope and skills of the support personnel

   _____ b. any activity directly supervized by the physical therapist

   _____ c. any activity other than the initial evaluation and discharge evaluation

   _____ d. any activity within the scope of the physical therapist assistant

2. Which of the following is LEAST appropriate when delegating patient-related tasks to support personnel?

   _____ a. use tasks with low breadth and scope of tasks

   _____ b. use very specialized tasks

   _____ c. use tasks requiring high autonomy

   _____ d. use tasks that are unskilled activities

3. Patient-related tasks have been delegated to support personnel other than physical therapist assistants. Which of the following levels of supervision is MOST appropriate when patient-related tasks are delegated to other support personnel?

   _____ a. direct personal supervision by a physical therapist assistant

   _____ b. general supervision by a physical therapist

   _____ c. supervision by telecommunications

   _____ d. indirect supervision by a physical therapist or physical therapist assistant

4. Which of the following situations is LEAST acceptable?

   _____ a. a physical therapist may delegate joint mobilization interventions to a qualified physical therapist assistant

   _____ b. a physical therapist may delegate for an aide to treat a person, alone in a satellite clinic, with telecommunication access to the physical therapist

   _____ c. a physical therapist may delegate routine tasks to an aide

   _____ d. a physical therapist may delegate a person to be treated solely by a physical therapist assistant for the next two visits at a satellite clinic

5. Which of the following individuals may be employed and practice with the same level of supervision as a licensed or registered physical therapist assistant?

   _____ a. students currently pursuing physical therapist education

   _____ b. licensed or registered graduates of accredited physical therapist assistant programs

   _____ c. physical therapy aides with more than three years of experience

   _____ d. certified athletic trainers with advanced clinically related continuing education

6. Considering the American Physical Therapy Association's position on utilizing physical therapy aides, which of the following is MOST appropriate?

 _____ a. an aide may be supervised by a physical therapist or student physical therapist

 _____ b. an aide may be supervised by a physical therapist indirectly when performing nonpatient related tasks

 _____ c. an aide may be supervised by a physical therapist assistant or supervisor

 _____ d. an aide may not be utilized after the year 2010

7. Which of the following is the MOST relevant criteria for determining if a patient-related task is appropriate for a physical therapy aide?

 _____ a. if the task requires extensive setup time

 _____ b. if the task requires physical assistance of another person

 _____ c. if the task requires an Associate's degree or higher

 _____ d. if the task requires clinical problem solving

8. Which statement is MOST appropriate regarding the use of support personnel by the physical therapist?

 _____ a. physical therapy support personnel should not record care without the cosignature of the physical therapist

 _____ b. physical therapy support personnel should sign their treatment notes with the credentials "PT,A"

 _____ c. physical therapy support personnel should sign their treatment notes with the credentials "PTT"

 _____ d. physical therapy support personnel should have weekly notes countersigned

9. Which of the following persons is MOST appropriate for directing support personnel in patient-related care?

 _____ a. physical therapist student

 _____ b. physical therapist assistant

 _____ c. supervisory physical therapist

 _____ d. physical therapy clinical supervisor

10. Which of the following activities is MOST appropriate for direction to physical therapy support personnel?

 _____ a. progression of strengthening exercises with a person, two weeks after rotator cuff repair

 _____ b. goniometry of a person with a total knee replacement

 _____ c. grade I-II manual joint traction to a person with a frozen shoulder

 _____ d. ice massage to a person with medial epicondylitis

INTERPERSONAL COMMUNICATION—PATIENTS, FAMILIES, CAREGIVERS, AND OTHERS

Fifteen Items

1. You are treating a person for weakness secondary to chronic renal failure. The patient states that her doctor has ordered dialysis starting next week. The patient is somewhat apprehensive about the treatment and asks you to explain dialysis. What SHOULD be your response?

    _____ a. explain to the patient what the procedure is, and why they should have it done

    _____ b. don't answer, but refer the patient back to the physician

    _____ c. give the patient a simple explanation, then explain that this is not your area of specialization, and recommend that they speak with their physician

    _____ d. call the patient's physician and inform them of the patient's confusion

2. When providing physical therapy interventions to address a person's pain, it is expected to monitor the effect of the intervention. Which of the following questions would NOT be considered leading?

    _____ a. Does this increase your symptoms?

    _____ b. Do your symptoms increase with activity?

    _____ c. Are your symptoms worse in the morning?

    _____ d. Does this alter your symptoms in any way?

3. Which forms of communication are MOST appropriate when treating and instructing a person who does not speak English?

    _____ a. nonverbal and visual

    _____ b. visual and verbal

    _____ c. nonverbal and listening

    _____ d. written and visual

4. Close-ended questions can be utilized to direct a person toward specific responses. Which of the following questions would be considered close-ended?

    _____ a. Which is the area of your neck that bothers you the MOST?

    _____ b. How would you describe the pain in your left shoulder?

    _____ c. Why don't you want to participate in physical therapy today?

    _____ d. Do you feel short of breath?

5. A physical therapist assistant should avoid which of the following statements to a patient due to legal implications?

    _____ a. you are making progress towards your goals

    _____ b. you can discuss pain control with your nurse and doctor

    _____ c. the physical therapist needs to reevaluate you today

    _____ d. if you work hard in therapy today, we can get you home sooner

6. A person in a nursing home is sitting bedside in a chair, in a slouched posture, apparently napping upon your arrival. Which of the following communication strategies is MOST appropriate for introducing yourself to this person?

_____ a. shut off the television, radio, and turn on the lights prior to verbally introducing yourself

_____ b. identify yourself prior to entering their space

_____ c. clearly identify the person by their first name

_____ d. allow the person to continue napping, as the elderly often need more rest

7. A physical therapist assistant is treating a child, younger than the legal age of consent. According to the Health Insurance Portability and Accountability Act, there are three situations when the parent would not be the minor's personal representative. Which of the following is NOT included in those exceptions?

_____ a. when the minor obtains care at the direction of the courts

_____ b. when the parent agrees that the minor may have a confidential relationship with the physician

_____ c. when the minor does not require parental consent based upon state or other law

_____ d. when the child has been sexually abused

8. A physical therapist assistant is treating a child in a physical therapy setting, with the parents present. During the treatment session, the parents ask a question about the child's prognosis, which the assistant knows does not have a very positive answer. Which of the following guidelines SHOULD the assistant use in responding to the parents of the child?

_____ a. the parents of a young child lack objectivity and should not be privy to specific negative information

_____ b. the parents of a young child rely upon health care professionals to shield them from negative information

_____ c. the parents of a young child depend upon health care professionals to be honest and empathetic

_____ d. the parents of a young child should only discuss health issues with qualified physicians

9. When instructing a person in a home exercise program, it is important to document patient comprehension and safety in performing the interventions. Which of the following MUST also be documented to eliminate potential patient abandonment?

_____ a. the current surgical precautions

_____ b. the need or absence of need for follow-up care

_____ c. any previous physical therapy care

_____ d. any safety concern

10. Which of the following amounts of space is generally regarded as a person's intimate space?

_____ a. from contact to 18"

_____ b. within a person's hospital room or bedroom

_____ c. from 18″ to 4′

_____ d. within a person's home dwelling

11. Clinicians occasionally respond to a person's explanation of their medical status or current experiences by overidentifying with the patient. Which of the following verbal responses is an example of overidentification?

_____ a. I know exactly how you feel

_____ b. I feel so sorry for you

_____ c. I would not want that to happen to me

_____ d. I understand what you are saying

12. Which of the following parameters is generally considered a social space for interpersonal interaction?

_____ a. from contact to 18″

_____ b. within a person's hospital room or bedroom

_____ c. from 18″ to 4′

_____ d. within a person's home dwelling

13. A physical therapist assistant is approaching an elder patient who is napping in their chair. After waking the person up, the assistant begins to introduce themself and explain why they are there. Which of the following communication strategies will facilitate getting the person's attention?

_____ a. gently touch the person during explanation

_____ b. use direct eye contact

_____ c. ask if the person can hear you clearly

_____ d. speaking with a firm voice

14. A physical therapist assistant is instructing a legal minor in several exercises to be performed at home. The child is performing the activities as instructed, with minimal cues and without corrections. During the instructions, the parent tells the child that they will have to get up an extra hour early for school to do these exercises, so that the parent can observe. The child complains that they already do not get enough sleep, and this is even more of a burden. Which of the following responses is MOST appropriate for the physical therapist assistant?

_____ a. inform the physical therapist that the child should not have to do the exercises because of the potential for lack of sleep

_____ b. inform the parent that sleep is more important than the parent watching the exercise

_____ c. inform the parent that the child can also wait to perform these exercises after school

_____ d. continue with the instructions without interfering

15. Which of the following distances is typically considered personal space for an individual?

_____ a. from contact to 18″

_____ b. from 18″ to 4′

_____ c. from 4′ to 12′

_____ d. from 3′ to 6′

INTERPERSONAL COMMUNICATION— COMMUNICATING WITH THE PHYSICAL THERAPIST AND OTHER HEALTH CARE PROFESSIONALS

Fourteen Items

1. A physical therapist assistant is providing information to a patient at the conclusion of a physical therapy treatment session. A physical therapist, who does not typically supervise the assistant and who is not the patient's primary therapist, approaches the assistant after the patient has left. The physical therapist provides the physical therapist assistant with some feedback regarding the information given to the patient. Which of the following is MOST appropriate?

   _____ a. listen to the physical therapist and discuss the feedback with the therapist supervising the patient's care

   _____ b. inform the therapist that you will not discuss any information regarding the patient or their plan of care

   _____ c. listen to the therapist and avoid discussing any personal health information about the patient

   _____ d. ask a supervisor to intervene on the assistant's behalf

2. Which of the following health care professionals is typically directly involved in arranging for home health services following discharge from a medical treatment center?

   _____ a. physical therapy

   _____ b. occupational therapy

   _____ c. home health aides

   _____ d. social services

3. During a team conference meeting, a physician asks a physical therapist assistant about a person's performance with recent physical therapy sessions. During the discussion, the physician assumes the role of being correct, and that the assistant is not. Which of the following conflict resolution strategies SHOULD be employed?

   _____ a. the assistant and physician should agree that they both want the BEST for the patient, and that it is not as important who wins the argument

   _____ b. the assistant and physician should bargain for which parts of the discussion they are correct about, and allow the other person to concede where they are wrong

   _____ c. the assistant and physician should continue the discussion until one of them clearly wins the argument

   _____ d. the assistant and physician should drop the discussion, and just agree to disagree

4. Which of the following team models is utilized when a physical therapist conducts an evaluation and delivers the therapy?

_____ a. intradisciplinary model

_____ b. multidisciplinary model

_____ c. interdisciplinary model

_____ d. transdisciplinary model

5. A physical therapist assistant is treating a person in an outpatient facility. After the patient is dismissed from the facility, the physical therapist asks to speak with the assistant about the patient. Which of the following is MOST appropriate for the assistant, when this therapist is not involved in this patient's care?

_____ a. avoid any conversation with the therapist

_____ b. inform the therapist when the patient is scheduled to return to the clinic so that the therapist can meet the patient personally

_____ c. inform the therapist that he cannot discuss anything specific regarding the patient

_____ d. inform the therapist that they should schedule an evaluation with the patient upon the next visit

6. A physical therapist assistant is working with several members of the interdisciplinary health care team. Which of the following health care members primarily promotes cost-effective solutions and interventions for the patient?

_____ a. physician

_____ b. social worker

_____ c. charge nurse

_____ d. case manager

7. A person in a neurological rehabilitation setting is having difficulty with visual perception which is affecting their balance and gait. Which of the following health care professionals SHOULD be included in the health care delivery team given the visual impairment?

_____ a. an ophthalmologist

_____ b. a rheumatologist

_____ c. an oncologist

_____ d. an endocrinologist

8. Which of the following health care professionals typically arranges for delivery of assistive or adaptive devices to a person's home following discharge from a medical facility?

_____ a. physical therapy

_____ b. nursing staff

_____ c. physician

_____ d. social service

9. In traditional medical facilities, physical therapy services are provided within which of the following team models?

_____ a. intradisciplinary model

_____ b. multidisciplinary model

_____ c. interdisciplinary model

_____ d. transdisciplinary model

10. A physical therapist and a physical therapist assistant are discussing the care of one of their patients. They are in disagreement about some aspects of the patient's care and progress to date. During the discussion the assistant states, "I guess you are the therapist, so it doesn't matter what I say." Which of the following types of conflict avoidance is demonstrated in this situation?

_____ a. conquest approach

_____ b. role player approach

_____ c. band-aid approach

_____ d. avoidance approach

11. A person in a hospital setting is having difficulty with getting dressed in time for their early morning therapy session, due to motor apraxia. The physical therapist assistant should discuss this issue with which of the following health care professionals FIRST?

_____ a. the physical therapist

_____ b. the nursing staff

_____ c. the neurologist

_____ d. the occupational therapist

12. Which of the following interdisciplinary health care team members coordinates and oversees the care planning and admissions for the patient?

_____ a. physician

_____ b. social worker

_____ c. charge nurse

_____ d. case manager

13. Two physical therapist assistants are discussing a patient with a physical therapist, whom they have each provided treatment to, on separate occasions. They disagree about whether the patient has been compliant with the home exercise program. During the discussion, one of the assistants states that they will agree that the person is in compliance, if the other assistant will agree that the patient should be discharged anyway. Which of the following conflict tactics is being employed in this situation?

_____ a. ineffective, conquest approach

_____ b. effective, bargaining approach

_____ c. ineffective, bargaining approach

_____ d. ineffective, band aid approach

14. Which of the following health care professionals is MOST specialized and skilled in providing adaptations and instructions in improving bathing and dressing skills for a patient?

_____ a. certified occupational therapy assistant

_____ b. certified nursing assistant

_____ c. licensed practical nurse

_____ d. occupational therapist

INTERPERSONAL COMMUNICATION— COMMUNICATING THE ROLE OF THE PHYSICAL THERAPIST AND PHYSICAL THERAPIST ASSISTANT

Twelve Items

1. A patient asks a physical therapist assistant regarding the method in which they were evaluated and diagnosed. Which of the following responses is MOST appropriate for the assistant?

   _____ a. ask the physical therapist to answer the patient's questions

   _____ b. explain the methods of testing and observation used to determine the person's diagnosis

   _____ c. ask the person why they are interested

   _____ d. demonstrate the methods recorded in the evaluation and answer questions as they arise

2. An experienced physical therapist assistant is working in a specialized rehabilitative setting. The physical therapist evaluates a patient and delegates them to the assistant. The therapist provides the assistant with a copy of the evaluation including the short-term goals. No specified interventions are included in the evaluation. Which of the following actions is MOST appropriate in this situation?

   _____ a. let the physical therapist know that they cannot initiate interventions until the therapist has provided a specified plan of care

   _____ b. review the short-term goals and initiate activities to address them

   _____ c. seek input for specific interventions from the patient's physician

   _____ d. seek input for specific interventions from other physical therapy staff

3. Which of the following data collection skills is considered by the normative model of Physical Therapist Assistant Education beyond entry-level for the physical therapist assistants?

   _____ a. measurement of vital signs

   _____ b. auscultation of heart sounds

   _____ c. auscultation of blood pressure

   _____ d. palpation of apical heart rate

4. A person is evaluated by the physical therapist in an outpatient setting. The physical therapist chooses to delegate the interventions to an entry-level physical therapist assistant. Which of the following actions is MOST appropriate?

   _____ a. the assistant should initiate a conference with the therapist to discuss the patient after the first treatment session

   _____ b. the therapist should provide short-term goals and general guidelines for the assistant to select specific interventions

_____ c. the assistant should initiate the interventions as documented

_____ d. the therapist should discuss and clarify the patient's condition, the interventions, and any potentially relevant precautions

5. Which of the following interventions is LEAST appropriate for an entry-level physical therapist assistant?

_____ a. pulsed ultrasound

_____ b. observe posture in a person with lumbosacral dysfunction

_____ c. pulsed electromagnetic fields

_____ d. sustained mechanical traction

6. Which of the following data collection skills is considered MOST appropriate based upon the normative model of Physical Therapist Assistant Education for entry-level physical therapist assistants?

_____ a. assessment of monofilament stimuli

_____ b. assessment of response to vestibular stimuli

_____ c. assessment of brachial plexus dermatomes

_____ d. assessment of cranial nerve dermatomes

7. Which of the following manual interventions is LEAST appropriate for application by an entry-level physical therapist assistant?

_____ a. manual cervical traction

_____ b. mechanical cervical traction

_____ c. home cervical traction instruction

_____ d. self-traction instruction

8. Which of the following data collection skills is considered by the normative model of physical therapist assistant education beyond entry-level for the physical therapist assistant?

_____ a. video analysis of a patient ambulating with an assistive device

_____ b. hamstring length test for a person with a posterior pelvic tilt

_____ c. observational gait analysis of a person with a Trendelenberg gait

_____ d. manual muscle testing for trace muscle contraction

9. A physical therapist assistant recently graduated from an accredited education program. A physical therapist delegates a patient to the assistant for wound care interventions. Which of the following interventions is MOST appropriate for an entry-level physical therapist assistant?

_____ a. autolytic wound debridement

_____ b. selective wound debridement

_____ c. portable hyperbaric oxygen chamber

_____ d. sharp wound debridement

10. Which of the following interventions is LEAST appropriate for an entry-level physical therapist assistant?

_____ a. therapeutic stretching of the knee

_____ b. joint mobilization of the knee

_____ c. tilt table with toe-touch weight bearing upon the knee

_____ d. standing frame with full weight bearing upon the knee

11. A physical therapist and an entry-level physical therapist assistant are discussing a newly evaluated patient. Which of the following technical skills is LEAST appropriate to be performed by an entry-level physical therapist assistant?

_____ a. manual lymphatic traction

_____ b. soft tissue mobilization

_____ c. passive joint motion

_____ d. active inhibition

12. Some states specify in their practice acts the level of supervision required by the physical therapist for the physical therapist assistant. Which of the following types of supervision is preferred in the model practice act by the American Physical Therapy Association?

_____ a. general supervision

_____ b. direct supervision

_____ c. personal supervision

_____ d. direct personal supervision

DOCUMENTATION—REVIEWING MEDICAL CHARTS

Three Items

1. Which of the following is NOT an intended purpose of the Health Insurance Portability and Accountability Act, in regards to medical records?

_____ a. generally limiting the release of information to the minimum necessary

_____ b. giving patient the right to examine and obtain copies of their health records

_____ c. allowing the patient to choose whether the services provided may be remunerated

_____ d. giving patients the right to have their medical records changed, or added to

2. In which of the following sections of a typical medical chart would you MOST likely expect to find a comprehensive discharge plan for a person immediately following a hospitalization?

_____ a. physician orders section

_____ b. social service section

_____ c. nursing section

_____ d. occupational therapy section

3. A person is hospitalized following a motor vehicle crash. A physical therapist assistant is preparing to treat this person as directed by the physical therapist. Which of the following types of medical information MUST be obtained during a review of the medical record prior to treatment?

_____ a. the person's current diagnosis and medical precautions

_____ b. the person's current occupation and age

_____ c. the person's current medical precautions and surgical report

_____ d. the person's current lab results and mechanism of injury

DOCUMENTATION—OBJECTIVELY DOCUMENTING RESULTS AND MEASUREMENTS

Eleven Items

1. Which of the following entries does NOT belong in the objective section of a SOAP note?

   _____ a. patient ambulated 150′ with a wheeled walker

   _____ b. patient complained of severe left anterior shoulder pain

   _____ c. patient required moderate assistance with supine to sit

   _____ d. patient performed fifteen repetitions of straight leg raises

2. Which of the following entries for a medical record is MOST appropriate?

   _____ a. range of motion has increased

   _____ b. the patient stated that they are feeling much better now

   _____ c. right middle trap strength has increased to 3/5

   _____ d. the patient needs assistance to ambulate

3. Which of the following medical record entries is a manual clinical observation used to describe the circulatory status of a person's limb?

   _____ a. peripheral pulse rate

   _____ b. girth measurement

   _____ c. 0−4+ pitting edema scale

   _____ d. capillary refill time

4. A person is cradled back into supine upon the edge of a treatment table. The clinician determines that the person has shortness of the iliopsoas and stiffness of the tensor fascia latae. Results of special tests are recorded in which section of a SOAP note?

   _____ a. subjective section

   _____ b. objective section

   _____ c. assessment section

   _____ d. problem section

5. Which of the following types of punctuation should be avoided with medical record entries?

   _____ a. hyphens

   _____ b. semicolons

_____ c. colons

_____ d. periods

6. Which of the following medical record entries does NOT belong in the objective section of a SOAP note?

_____ a. explanation of why the person has missed the last three visits

_____ b. results of left shoulder goniometry

_____ c. observations of a person's posture while standing in the parallel bars

_____ d. sequential list of interventions applied during a treatment session

7. Which of the following types of punctuation is used to connect two related statements in the subjective portion of a SOAP note?

_____ a. hyphens

_____ b. semicolons

_____ c. colons

_____ d. periods

8. A physical therapist assistant is recording observations after a patient care session. Which of the following entries BEST reflects a person's muscle strength?

_____ a. available range of motion degrees

_____ b. manual muscle test results

_____ c. palpable substitutions during active movement

_____ d. active range of motion degrees

9. A person is participating in cardiac rehabilitation in a physical therapy setting. After completing an exercise session with the patient, the physical therapist assistant begins recording the person's vital signs in the medical record. Which of the following observations is NOT an objective descriptor for documenting a person's vital signs?

_____ a. pulse rate

_____ b. rate of perceived exertion

_____ c. pulse rhythm

_____ d. beats per minute

10. Which of the following is in an appropriate format for entry into a medical record?

_____ a. the patient asked for advice regarding their medication, which I deferred to their physician

_____ b. the patient is to phone if they have any questions

_____ c. I advised the patient to return to the clinic three times a week for the current plan of care

_____ d. during goniometric measurement, I was only able to achieve 92° of passive right knee flexion

11. Which of the following types of information does not belong to the objective section of a SOAP note?

_____ a. medical diagnosis is discogenic causalgia

_____ b. active range of motion within normal limits

_____ c. per patient, 14 year history of diabetes

_____ d. patient rubbed left proximal forearm after exercise today

DOCUMENTATION—OBJECTIVELY DOCUMENTING ALL ASPECTS OF PATIENT CARE, INCLUDING INTERVENTIONS, RESPONSES, PROGRESS, AND OUTCOMES

Eighteen Items

1. This is your fifth bedside visit with a person who has been ambulating twice a day with standby assistance of one person for 20′. On this visit, they ambulated 100′. Where in the SOAP note would you state that the patient is progressing toward their ambulation goals?

   _____ a. subjective section

   _____ b. objective section

   _____ c. assessment section

   _____ d. plan section

2. It is your facility's policy that documentation occurs in the SOAP format. Your patient tells you that their chief complaint is limited function or loss of range of motion in the left shoulder. In which portion of the SOAP note SHOULD you quantify this observation?

   _____ a. subjective section

   _____ b. objective section

   _____ c. assessment section

   _____ d. plan section

3. A person attends physical therapy three times a week for therapeutic exercise. The person has been performing straight leg raises with a 6 pound weight for three sets of 30 repetitions. You want them to increase the weight and decrease the repetitions on the next visit. Where SHOULD you record that information?

   _____ a. subjective section

   _____ b. objective section

   _____ c. assessment section

   _____ d. plan section

4. Your patient is a woman, 37 years of age, who is a professional firefighter. Today, prior to the treatment, the physical therapist has asked you to take range of motion measurements. She has full active range of motion in her left knee and 5°–110° active range of motion with her right. Where does this information belong in a SOAP note?

   _____ a. subjective section

   _____ b. objective section

_____ c. assessment section

_____ d. plan section

5. A person explains that they have been performing their home exercise program daily, with the exception of yesterday, when they attended a funeral for a close friend. In which part of a standard SOAP note will you record this information?

_____ a. subjective section

_____ b. objective section

_____ c. assessment section

_____ d. plan section

6. Which of the following is LEAST accurate regarding medical record entries?

_____ a. only facility approved abbreviations should be used in documentation

_____ b. clear and concise language is preferred over elaborate descriptions

_____ c. erasable ink is preferred, to maintain neatness in permanent records, for future photocopying

_____ d. a dark ink pen is preferred over a pencil

7. Which of the following adjustments is the correct method for correcting entry errors recorded in a person's hospital records?

_____ a. use correction fluid to neatly cover any error, place a single line over the dried correction fluid mark, initial and date to the immediate right, and write the correct entry

_____ b. discard all attached documents and replace with newer corrected versions

_____ c. place a single line through the error, initial and date, and write the correct entry

_____ d. mark completely over the error with dark blue or black ink, so that it cannot be read, initial and date, and write the correct entry

8. Immediately after recording the statement, "Patient ambulated 150' with a wheeled walker," you realize your error that the device used by the patient was a standard walker. Which of the following actions would be MOST appropriate?

_____ a. mark through the error completely and emphasize the correct assistive device in the next progress note

_____ b. apply correction fluid to the mistake, initial the entry, and write the word "standard" immediately above the error

_____ c. mark a single line through the word "wheeled," write your initials, time and date of correction, and write the word "standard" as close to the error as possible

_____ d. place a double line through the entire incorrect statement, write the word error, include your initials and date of correction, and write the correct assistive device in the nearest margin of the document

9. Which of the following types of information is MOST appropriate for inclusion in the objective portion of a SOAP note?

_____ a. mechanism

_____ b. typical daily activities of the patient

_____ c. activities that exacerbate the patient's symptoms

_____ d. number of treatment sessions provided

10. Which of the following medical record entries is MOST appropriate for a physical therapist assistant documenting a patient's refusal to participate in a physical therapy session?

_____ a. patient refused treatment

_____ b. patient was noncompliant

_____ c. patient declined treatment against medical advice

_____ d. patient refused to participate in therapy session, physical therapist advised

11. Which of the following statements is inappropriate for a physical therapist assistant to record in the plan section of a SOAP note?

_____ a. will increase resistance to 2 pounds for the next treatment session

_____ b. will have handouts of the patient's home exercise available for the next visit

_____ c. physical therapist will evaluate the patient on the next visit

_____ d. will inform physical therapist that the patient is malingering

12. Physical therapy services are directed towards specific, reasonable goals and functional outcomes. Which of the following short-term goals is MOST appropriate for a person recovering from a cerebral vascular accident?

_____ a. patient will ambulate with a hemiaide 45' with minimal assistance of one person

_____ b. patient will increase occurrence of heel strike during initial contact phase by 20% in one week

_____ c. patient will increase left deltoid strength from 3/5 to 5/5 in two days

_____ d. patient will improve strength and functional mobility

13. Which of the following categories of organizing subjective information is NOT typically used in the subjective section of a SOAP note?

_____ a. history

_____ b. palpable tenderness

_____ c. complaints

_____ d. patient's goals

14. Which of the following statements is MOST true regarding the writing utensil used for medical record entries?

_____ a. only permanent black ink pens are an acceptable writing utensil

_____ b. permanent blue ink pens are used to designate the original from later photocopies

_____ c. pencils are preferred over permanent ink pens for entries in the medical record

_____ d. only permanent black or blue ink pens should be used for medical record entries

15. Which of the following types of information is NOT appropriate for inclusion in the objective section of a SOAP note?

    _____ a. description of a person's function

    _____ b. current status of goals

    _____ c. observations made by the physical therapist assistant

    _____ d. results of manual muscle test

16. Which of the following descriptions is NOT necessary for documenting interventions, in order for the session to be reproducible?

    _____ a. dosage

    _____ b. complicating factors

    _____ c. positioning

    _____ d. all of the above are necessary

17. Which of the following SOAP note entries is MOST appropriate for documenting a treatment session?

    _____ a. instructed patient in crutch walking, weight bearing as tolerated

    _____ b. patient issued crutches and handout for fit and use of crutches, weight bearing as tolerated with their left lower extremity

    _____ c. instructed patient in crutch walking, using axillary crutches for 125′

    _____ d. patient ambulated with axillary crutches 75′ with minimal assistance, and verbal cueing to hold their head erect

18. Which of the following statements is MOST accurate regarding the use of abbreviations?

    _____ a. the use of abbreviations is intended to protect the document from non health care professionals

    _____ b. the use of abbreviations should be maximized in documentation for universal clarity

    _____ c. the use of abbreviations facilitates brevity in documentation

    _____ d. the use of abbreviations is not allowed in narrative forms of documentation

KNOWLEDGE OF MEDICAL AND PHYSICAL THERAPY TERMINOLOGY

Fourteen Items

1. A child who has trauma to the upper extremities often does not experience a full thickness fracture. Which of the following terms BEST describes this type of fracture?

    _____ a. spiral

    _____ b. nondisplaced

    _____ c. greenstick

    _____ d. comminuted

2. A person who had a trauma to their left lower extremity is diagnosed with having the type of injury where part of the bone is pulled out by a muscle tendon. Which type of lesion does this describe?

   ____ a. propulsion

   ____ b. avulsion

   ____ c. divulsion

   ____ d. revision

3. Which form of arthritis typically affects in the weight bearing joints FIRST?

   ____ a. rheumatoid arthritis

   ____ b. osteoarthritis

   ____ c. degenerative polymyositis

   ____ d. gout

4. A person whom you observe ambulating, avoids bearing weight upon their right lower extremity secondary to pain. When you document this decrease in stance period, which of the following gait terms would be MOST accurate?

   ____ a. antalgic gait

   ____ b. steppage gait

   ____ c. festination gait

   ____ d. limb gait

5. Which of the following conditions is tested by tucking the thumb under the fingers of the same hand, and ulnar deviating, then comparing the results to the other extremity?

   ____ a. Thompson's

   ____ b. DeQuervain's

   ____ c. Finkelstein's

   ____ d. Hawkin's

6. Upon reviewing a patient's medical chart, you find that their physical therapist is attempting to rule out a basilar artery lesion. Which of the following vascular structures converge into the basilar artery?

   ____ a. anterior communicating artery

   ____ b. circle of Willis

   ____ c. posterior communicating artery

   ____ d. vertebral artery

7. You receive orders for a patient who needs preoperative instruction in exercises and ambulation. On the therapist's evaluation form they have noted that the patient has a positive Lachman's test. Which condition does this mostly indicate?

   ____ a. increase in laxity of the anterior cruciate ligament

   ____ b. decrease in laxity of the anterior cruciate ligament

   ____ c. impingement of the medial meniscus

   ____ d. no medial meniscal involvement

8. Diabetes type I is BEST described by which of the following?

    _____ a. deficiency of insulin

    _____ b. overproduction of insulin

    _____ c. unrelated to diet

    _____ d. increase of serum sugar levels after exercise

9. A person who is 36 years of age is an office worker whose chief complaint is pain at the base of the neck radiating down the left upper extremity. The patient has been evaluated and diagnosed with thoracic outlet syndrome. Which of the following terms in NOT a classification of thoracic outlet syndrome?

    _____ a. cervical rib syndrome

    _____ b. scaleneus anticus syndrome

    _____ c. costoclavicular syndrome

    _____ d. hyperadduction syndrome

10. A person's condition is described as a disease of the palmar fascia of the right hand, in which a progressive contracture of the fascia occurs. This results in a flexion deformity of the distal palm and fingers. What is the name of this condition?

    _____ a. tenosynovitis

    _____ b. ganglion contracture

    _____ c. hypothenar hammer syndrome

    _____ d. Dupuytren's contracture

11. You are reviewing a person's physical therapy record prior to their appointment. In their record, you read that they have been diagnosed three years ago with ankylosing spondylitis. What is the main difference between ankylosing spondylitis and ankylosing spondylolithesis?

    _____ a. ankylosing spondylitis involves inflammation of the vertebrae without fusing of the spine

    _____ b. ankylosing spondylolithesis involves forward displacement of the lumbar vertebrae on the one below it with fusing of the spine

    _____ c. ankylosing spondylitis and spondylolithesis are the same thing

    _____ d. ankylosing spondylitis is valid, but not spondylolithesis

12. Which of the following neurological disorders is considered as an upper motor neuron lesion?

    _____ a. amyotrophic lateral sclerosis

    _____ b. Guillian-Barre

    _____ c. Parkinson's disease

    _____ d. carpal tunnel

13. Which of the following terms would be an accurate classification of a peripheral nerve injury? This is often a result of transient ischemia, or temporary compression, without loss of autonomic function. In addition, there is a decrease in strength and loss of sensation with the potential for spontaneous recovery in less than three months.

_____ a. axonotmesis

_____ b. neurotmesis

_____ c. neuropraxia

_____ d. axonal degeneration

14. What is the MOST common mechanism of injury for a Brown-Sequard lesion?

_____ a. infection

_____ b. meningitis

_____ c. tumor

_____ d. gun shot wound

PATIENT INSTRUCTION: DEMONSTRATING AND EXPLAINING TREATMENT PROCEDURES

Nine Items

1. Which of the following would be a primary precaution to consider with patient positioning?

_____ a. angina

_____ b. age

_____ c. recent cancers

_____ d. recent hip surgery

2. After a person is evaluated by a physical therapist, the therapist directs a physical therapist assistant to perform some of the interventions. The physical therapist will reevaluate the person in three days or sooner if needed. Who is responsible for ensuring that the person does not have contraindications to the interventions?

_____ a. the treating physical therapist assistant

_____ b. the supervising physical therapist

_____ c. the individual clinician applying the intervention

_____ d. the physician

3. A physical therapist assistant is preparing to work with a patient in an inpatient orthopedic setting to improve their mobility. Prior to visiting the person, the assistant reviews the person's medical record. Which of the following information is MOST critical to determine prior to entering the patient's room?

_____ a. weight-bearing status

_____ b. vital signs

_____ c. previous ambulation distance

_____ d. length of stay

4. A person can reduce their risk for postoperative deep vein thrombosis by performing all of the following EXCEPT which?

_____ a. dependently positioning their lower extremities

_____ b. isometrically contracting their lower extremity muscles

_____ c. actively participating in bed mobility

_____ d. Valsalva manuever

5. A person you are treating recently underwent lumbar spine surgery. The physical therapist has requested that you review lumbar spine precautions with the patient during today's treatment. Which of the following instructions should be avoided?

_____ a. bend at your hips only to 90°

_____ b. log roll in bed or on the mat table

_____ c. use a trapeze bar to transfer from supine to sit

_____ d. do not arch your back

6. A physical therapist has asked you to instruct a patient in basic activities of daily living. Which of the following activities is LEAST appropriate to include in patient education?

_____ a. brushing their teeth

_____ b. doing their laundry

_____ c. eating

_____ d. dressing

7. A physical therapist assistant is reviewing patient education with a person who will soon be discharged to a home setting. Which of the following patient education content is not considered to be an instrumental activity of daily living?

_____ a. washing their face

_____ b. taking their medications

_____ c. managing their finances

_____ d. cleaning their house

8. A person who injured their left wrist within the past two weeks is currently participating in physical therapy. Which of the following is LEAST appropriate for inclusion in the current education plan?

_____ a. inform the person of the anticipated healing time

_____ b. teach the person home exercises

_____ c. modify functional activities within the current precautions

_____ d. teach resisted eccentric activities for strengthening

9. A physical therapist assistant is preparing to apply an intervention to a person with Osgood-Schlatter's. Which question must the assistant ask that MOST directly and specifically relates to the application of short-wave diathermy in this situation?

_____ a. Do they have metal implants near their shoulder?

_____ b. Do they have a pacemaker?

_____ c. Do they have diabetes?

_____ d. Do they have an acute injury?

INSTRUCTING AND DEMONSTRATING SAFE APPLICATION OF PATIENT CARE TECHNIQUES WITH THE PATIENT AND THEIR FAMILY, INCLUDING WRITTEN INSTRUCTIONS

Six Items

1. When teaching a person how to ambulate using axillary crutches and a three-point gait pattern, which of the following would be MOST effective to incorporate into patient education?
   _____ a. explain step by step the components of the three-point placement and sequence
   _____ b. give a handout with a picture and description of the three-point pattern
   _____ c. give basic explanation and provide feedback during and after their performance
   _____ d. explain the differences between the two-point, three-point, and four-point gait patterns

2. A person, 23 years of age, fractured their left femur two weeks ago. On the same day as the accident, they had an open reduction with internal fixation, and their left lower extremity was placed in a straight leg immobilizer. Which of the following components of bed mobility would be MOST difficult for this person?
   _____ a. sit to supine
   _____ b. rolling right
   _____ c. scooting up in bed
   _____ d. bridging

3. Which of the following interventions would be MOST appropriate for a person who underwent a left quadriceps tendon repair two days ago and is required to wear a knee immobilizer at all times?
   _____ a. ankle pumps
   _____ b. quad sets
   _____ c. straight leg raises
   _____ d. short-arc quads

4. Which of the following sequences of application is MOST appropriate for applying peripheral joint mobilization?
   _____ a. warm the tissues, perform passive range of motion, perform self-stretching, and then perform joint mobilization
   _____ b. warm the tissues, perform self-stretching, perform passive range of motion, and then perform joint mobilization
   _____ c. warm the tissues, perform hold-relax technique, perform joint mobilization, and then perform reciprocal inhibition
   _____ d. warm the tissues, perform joint mobilization, and then perform passive range of motion

5. An important aspect of patient education is providing written instructions. What is the appropriate reading level for developing written handouts for a patient?

_____ a. sixth to eighth grade reading level

_____ b. eighth to tenth grade reading level

_____ c. tenth to twelfth grade reading level

_____ d. at least twelfth grade reading level

6. A person is participating in physical therapy to address recurrent postural pain. Included in the plan of care is patient education directed at reducing mechanical stress upon the spine. Which of the following instructional techniques is MOST appropriate in this situation?

_____ a. use a question and answer exchange with the person

_____ b. simulate their work activities and provide feedback

_____ c. provide written instructions with recommendations

_____ d. give verbal instructions reinforced with pictures

PATIENT INSTRUCTION: DETERMINING EFFECTIVENESS OF INSTRUCTION AND MODIFYING AS NEEDED

Eleven Items

1. A person is performing a strengthening exercise in the quadruped position. The person is instructed to simultaneously lift one arm and the contralateral leg, without moving their back. The physical therapist assistant is observing the patient during the exercise. The assistant observes that the patient tends to extend and rotate their spine when they lift their leg. Which of the following is MOST appropriate?

_____ a. touch their abdominals to increase proprioception and verbally cue the patient on the deviation

_____ b. instruct the patient to tighten their abdominals

_____ c. instruct the patient not to move their back

_____ d. touch their paraspinals muscles to increase proprioception and verbally cue the patient on the deviation

2. When instructing a person in taking their pulse on a treadmill, which of the following would NOT be an effective sight for them to practice this skill?

_____ a. apical

_____ b. pedal

_____ c. carotid

_____ d. radial

3. A person recently had abdominal surgery, and is sitting upon the edge of the mat table preparing to lay down supine. The person is a male, 14 years of age, and is having difficulty with the transfer technique. He currently has the medical precaution of avoiding activation of the abdominal muscles during transfers. Which of the following instructions is MOST appropriate to facilitate this transfer?

   _____ a. instruct the person to lay their hands upon their abdomen during the transfer

   _____ b. instruct the person to lay onto their side and elbow, ease their feet onto the table, and then roll onto their back

   _____ c. instruct the person to act as if they are pregnant, to avoid using the trunk flexors, and rest back onto their elbows

   _____ d. instruct the person to attempt to lay down, observe, and correct after he has achieved the supine position.

4. A person is participating in gait training after a stroke primarily affecting their left cerebrum. During ambulation using a wheeled walker, the person requires 50% assistance to reduce loss of balance. The physical therapist assistant has instructed the person to widen their base of support and shift their weight onto their left. The person continues to lose their balance towards their right during right initial contact. Which of the following is appropriate?

   _____ a. modify the instructions to have the person shift their weight onto their right during right limb swing

   _____ b. modify the instructions to have the person shift their weight forward to the left

   _____ c. demonstrate the differences between their current movement and the desired movement

   _____ d. demonstrate the correct movement and modify the instructions to have the person shift their weight forward to the left

5. A person is participating in an outpatient physical therapy setting to address subacute strain of their scapular musculature. The physical therapist assistant explains the technique and rationale for applying interferrential stimulation and moist heat pad to their thoracic spine in semirecumbent. The patient acknowledges comprehension prior to application of the two interventions. While increasing the intensity of the interferrential unit, the person appears to grimace. Which of the following responses is MOST appropriate?

   _____ a. clarify to the person that a sensory input is desired and that maximal posterior input is not required to block the gate for pain control

   _____ b. clarify to the person that the electrical current should not be uncomfortable, and offer to discontinue the intervention

   _____ c. clarify to the person that the stimulation may be uncomfortable for a few minutes, but that they will accommodate

   _____ d. clarify to the person that the intensity is effective when they feel it, and that they do not have to tolerate the stimulation at an uncomfortable setting

6. A patient is working with a physical therapist assistant on exercises to reduce the person's anterior pelvic tilted posture. Which of the following should the assistant observe to determine if the person is performing the activity correctly?

_____ a. contraction of the gluteus maximus

_____ b. contraction of the abdominals

_____ c. contraction of the paraspinal muscles with lack of abdominal contraction

_____ d. lack of gluteal contraction, with contraction of abdominals

7. After a person recently had a total hip replacement, they are participating in physical therapy to address their level of function. Which of the following activities must be observed the closest to determine if the person comprehends and can comply with their hip precautions?

_____ a. bed mobility and transfers

_____ b. home exercise program

_____ c. ambulation

_____ d. upper extremity exercises

8. A person is participating in therapeutic exercises with a physical therapist assistant. The assistant takes them passively through a diagonal pattern for the proprioceptive neuromuscular facilitation technique. While attempting to verbally and manually facilitate the upper extremity motion, the person has difficulty with the correct radioulnar timing and movement. Which of the following actions is MOST appropriate for the assistant?

_____ a. take the person through the motion passively again, and verbally reinforce the synergy

_____ b. have the person watch the extremity during the motion

_____ c. using timing for emphasis during the forearm component of the pattern

_____ d. take the person through the motion passively again, with verbal and visual reinforcement, using timing for emphasis during the forearm component of the pattern

9. When ambulating with a person who is more than 80 years of age, you observe that they occasionally tend to hold their head down, looking at the floor. When you remind them to hold their head erect more often, it appears that they did not hear you. Which of the following is MOST appropriate?

_____ a. attempt to speak directly in their ear, and louder

_____ b. attempt to speak clearer and provide tactile cues

_____ c. attempt to speak louder and provide verbal cues

_____ d. do not address their posture until after ambulation is finished

10. Which of the following interventions would be considered MOST appropriate when treating a person who had a left transtibial amputation one week ago?

_____ a. teach the person to stand-pivot transfer from the mat to wheelchair, with the wheelchair on the left

_____ b. teach the person to sliding board transfer from the mat to the wheelchair, with the wheelchair on the left

_____ c. teach the person to sliding board transfer from the wheelchair to the mat, with the mat on the right

_____ d. teach the person to ambulate with a small-base quad cane in their right hand, left lower extremity non weight-bearing

11. After instructing a person in the technique for strengthening the transverse abdominus muscle, the physical therapist assistant observes to ensure proper performance by the patient. Which observation indicates that the person is performing the Valsalva maneuver?

_____ a. the person does not appear to be holding their breath

_____ b. the person appears to be contracting their abdominals

_____ c. the person closes their mouth and gasps at the completion of the muscle contraction

_____ d. the person clinches their teeth for the duration of the muscle contraction

SELECTING EFFECTIVE TEACHING ENVIRONMENTS AND PROVIDING PATIENT EDUCATION BASED ON EDUCATIONAL THEORIES

Fourteen Items

1. The physical therapist assistant treating a person, 26 years of age, with traumatic brain injury, wants to use behavior modification to achieve more focus on the task at hand. Which of the following strategies would BEST address this goal?

_____ a. provide negative feedback when the person lacks focus

_____ b. use multidisciplinary approach to provide patient education on proper and improper behaviors

_____ c. wait for the person to self-correct lack of focus

_____ d. employ frequent reinforcement of the desired behavior

2. A person recently admitted to skilled nursing facility has been diagnosed with Alzheimer's disease. Which of the following would BEST benefit this person?

_____ a. provide maximum opportunities for their input, to maintain patient autonomy

_____ b. offer a variety of activities in their daily schedule, and vary from day to day, to reduce boredom and depression

_____ c. provide a highly structured environment to reduce anxiety and confusion

_____ d. provide moderate stimulation to maintain patient interest

3. The physical therapist has requested that you teach a person with receptive aphasia on how to perform diaphragmatic breathing exercises. Which of the following is MOST effective in achieving comprehension by the patient?

_____ a. ask the person if they understand the technique

_____ b. demonstrate the desired breathing pattern to the person

_____ c. manually facilitate prolonged expiration

_____ d. manually facilitate use of abdominals and internal intercostals during expiration

4. A teenage patient has been reluctant to ask questions, or offer subjective information to the physical therapist assistant. The patient appears to lack confidence and assertiveness. Which of the following strategies will facilitate the person's comfort through increased confidence with the patient–clinician interaction?

_____ a. share several jokes with the patient to help them relax

_____ b. offer the patient a choice in the sequence or application of interventions during a treatment session, within the plan of care

_____ c. explain to the patient that they have no reason to be uptight, and they should try to relax

_____ d. gain the patient's trust through sharing a personal story

5. A physical therapist assistant is instructing a person to perform isometric postural stabilization activities. The assistant instructs the person to perform the activity while driving to work. The assistant directs the person to repeat the activity at every intersection. Which of the following educational strategies is the assistant employing?

_____ a. operant conditioning

_____ b. classical conditioning

_____ c. two-step commands

_____ d. directive learning

6. You are to instruct a person, who is legally blind in both eyes, in a home exercise program. The person has also been diagnosed with early Alzheimer's disease. Which of the following teaching strategies would be MOST appropriate to ensure compliance with the home program?

_____ a. just issue the patient a printed copy of the exercises with pictures and typed instructions

_____ b. just show the exercises that the patient prefers

_____ c. educate the patient with the family, issue a type and pictorial instructions, and focus on the exercises the patient prefers

_____ d. educate the patient with the family

7. Which of the following presentation tips should not be employed with patient instruction?

_____ a. be brief and emphasize the main point

_____ b. provide specific instruction

_____ c. present at the level of the learner

_____ d. present the most important content last, for memory

8. A physical therapist assistant is preparing to teach and practice functional activities with a person who has moderate cognitive impairment. After knocking on the door, the patient verbalizes for them to enter. Upon entering a person's room, the assistant observes that the patient appears to be masturbating. Which of the following responses is appropriate in this situation?

_____ a. leave the room until they are done

_____ b. attempt to distract the patient from the activity

_____ c. yell from the patient's room for the nurse or physician

_____ d. ask the person what they are doing

9. A physical therapist assistant is preparing to teach exercises to a patient. Which of the following single strategies is MOST important for achieving effective learning by the patient?

_____ a. demonstrate the exercises and have the patient return demonstration

_____ b. explain the purpose and anatomical justification for the exercises

_____ c. explain the correct technique and common muscle substitutions of the exercise

_____ d. issue a home exercise program and instruct them to return to the clinic as needed

10. When communicating with the patient, which of the following aspects of communication has the greatest impact on the message being delivered?

_____ a. eye contact

_____ b. body language

_____ c. tone of voice

_____ d. verbal content

11. When communicating with patients and co-workers, it is important to listen actively at times to ensure comprehension of their message. Which of the following techniques of active listening is an example of clarification technique?

_____ a. paraphrase what the person said and your understanding

_____ b. repeat what was said in shorter, simpler terms, attempting to clarify the feelings behind their message

_____ c. listen without interruption

_____ d. repeat the words to the person that you heard

12. When communicating with patients and co-workers, it is important at times to listen actively to ensure comprehension of their message. Which of the following techniques of active listening is an example of the reflection technique?

_____ a. paraphrase what the person said and your understanding of their intent

_____ b. repeat what was said in shorter, simpler terms

_____ c. listen without interruption

_____ d. repeat the words to the person that you heard

13. When communicating with patients and co-workers, it is important at times to listen actively to ensure comprehension of their message. Which of the following techniques of active listening is an example of the restating technique?

_____ a. paraphrase what the person said and your understanding

_____ b. repeat what was said in shorter, simpler terms

_____ c. listen without interruption

_____ d. repeat the words to the person that you heard

14. When communicating with patients and co-workers, it is important at times to listen actively to ensure comprehension of their message. Which of the following techniques of active listening is used only in the initial stages of communication to demonstrate to the person that you are hearing their words?

_____ a. reflection

_____ b. clarification

_____ c. restatement

_____ d. passive listening

PATIENT INSTRUCTION—CONSIDERING THE DEVELOPMENTAL LEVEL, CULTURAL BACKGROUND, SOCIAL HISTORY, HOME SITUATION, AND GEOGRAPHIC BARRIERS OF THE PATIENT

Nine Items

1. A person is experiencing low back stiffness secondary to lack of lumbar extension and hypomobility of the lumbar spine. Which of the following interventions is MOST appropriate for a resident at an extended care facility, 57 years of age, with this condition?

_____ a. intermittent lumbar traction in prone, 3 days a week, as an outpatient

_____ b. intermittent lumbar traction in supine, 3 days a week, as an outpatient

_____ c. continuous ultrasound in prone, 3 days a week, at residence

_____ d. home-issue transcutaneous electrical nerve stimulation unit

2. A person who is recovering from a brain injury, currently exhibits psychotic behavior, is frequently suspicious, and resentful of their family and medical staff members. Which of the following terms do these behaviors describe?

_____ a. hypochondria

_____ b. hysteria

_____ c. depression

_____ d. paranoia

3. Which of the following behaviors would you LEAST expect to see from someone who is experiencing a recent loss of physical function?

_____ a. denial

_____ b. anger

_____ c. bargaining

_____ d. acceptance

4. You are assisting in discharge planning for a middle-aged adult. Which of the following are key issues facing middle-aged adults?

_____ a. parenting, education, and relationships

_____ b. careers and education

_____ c. relationships and retirement

_____ d. careers, parenting, and relationships

5. A person is suffering from a fatal condition, with a poor prognosis. Which of the following traditional cultural values views death as something that should occur in the home?

_____ a. Chinese

_____ b. Filipino

_____ c. Korean

_____ d. Mexican

6. When instructing a person with cognitive impairments in functional activities which of the following statements is MOST appropriate?

_____ a. if you are ready, and all is right with the world, let's get started on some walking

_____ b. its time to start your therapy

_____ c. first, let's work on getting you out of the bed

_____ d. first, we are going to work together on getting out of bed, then walking towards the nurses' station, and then we can practice the stairs

7. When treating a person, it is important to recognize and respect their personal space. Which of the following cultures, traditionally, are LEAST comfortable with being very close to someone with whom they are speaking?

_____ a. Indonesian

_____ b. African

_____ c. British

_____ d. Arabic

8. A physical therapist assistant introduces himself or herself to a Hispanic patient. During the initial interaction, which of the following guidelines SHOULD be observed?

_____ a. greet the person, shake their hand, and position yourself close during communication

_____ b. avoid shaking hands, as it is considered a sign of physical aggression

_____ c. avoid sitting too close while gathering subjective information

_____ d. avoid shaking their hand until they have gotten to know you well

9. Which of the following actions is typically LEAST appropriate when providing physical therapy to a person of Arabic culture?

_____ a. scheduling them with female physical therapy staff

_____ b. forcing the patient to remain autonomous and responsible for decision making

_____ c. scheduling the person with someone of the same gender

_____ d. giving the specific rationale for the plan of care

ANSWERS AND RATIONALE

COORDINATION OF CARE—COMMUNICATION WITH THE PHYSICAL THERAPIST

Twelve Items

1. Correct answer: (c)

   Rationale: Physical therapist assistants make recommendations to the therapist and the interdisciplinary team regarding seat cushions.

   Reference: (1999). *A normative model of physical therapist assistant education: Version 99* (p. 94). Alexandria, VA: American Physical Therapy Association.

2. Correct answer: (b)

   Rationale: The physical therapist is not typically required to sign every progress note written by a physical therapist assistant.

   Reference: Scott, R. (2002). *Foundations of physical therapy, a 21st century-focused view of the profession* (p. 339). New York: McGraw-Hill.

3. Correct answer: (d)

   Rationale: The physical therapist must see the patient prior to discharge.

   Reference: Pagliarulo, M. (2001). *Introduction to physical therapy* (2nd ed., p. 58). St. Louis: Mosby.

4. Correct answer: (d)

   Rationale: This is considered beyond the scope of an entry-level physical therapist assistant.

   Reference: (1999). *A normative model of physical therapist assistant education: Version 99* (p. 94, 95). Alexandria, VA: American Physical Therapy Association.

5. Correct answer: (c)

   Rationale: Each of these should at least be informally communicated to the therapist, but it is most important to report the increase in crepitus.

   Reference: (1999). *A normative model of physical therapist assistant education: Version 99* (pp. 56–79). Alexandria, VA: American Physical Therapy Association.

6. Correct answer: (c)

   Rationale: Additional subjective information will be more useful for the physical therapist to determine any action needed.

   Reference: (1999). *A normative model of physical therapist assistant education: Version 99* (pp. 56–79). Alexandria, VA: American Physical Therapy Association.

7. Correct answer: (a)

   Rationale: Recommending a patient apply protective taping is the least appropriate choice and beyond the scope of the entry-level physical therapist assistant.

Reference: (1999). *A normative model of physical therapist assistant education: Version 99* (p. 95). Alexandria, VA: American Physical Therapy Association.

8. Correct answer: (c)

   Rationale: Proxemics is the use of personal space for communication, and each of these are appropriate explanations of the benefits.

   Reference: Luckman, J. (2000). *Transcultural communication in health care* (p. 54, 55). Albany: Delmar.

9. Correct answer: (d)

   Rationale: Appropriate return of range of motion is a critical outcome after a total knee replacement. A lack of progress with range of motion should be reported to the physical therapist. The other activities do not specifically state any lack of progress.

   Reference: (1999). *A normative model of physical therapist assistant education: Version 99* (pp. 56–79). Alexandria, VA: American Physical Therapy Association.

10. Correct answer: (d)

    Rationale: This skill is considered beyond the domain of the physical therapist assistant.

    Reference: (1999). *A normative model of physical therapist assistant education: Version 99* (p. 94). Alexandria, VA: American Physical Therapy Association.

11. Correct answer: (b)

    Rationale: There is not a commonly defined number of visits for indicating need for reevaluation.

    Reference: Pagliarulo, M. (2001). *Introduction to physical therapy* (2nd ed., p. 58). St. Louis: Mosby.

12. Correct answer: (d)

    Rationale: Neurogenic symptoms may cause concern about reflex sympathetic dystrophy.

    Reference: Lesh, S. (2000). *Clinical orthopedics for the physical therapist assistant* (p. 447). Philadelphia: FA Davis.

COORDINATION OF CARE—PROGRESSING TREATMENT WITHIN THE PLAN OF CARE

Ten Items

1. Correct answer: (d)

   Rationale: A cardex is often recorded in pencil to allow for ongoing updates.

   Reference: Lukan, M. (2001). *Documentation for physical therapist assistants* (2nd ed., p. 34). Philadelphia: FA Davis.

2. Correct answer: (a)

   Rationale: This activity provides a progression, beginning with a more achievable task.

   Reference: Sine, R., et al. (2000). *Basic rehabilitation techniques* (4th ed., p. 174, 175). Maryland: Aspen.

3. Correct answer: (c)

   Rationale: Improving physical endurance requires physiological adaptation.

   Reference: Kisner, C., & Colby, L. (2002). *Therapeutic exercise: Foundations and techniques* (4th ed., pp. 150–152). Philadelphia: FA Davis.

4. Correct answer: (c)

   Rationale: Progression in duration will improve functional muscular endurance.

   Reference: Kisner, C., & Colby, L. (2002). *Therapeutic exercise: Foundations and techniques* (4th ed., p. 191, 192). Philadelphia: FA Davis.

5. Correct answer: (c)

   Rationale: Weight shifting and hip hiking are required prior to stepping. Stepping forward is required to transition into gait training. Side stepping is a progression of basic gait training.

   Reference: O'Sullivan. (2001). *Physical rehabilitation assessment and treatment* (4th ed., pp. 422–424). Philadelphia: FA Davis.

6. Correct answer: (d)

   Rationale: The IEP meets several requirements established by congress; meetings are conducted at least once every six months. Regarding the second choice, it is not intended to directly communicate to the physical therapist assistant.

   Reference: Lukan, M. (2001). *Documentation for physical therapist assistants* (2nd ed., p. 34). Philadelphia: FA Davis.

7. Correct answer: (b)

   Rationale: Avoid exacerbating the patient's symptoms.

   Reference: Kisner, C., & Colby, L. (2002). *Therapeutic exercise: Foundations and techniques* (4th ed., p. 227). Philadelphia: FA Davis.

8. Correct answer: (b)

   Rationale: Lateral weight shifts are more basic than the other tasks.

   Reference: O'Sullivan. (2001). *Physical rehabilitation assessment and treatment* (4th ed., p. 424). Philadelphia: FA Davis.

9. Correct answer: (c)

   Rationale: Gentle plantarflexion and dorsiflexion of the ankle should be initiated first.

   Reference: Prentice, W. (1998). *Rehabilitation techniques in sports medicine* (2nd ed., p. 442). St. Louis: Mosby.

10. Correct answer: (b)

    Rationale: Each of the other methods is appropriate when steps are taken to protect the contents of the faxed or mailed documents, and the discussions are directly related to the care of the patient.

    Reference: Lukan, M. (2001). *Documentation for physical therapist assistants* (2nd ed., p. 34). Philadelphia: FA Davis.

COORDINATION OF CARE—DIRECTING TASKS TO SUPPORT PERSONNEL

Ten Items

1. Correct answer: (b)

   Rationale: Only the physical therapist can determine which tasks can be delegated to support personnel. The physical therapist may directly supervise the performance of tasks when delegated.

   Reference: Pagliarulo, M. (2001). *Introduction to physical therapy* (2nd ed., p. 55). St. Louis: Mosby.

2. Correct answer: (c)

   Rationale: The patient-related tasks for unskilled positions should be performed with limited autonomy.

   Reference: Nosse, L., et al. (1999). *Managerial and supervisory principles for physical therapists* (p. 105, 106). Baltimore: Williams & Wilkins.

3. Correct answer: (a)

   Rationale: Direct personal supervision by either the physical therapist or physical therapist assistant where allowable by law is most appropriate.

   Reference: Pagliarulo, M. (2001). *Introduction to physical therapy* (2nd ed., p. 59). St. Louis: Mosby.

4. Correct answer: (b)

   Rationale: Telecommunication access is insufficient supervision for support personnel.

   Reference: Scott, R. (2002). *Foundations of physical therapy, a 21st century-focused view of the profession* (p. 339). New York: McGraw-Hill.

5. Correct answer: (d)

   Rationale: Physical therapist assistants require a two-year college degree in physical therapy. Other persons, regardless of their level of education, do not qualify to practice as assistants. The American Physical Therapy Association defines three personnel in physical therapy as the physical therapist, the physical therapist assistant, and support personnel.

   Reference: Anemaet, W., et al. (2000). *Home rehabilitation: Guide to clinical practice* (p. 30). St. Louis: Mosby.

6. Correct answer: (b)

   Rationale: Direct personal supervision is only required for patient-related tasks.

   Reference: Pagliarulo, M. (2001). *Introduction to physical therapy* (2nd ed., p. 57, 58). St. Louis: Mosby.

7. Correct answer: (d)

   Rationale: Only tasks that do not require clinical decision making are appropriate for direction to support personnel.

   Reference: Pagliarulo, M. (2001). *Introduction to physical therapy* (2nd ed., p. 59). St. Louis: Mosby.

8. Correct answer: (a)

   Rationale: The use of credentials by support personnel is discouraged.

Reference: Scott, R. (2002). *Foundations of physical therapy, a 21st century-focused view of the profession* (p. 382, 383). New York: McGraw-Hill.

9. Correct answer: (c)

   Rationale: In some states, the assistant is not allowed to direct or supervise the actions of support personnel. In all states, it is appropriate for the supervisory physical therapist to direct and supervise the provision of physical therapy.

   Reference: Scott, R. (2002). *Foundations of physical therapy, a 21st century-focused view of the profession* (p. 205). New York: McGraw-Hill.

10. Correct answer: (d)

    Rationale: Physical therapy aides should not be expected to apply to clinical problem solving, or reasoning, as demanded from the other three activities.

    Reference: Scott, R. (2002). *Foundations of physical therapy, a 21st century-focused view of the profession* (p. 339–345). New York: McGraw-Hill.

INTERPERSONAL COMMUNICATION—PATIENTS, FAMILIES, CAREGIVERS, AND OTHERS

Fifteen Items

1. Correct answer: (c)

   Rationale: The scope of the physical therapist assistant does not include specialization in dialysis.

   Reference: (1999). *A normative model of physical therapist assistant education: Version 99* (p. 3). Alexandria, VA: American Physical Therapy Association.

2. Correct answer: (d)

   Rationale: The first three choices result in a yes or no answer, and are suggestive. The last question is an open-ended question that allows for more patient input.

   Reference: Hanna, M., & Gibson, J. (1987). *Public speaking for personal success* (p. 82). Dubuque, IA: William C. Brown Publishers.

3. Correct answer: (a)

   Rationale: Nonverbal and visual are not as limited by spoken language.

   Reference: Hanna, M., & Gibson, J. (1987). *Public speaking for personal success* (p. 171). Dubuque, IA: William C. Brown Publishers.

4. Correct answer: (d)

   Rationale: Close-ended questions limit the responses available to the person, often to two or three choices only. Open-ended questions allow the person to respond in a variety of ways, and do not limit them to their choices.

Reference: Hanna, M., & Gibson, J. (1987). *Public speaking for personal success* (p. 82). Dubuque, IA: William C. Brown Publishers.

5. Correct answer: (d)

   Rationale: The communication of therapeutic promises may create legal obligations to the patient.

   Reference: Navarra, T., et al. (1990). *Therapeutic communication, a guide to effective interpersonal skills for health care professionals* (p. 137). Thorofare, NJ: Slack.

6. Correct answer: (b)

   Rationale: Address patients by their last name and clearly identify yourself. Manipulating their environment is intrusion on their rights. The choice to ignore the person is based upon stereotypes.

   Reference: O'Sullivan. (2001). *Physical rehabilitation assessment and treatment* (4th ed., p. 163). Philadelphia: FA Davis.

7. Correct answer: (d)

   Rationale: This choice has nothing to do with the HIPAA. Although abuse by a parent may prevent them from representing the child in the future, it was not described in this item.

   Reference: www.hhs.gov

8. Correct answer: (c)

   Rationale: Parents of young children rely upon health care professionals to be respectful, empathetic, responsive, and honest. Do not withhold information from parents, but respond with tact and sensitivity.

   Reference: Scott, R. (2002). *Foundations of physical therapy, a 21st century-focused view of the profession* (p. 144, 145). New York: McGraw-Hill.

9. Correct answer: (b)

   Rationale: The lack of documenting this item may constitute patient abandonment. Each of the other choices should be documented, but do not specifically relate to patient abandonment.

   Reference: Scott, R. (1994). *Legal aspects of documenting patient care* (2nd ed., p. 67). Maryland: Aspen.

10. Correct answer: (a)

    Rationale: This immediate space is generally considered intimate and must be utilized appropriately.

    Reference: Luckman, J. (2000). *Transcultural communication in health care* (p. 54, 55). Albany: Delmar.

11. Correct Answer: (a)

    Rationale: The effort to avoid overidentification begins with seeing the person as a unique individual.

    Reference: Purtillo, R., & Haddad, A. (2002). *Health professional and patient interaction* (6th ed., p. 216, 217). Philadelphia: WB Saunders.

12. Correct answer: (c)

    Rationale: This distance is generally considered as an appropriate range of social space for common interactions.

    Reference: Luckman, J. (2000). *Transcultural communication in health care* (p. 54, 55). Albany: Delmar.

13. Correct answer: (c)

    Rationale: Asking a person if they can hear you clearly is appropriate for various ages and cultures. The other three answers may not be appropriate at times.

    Reference: O'Sullivan. (2001). *Physical rehabilitation assessment and treatment* (4th ed., p. 163). Philadelphia: FA Davis.

14. Correct answer: (d)

    Rationale: It is important to respect the family unit, and not to interfere with family dynamics, even if they differ from the values of the assistant.

    Reference: Scott, R. (2002). *Foundations of physical therapy, a 21st century-focused view of the profession* (p. 144, 145). New York: McGraw-Hill.

15. Correct answer: (b)

    Rationale: This space is commonly reserved for friends, or with appropriate interactions with health care providers.

    Reference: Luckman, J. (2000). *Transcultural communication in health care* (p. 54, 55). Albany: Delmar.

INTERPERSONAL COMMUNICATION— COMMUNICATING WITH THE PHYSICAL THERAPIST AND OTHER HEALTH CARE PROFESSIONALS

Fourteen Items

1. Correct answer: (a)

    Rationale: A physical therapist assistant is expected to be open and responsive to constructive feedback on clinical performance. Since the therapist has some experience with the patient, their insight may improve or contribute to the well being of the patient.

    Reference: (1999). *A normative model of physical therapist assistant education: Version 99* (p. 43). Alexandria, VA: American Physical Therapy Association.

2. Correct answer: (d)

    Rationale: Social services typically arrange home health care following discharge from a medical treatment center.

    Reference: Anemaet, W., et al. (2000). *Home rehabilitation: Guide to clinical practice* (p. 29). St. Louis: Mosby.

3. Correct answer: (a)

    Rationale: This is using the "we" versus "me" approach to resolving conflict, demonstrating a shared interest in doing what is best for the patient.

    Reference: Nosse, L., et al. (1999). *Managerial and supervisory principles for physical therapists* (p. 85). Baltimore: Williams & Wilkins.

4. Correct answer: (a)

   Rationale: The intradisciplinary model functions without the input or collaboration of other disciplines.

   Reference: Scott, R. (2002). *Foundations of physical therapy, a 21st century-focused view of the profession* (p. 146). New York: McGraw-Hill.

5. Correct answer: (c)

   Rationale: Any person not directly involved in the person's care is not privy to information specific to the patient. This assertive and polite response is most appropriate.

   Reference: Purtillo, R. (1999). *Ethical dimensions in the health professions* (3rd ed., p. 154). Philadelphia: WB Saunders.

6. Correct answer: (d)

   Rationale: The case manager oversees the cost-effective implementation of the total plan of care.

   Reference: Anemaet, W., et al. (2000). *Home rehabilitation: Guide to clinical practice* (p. 28). St. Louis: Mosby.

7. Correct answer: (a)

   Rationale: An ophthalmologist is a specialist for eye disorders.

   Reference: Chabner, D. (2003). *Medical terminology: A short course* (3rd ed., p. 150). Philadelphia: WB Saunders.

8. Correct answer: (d)

   Rationale: Social services often arrange for the delivery of durable medical equipment following discharge from a medical facility.

   Reference: Anemaet, W., et al. (2000). *Home rehabilitation: Guide to clinical practice* (p. 29). St. Louis: Mosby.

9. Correct answer: (b)

   Rationale: The multidisciplinary model is the most common in traditional medical facilities. An example of this model is the physical therapist evaluating and treating the patient, while seeking input from other disciplines.

   Reference: Scott, R. (2002). *Foundations of physical therapy, a 21st century-focused view of the profession* (p. 146). New York: McGraw-Hill.

10. Correct answer: (b)

    Rationale: The role player approach avoids resolving the conflict through portraying perceived or actual professional or social roles, such as parent versus child.

    Reference: Nosse, L., et al. (1999). *Managerial and supervisory principles for physical therapists* (p. 84). Baltimore: Williams & Wilkins.

11. Correct answer: (a)

    Rationale: The physical therapist should be informed first, followed by the occupational therapist.

    Reference: Anemaet, W., et al. (2000). *Home rehabilitation: Guide to clinical practice* (p. 29). St. Louis: Mosby.

12. Correct answer: (d)

Rationale: The case manager oversees the cost-effective implementation of the total plan of care.

Reference: Anemaet, W., et al. (2000). *Home rehabilitation: Guide to clinical practice* (p. 28). St. Louis: Mosby.

13. Correct answer: (c)

Rationale: To make demands to resolve conflict or trade-offs is typically ineffective.

Reference: Nosse, L., et al. (1999). *Managerial and supervisory principles for physical therapists* (p. 84). Baltimore: Williams & Wilkins.

14. Correct answer: (d)

Rationale: The occupational therapist is most specialized and skilled for bathing and dressing activities.

Reference: (1997). *Stedman's concise medical dictionary for the health professions* (3rd ed.). Baltimore: Williams & Wilkins.

INTERPERSONAL COMMUNICATION— COMMUNICATING THE ROLE OF THE PHYSICAL THERAPIST AND PHYSICAL THERAPIST ASSISTANT

Twelve Items

1. Correct answer: (a)

Rationale: It is within the role of the physical therapist to explain testing and diagnostic procedures.

Reference: (1999). *A normative model of physical therapist assistant education: Version 99* (p. 42). Alexandria, VA: American Physical Therapy Association.

2. Correct answer: (b)

Rationale: It is appropriate for an experienced physical therapist assistant to initiate interventions consistent with the goals, when delegated by the physical therapist.

Reference: Pagliarulo, M. (2001). *Introduction to physical therapy* (2nd ed., p. 68). St. Louis: Mosby.

3. Correct answer: (b)

Rationale: This data collection skill is considered beyond the scope of an entry-level physical therapist assistant.

Reference: (1999). *A normative model of physical therapist assistant education: Version 99* (p. 203, 204). Alexandria, VA: American Physical Therapy Association.

4. Correct answer: (d)

Rationale: It is most appropriate to clarify these issues prior to delegating the patient to the entry-level assistant.

Reference: Pagliarulo, M. (2001). *Introduction to physical therapy* (2nd ed., p. 68). St. Louis: Mosby.

5. Correct answer: (b)

   Rationale: This intervention is considered beyond the scope of an entry-level physical therapist assistant.

   Reference: (1999). *A normative model of physical therapist assistant education: Version 99* (pp. 90–100). Alexandria, VA: American Physical Therapy Association.

6. Correct answer: (c)

   Rationale: The other data collection skills are considered beyond the scope of an entry-level physical therapist assistant.

   Reference: (1999). *A normative model of physical therapist assistant education: Version 99* (p. 203, 204). Alexandria, VA: American Physical Therapy Association.

7. Correct answer: (a)

   Rationale: Manual traction is considered beyond an entry-level skill for physical therapist assistants.

   Reference: (1999). *A normative model of physical therapist assistant education: Version 99* (p. 209, 210). Alexandria, VA: American Physical Therapy Association.

8. Correct answer: (a)

   Rationale: This data collection skill is considered beyond the scope of an entry-level physical therapist assistant.

   Reference: (1999). *A normative model of physical therapist assistant education: Version 99* (p. 203, 204). Alexandria, VA: American Physical Therapy Association.

9. Correct answer: (a)

   Rationale: The other choices are considered technical skills not to be performed by entry-level physical therapist assistants.

   Reference: (1999). *A normative model of physical therapist assistant education: Version 99* (pp. 201–209). Alexandria, VA: American Physical Therapy Association.

10. Correct answer: (b)

   Rationale: This intervention is considered within full competency level for an entry-level physical therapist assistant.

   Reference: (1999). *A normative model of physical therapist assistant education: Version 99* (pp. 90–100). Alexandria, VA: American Physical Therapy Association.

11. Correct answer: (a)

   Rationale: This technical skill is excluded from entry-level skills for the physical therapist assistant.

   Reference: (1999). *A normative model of physical therapist assistant education: Version 99* (pp. 201–209). Alexandria, VA: American Physical Therapy Association.

12. Correct answer: (a)

   Rationale: General supervision allows for off-site and telecommunication availability of the therapist.

   Reference: Scott, R. (2002). *Foundations of physical therapy, a 21st century-focused view of the profession* (p. 400). New York: McGraw-Hill.

DOCUMENTATION—REVIEWING MEDICAL CHARTS

Three Items

1. Correct answer: (c)

   Rationale: All of the other choices are valid.

   Reference: www.hhs.gov

2. Correct answer: (b)

   Rationale: One of the primary functions of social services is to coordinate placement of a patient after hospitalization. All members of the health care team should contribute to the discharge plan.

   Reference: (1997). *Stedman's concise medical dictionary for the health professions* (3rd ed.). Baltimore: Williams & Wilkins.

3. Correct answer: (a)

   Rationale: A person's current diagnosis and medical precautions must be known before treating the person.

   Reference: Lukan, M. (2001). *Documentation for physical therapist assistants* (2nd ed., p. 62). Philadelphia: FA Davis.

DOCUMENTATION—OBJECTIVELY DOCUMENTING RESULTS AND MEASUREMENTS

Eleven Items

1. Correct answer: (b)

   Rationale: This information, reported by the patient, belongs in the subjective section of a SOAP note.

   Reference: Kettenbach, G. (1995). *Writing SOAP notes* (2nd ed., p. 44). Philadelphia: FA Davis.

2. Correct answer: (c)

   Rationale: This entry is specific and concise with clarity.

   Reference: Kettenbach, G. (1995). *Writing SOAP notes* (2nd ed., p. 9). Philadelphia: FA Davis.

3. Correct answer: (b)

   Rationale: These observations represent the presence of edema, and arterial supply for a limb; girth measurements are not a manual technique.

   Reference: Kettenbach, G. (1995). *Writing SOAP notes* (2nd ed., p. 49). Philadelphia: FA Davis.

4. Correct answer: (b)

   Rationale: Results of special tests are recorded in the objective section of a SOAP note.

   Reference: Lukan, M. (2001). *Documentation for physical therapist assistants* (2nd ed., p. 76). Philadelphia: FA Davis.

5. Correct answer: (a)

   Rationale: The use of a hyphen can be confusing. Several symbols such as minus or negative can be confused with a hyphen.

   Reference: Kettenbach, G. (1995). *Writing SOAP notes* (2nd ed., p. 10). Philadelphia: FA Davis.

6. Correct answer: (a)

   Rationale: This information belongs to the subjective section of the SOAP note, if provided by another person. If the recorder is commenting on the absence, it may be more appropriate in the assessment section of the note.

   Reference: Lukan, M. (2001). *Documentation for physical therapist assistants* (2nd ed., p. 76). Philadelphia: FA Davis.

7. Correct answer: (b)

   Rationale: The semicolon can be used similar to its function in nontechnical grammar.

   Reference: Kettenbach, G. (1995). *Writing SOAP notes* (2nd ed., p. 10). Philadelphia: FA Davis.

8. Correct answer: (b)

   Rationale: Manual muscle testing is the best choice that reflects a person's strength. Substitutions during active motion could be due to weakness or improper motor recruitment. Available range of motion does not reflect strength.

   Reference: Kettenbach, G. (1995). *Writing SOAP notes* (2nd ed., p. 49). Philadelphia: FA Davis.

9. Correct answer: (b)

   Rationale: Rate of perceived exertion or perceived level of exertion is a subjective measurement of tolerance to physical activity.

   Reference: Kettenbach, G. (1995). *Writing SOAP notes* (2nd ed., p. 50). Philadelphia: FA Davis.

10. Correct answer: (b)

    Rationale: The other choices are written in first-person perspective. Medical record SHOULD be written about the patient.

    Reference: Kettenbach, G. (1995). *Writing SOAP notes* (2nd ed., p. 11). Philadelphia: FA Davis.

11. Correct answer: (c)

    Rationale: Information based upon the patient, family, or another caregiver is recorded in the subjective section of a SOAP note.

    Reference: Kettenbach, G. (1995). *Writing SOAP notes* (2nd ed., p. 53). Philadelphia: FA Davis.

DOCUMENTATION—OBJECTIVELY DOCUMENTING ALL ASPECTS OF PATIENT CARE, INCLUDING INTERVENTIONS, RESPONSES, PROGRESS, AND OUTCOMES

Eighteen Items

1. Correct answer: (c)

    Rationale: Progress is documented in the assessment section of a SOAP note.

    Reference: Pagliarulo, M. (2001). *Introduction to physical therapy* (2nd ed., p. 34). St. Louis: Mosby.

2. Correct answer: (a)

    Rationale: The subjective section of the SOAP note is where second-hand information is recorded.

    Reference: Pagliarulo, M. (2001). *Introduction to physical therapy* (2nd ed., p. 34). St. Louis: Mosby.

3. Correct answer: (d)

    Rationale: The plan section of a SOAP note is where future activities or intended adjustments are recorded.

    Reference: Lukan, M. (2001). *Documentation for physical therapist assistants* (2nd ed., p. 115). Philadelphia: FA Davis.

4. Correct answer: (b)

    Rationale: The results of measurements and tests are recorded in the objective section of a SOAP note. Goniometry is a clinical measurement.

    Reference: Lukan, M. (2001). *Documentation for physical therapist assistants* (2nd ed., p. 77). Philadelphia: FA Davis.

5. Correct answer: (a)

    Rationale: This is second-hand (subjective) information, and is recorded in the subjective portion of the note.

    Reference: Lukan, M. (2001). *Documentation for physical therapist assistants* (2nd ed., p. 62). Philadelphia: FA Davis.

6. Correct answer: (c)

    Rationale: Documentation should not be erasable; it compromises the legitimacy of the document.

    Reference: Lukan, M. (2001). *Documentation for physical therapist assistants* (2nd ed., p. 55). Philadelphia: FA Davis.

7. Correct answer: (c)

    Rationale: Medical records are legal documents and should not be destroyed. A single line allows the error to be viewed later as needed, without the appearance of fraud.

    Reference: Scott, R. (1994). *Legal aspects of documenting patient care* (2nd ed., p. 47). Maryland: Aspen.

8. Correct answer: (c)

   Rationale: Do not attempt to hide errors. The original entry should be clearly designated as an error. Avoid overwriting or using correction fluid in medical records. Include date and time.

   Reference: Scott, R. (1994). *Legal aspects of documenting patient care* (2nd ed., p. 49). Maryland: Aspen.

9. Correct answer: (d)

   Rationale: This is the only objective type data of the choices. Other appropriate information would be description of the person's function, interventions applied, and results of measurements and tests.

   Reference: Lukan, M. (2001). *Documentation for physical therapist assistants* (2nd ed., p. 76). Philadelphia: FA Davis.

10. Correct answer: (d)

    Rationale: Refusal of interventions should be documented, along with their reason, and actions taken by the clinician. In addition, refusals given to the physical therapist assistant SHOULD include a statement recording informing the physical therapist.

    Reference: Lukan, M. (2001). *Documentation for physical therapist assistants* (2nd ed., p. 122, 123). Philadelphia: FA Davis.

11. Correct answer: (d)

    Rationale: It is acceptable to state intended discussions with the physical therapist, but the physical therapist assistant should avoid stating conclusions in the plan section of a SOAP note.

    Reference: Lukan, M. (2001). *Documentation for physical therapist assistants* (2nd ed., p. 115). Philadelphia: FA Davis.

12. Correct answer: (b)

    Rationale: This goal is directed at a specific function, is quantifiable, and has a specific and reasonable timeline.

    Reference: Lukan, M. (2001). *Documentation for physical therapist assistants* (2nd ed., p. 97). Philadelphia: FA Davis.

13. Correct answer: (b)

    Rationale: Palpation observations are recorded in the objective portion of the SOAP note.

    Reference: Lukan, M. (2001). *Documentation for physical therapist assistants* (2nd ed., p. 65). Philadelphia: FA Davis.

14. Correct answer: (d)

    Rationale: Permanent black or blue ink pens are the only current acceptable writing utensils. Blue ink is used to indicate original copies.

    Reference: Lukan, M. (2001). *Documentation for physical therapist assistants* (2nd ed., p. 54). Philadelphia: FA Davis.

15. Correct answer: (b)

    Rationale: The current goals are addressed in either the assessment or plan section of a SOAP note.

Reference: Lukan, M. (2001). *Documentation for physical therapist assistants* (2nd ed., p. 76). Philadelphia: FA Davis.

16. Correct answer: (d)

Rationale: Each of these is necessary for establishing reproducible documentation.

Reference: Lukan, M. (2001). *Documentation for physical therapist assistants* (2nd ed., p. 78, 79). Philadelphia: FA Davis.

17. Correct answer: (d)

Rationale: The last choice records the patient response and performance during the treatment session. Additional information could specify tolerance to activity, vital signs, why the person ambulated only 75', and other data would further improve the entry.

Reference: Lukan, M. (2001). *Documentation for physical therapist assistants* (2nd ed., p. 80). Philadelphia: FA Davis.

18. Correct answer: (c)

Rationale: The use of abbreviations does contribute to brevity, but also compromises the accuracy of the entry.

Reference: Lukan, M. (2001). *Documentation for physical therapist assistants* (2nd ed., p. 53). Philadelphia: FA Davis.

KNOWLEDGE OF MEDICAL AND PHYSICAL THERAPY TERMINOLOGY

Fourteen Items

1. Correct answer: (c)

Rationale: Because of the spongy ratio of bone material in children, fractures often splinter resulting in incomplete fracture.

Reference: (1997). *Taber's cyclopedic medical dictionary* (19th ed.). Philadelphia: FA Davis.

2. Correct answer: (b)

Rationale: An avulsion is a forcible tearing of a structure.

Reference: (1997). *Taber's cyclopedic medical dictionary* (19th ed.). Philadelphia: FA Davis.

3. Correct answer: (b)

Rationale: Osteoarthritis typically affects larger, weight-bearing joints.

Reference: (1997). *Taber's cyclopedic medical dictionary* (19th ed.). Philadelphia: FA Davis.

4. Correct answer: (a)

Rationale: A person will typically demonstrate a decreased stance time upon a painful lower limb.

Reference: Rothstein, J., et al. (1998). *The rehabilitation specialist's handbook* (2nd ed., p. 816). Philadelphia: FA Davis.

5. Correct answer: (c)

Rationale: Finkelstein's test detects tenosynovitis of the thumb abductor and extensor tendons.

Reference: Rothstein, J., et al. (1998). *The rehabilitation specialist's handbook* (2nd ed., p. 176). Philadelphia: FA Davis.

6. Correct answer: (d)

Rationale: The vertebral arteries converge into the basilar artery. These structures supply the circle of Willis which maintains distribution of the cerebral vascular supply.

Reference: O'Sullivan. (2001). *Physical rehabilitation assessment and treatment* (4th ed., p. 523). Philadelphia: FA Davis.

7. Correct answer: (a)

Rationale: Lachman's test detects laxity of the anterior cruciate ligament in the knee.

Reference: Rothstein, J., et al. (1998). *The rehabilitation specialist's handbook* (2nd ed., p. 184). Philadelphia: FA Davis.

8. Correct answer: (a)

Rationale: Diabetes type I is an absolute deficiency of insulin.

Reference: (1997). *Taber's cyclopedic medical dictionary* (19th ed.). Philadelphia: FA Davis.

9. Correct answer: (d)

Rationale: Each of the first three choices and hyperabduction syndrome are related classifications of thoracic outlet syndrome.

Reference: Kisner, C., & Colby, L. (2002). *Therapeutic exercise: Foundations and techniques* (4th ed., p. 359). Philadelphia: FA Davis.

10. Correct answer: (d)

Rationale: A Dupuytren's contracture is a flexion deformity of the fourth or fifth finger.

Reference: (1997). *Taber's cyclopedic medical dictionary* (19th ed.). Philadelphia: FA Davis.

11. Correct answer: (b)

Rationale: Ankylosis means fusion, spondylitis is inflammation of the spine, and spondylolisthesis is displacement of one vertebrae upon another.

Reference: (1997). *Taber's cyclopedic medical dictionary* (19th ed.). Philadelphia: FA Davis.

12. Correct answer: (d)

Rationale: Parkinson's disease is the only upper motor neuron condition in these choices. Amyotrophic lateral sclerosis affects both upper motor neurons. Guillian-Barre and carpal tunnel are lower motor neuron impairments.

Reference: O'Sullivan. (2001). *Physical rehabilitation assessment and treatment* (4th ed., p. 748, 749). Philadelphia: FA Davis.

13. Correct answer: (c)

Rationale: Neuropraxia is the transient impairment of peripheral nerves.

Reference: O'Sullivan. (2001). *Physical rehabilitation assessment and treatment* (4th ed., p. 233). Philadelphia: FA Davis.

14. Correct answer: (d)

Rationale: Gun shot, stabbing, or motor vehicle accidents account for the majority of lateral cord syndromes.

Reference: Somers, M. (2001). *Spinal cord injury: Functional rehabilitation* (2nd ed., p. 28). New Jersey: Prentice Hall.

PATIENT INSTRUCTION: DEMONSTRATING AND EXPLAINING TREATMENT PROCEDURES

Nine Items

1. Correct answer: (d)

Rationale: All of the above are important precautions to consider, but of these choices, recent hip surgery is the most limiting in terms of positioning.

Reference: Placzek, J., & Boyce, D. (2001). *Orthopedic physical therapy secrets* (p. 399). Philadelphia: Hanley & Belfus, Inc.

2. Correct answer: (c)

Rationale: All persons applying interventions are responsible for ensuring that they are not contraindicated.

Reference: Scott, R. (2002). *Foundations of physical therapy, a 21st century-focused view of the profession* (p. 339). New York: McGraw-Hill.

3. Correct answer: (a)

Rationale: The assistant must know the weight-bearing status of the lower extremities prior to teaching bed mobility. The weight-bearing status will affect the techniques utilized for mobility. Vital signs are also very relevant, but not specifically prior to entering the person's room. The last two choices are also important, but less critical before entering the person's room.

Reference: Pierson, F. (2002). *Principles and techniques of patient care* (3rd ed., p. 223). Philadelphia: WB Saunders.

4. Correct answer: (a)

Rationale: Dependent positioning occurs with positioning body parts lower than the heart, which is more likely to result in edema and thrombus formation.

Reference: Kisner, C., & Colby, L. (2002). *Therapeutic exercise: Foundations and techniques* (4th ed., p. 717). Philadelphia: FA Davis.

5. Correct answer: (c)

   Rationale: A person with lumbar spine precautions should not pull or push their body weight with the risk of excess trauma or motion to the lumbar spine.

   Reference: Somers, M. (2001). *Spinal cord injury: Functional rehabilitation* (2nd ed., p. 176). New Jersey: Prentice Hall.

6. Correct answer: (b)

   Rationale: Doing laundry is considered an instrumental activity of daily living.

   Reference: Anemaet, W., et al. (2000). *Home rehabilitation: Guide to clinical practice* (p. 279). St. Louis: Mosby.

7. Correct answer: (a)

   Rationale: Grooming is considered a basic activity of daily living.

   Reference: Anemaet, W., et al. (2000). *Home rehabilitation: Guide to clinical practice* (p. 279). St. Louis: Mosby.

8. Correct answer: (d)

   Rationale: Resisted eccentric activity is the least appropriate choice during the subacute phase of healing.

   Reference: Kisner, C., & Colby, L. (2002). *Therapeutic exercise: Foundations and techniques* (4th ed., p. 291). Philadelphia: FA Davis.

9. Correct answer: (b)

   Rationale: Short-wave diathermy emits an electromagnetic field which may interfere with the function of electronic implanted devices.

   Reference: Cameron, M. (1999). *Physical agents in rehabilitation: From research to practice* (p. 328). Philadelphia: WB Saunders.

INSTRUCTING AND DEMONSTRATING SAFE APPLICATION OF PATIENT CARE TECHNIQUES WITH THE PATIENT AND THEIR FAMILY, INCLUDING WRITTEN INSTRUCTIONS

Six Items

1. Correct answer: (c)

   Rationale: Verbal and written explanations are useful, but feedback directed at their performance will achieve the particular results necessary for this intervention.

   Reference: Davis, C. (1998). *Patient practitioner interaction: An experiential manual for developing the art of health care* (3rd ed., p. 209). Thorofare, NJ: Slack, Inc.

2. Correct answer: (d)

   Rationale: This activity requires lift of the straightened limb, with a greater lever arm of resistance.

   Reference: O'Sullivan. (2001). *Physical rehabilitation assessment and treatment* (4th ed., p. 416). Philadelphia: FA Davis.

3. Correct answer: (a)

   Rationale: The quadriceps should not be actively contracted until healing has occurred and the precautions are removed by the physician.

   Reference: Rothstein, J., et al. (1998). *The rehabilitation specialist's handbook* (2nd ed., p. 138). Philadelphia: FA Davis.

4. Correct answer: (c)

   Rationale: This is the correct sequence of application for peripheral joint mobilization. Other interventions can be incorporated into the sequence.

   Reference: Kisner, C., & Colby, L. (2002). *Therapeutic exercise: Foundations and techniques* (4th ed., p. 227). Philadelphia: FA Davis.

5. Correct answer: (a)

   Rationale: This is an appropriate level for written handouts, which should avoid the use of jargon.

   Reference: Davis, C. (1998). *Patient practitioner interaction: An experiential manual for developing the art of health care* (3rd ed., p. 212). Thorofare, NJ: Slack, Inc.

6. Correct answer: (b)

   Rationale: Simulations are valuable for feedback and improvement of physical skills.

   Reference: Davis, C. (1998). *Patient practitioner interaction: An experiential manual for developing the art of health care* (3rd ed., p. 212). Thorofare, NJ: Slack, Inc.

PATIENT INSTRUCTION: DETERMINING EFFECTIVENESS OF INSTRUCTION AND MODIFYING AS NEEDED

Eleven Items

1. Correct answer: (a)

   Rationale: Tactile and proprioceptive cues can reinforce the correct motor recruitment.

   Reference: Kisner, C., & Colby, L. (2002). *Therapeutic exercise: Foundations and techniques* (4th ed., p. 662). Philadelphia: FA Davis.

2. Correct answer: (b)

   Rationale: The apical, carotid, and radial sites are easily accessible. It would not be reasonable for a person to remove their shoe to monitor their heart rate during ambulation.

Reference: Pierson, F. (1994). *Principles and techniques of patient care* (p. 188). Philadelphia: WB Saunders.

3. Correct answer: (b)

   Rationale: This is the correct technique for the precaution. It may not be beneficial to relate pregnancy to the teenage male.

   Reference: Long, T., & Cintas, H. (1995). *Handbook of pediatric physical therapy* (pp. 46–50). Philadelphia: Williams & Wilkins.

4. Correct answer: (d)

   Rationale: Both the correction and technique are appropriate for facilitating improved performance during gait training through the total communication concept.

   Reference: Long, T., & Cintas, H. (1995). *Handbook of pediatric physical therapy* (p. 270). Philadelphia: Williams & Wilkins.

5. Correct answer: (d)

   Rationale: These instructions are accurate and patient-appropriate regarding the level of communication.

   Reference: Cameron, M. (1999). *Physical agents in rehabilitation: From research to practice* (p. 387). Philadelphia: WB Saunders.

6. Correct answer: (d)

   Rationale: Posterior tilts should be performed primarily by the abdominals, without the use of the gluteus maximus, which is observed to ensure it is relaxed.

   Reference: Kisner, C., & Colby, L. (2002). *Therapeutic exercise: Foundations and techniques* (4th ed., p. 470). Philadelphia: FA Davis.

7. Correct answer: (a)

   Rationale: During bed mobility and transfers, the person is most likely to exceed their hip precautions, which is a primary concern after a hip replacement.

   Reference: Kisner, C,. & Colby, L. (2002). *Therapeutic exercise: Foundations and techniques* (4th ed., p. 476). Philadelphia: FA Davis.

8. Correct answer: (d)

   Rationale: Each of these is an effective facilitation technique, especially when used concurrently.

   Reference: Kisner, C., & Colby, L. (2002). *Therapeutic exercise: Foundations and techniques* (4th ed., p. 115). Philadelphia: FA Davis.

9. Correct answer: (b)

   Rationale: Avoid speaking excessively loud, or directly into someone's ear, as it may cause discomfort or a compromise in speech clarity. Using more than one method of communication concurrently represents the total communication approach.

   Reference: Long, T., & Cintas, H. (1995). *Handbook of pediatric physical therapy* (p. 270). Philadelphia: Williams & Wilkins.

10. Correct answer: (c)

Rationale: Initially sliding towards the nonoperative side is easier.

Reference: Pierson, F. (2002). *Principles and techniques of patient care* (3rd ed., p. 146, 147). Philadelphia: WB Saunders.

11. Correct answer: (c)

Rationale: Gasping after completing a contraction is an indication that a person is holding their breath.

Reference: Kisner, C., & Colby, L. (2002). *Therapeutic exercise: Foundations and techniques* (4th ed., p. 98, 99). Philadelphia: FA Davis.

SELECTING EFFECTIVE TEACHING ENVIRONMENTS AND PROVIDING PATIENT EDUCATION BASED ON EDUCATIONAL THEORIES

Fourteen Items

1. Correct answer: (d)

Rationale: Focus on task should be improved through use of positive reinforcement.

Reference: Campbell, M. (2000). *Rehabilitation for traumatic brain injury: Physical therapy practice in context* (p. 227). Philadelphia: Churchill Livingstone.

2. Correct answer: (c)

Rationale: A structured environment will reduce stress and confusion, thereby facilitating participation.

Reference: Goodman, C., et al. (2003). *Pathology implications for the physical therapist* (2nd ed., p. 1031, 1032). Philadelphia: WB Saunders.

3. Correct answer: (b)

Rationale: The last two choices cause contraction of accessory muscles. A person with receptive aphasia may have difficulty expressing their thoughts verbally.

Reference: O'Sullivan. (2001). *Physical rehabilitation assessment and treatment* (4th ed., p. 534). Philadelphia: FA Davis.

4. Correct answer: (b)

Rationale: Offering a person a choice will help build their confidence and trust.

Reference: Ramsden, E. (1999). *The person as patient, psychosocial perspectives for the health care professional* (p. 90). Philadelphia: WB Saunders.

5. Correct answer: (b)

Rationale: The assistant is attempting to associate intersection with the isometric exercises. This is an application of classical conditioning.

Reference: Ramsden, E. (1999). *The person as patient, psychosocial perspectives for the health care professional* (p. 32). Philadelphia: WB Saunders.

6. Correct answer: (c)

   Rationale: This comprehensive strategy is most appropriate to communicate with a person who has visual and memory impairments.

   Reference: Navarra, T., et al. (1990). *Therapeutic communication, a guide to effective interpersonal skills for health care professionals* (pp. 88–91). Thorofare, NJ: Slack.

7. Correct answer: (d)

   Rationale: The most important content should be presented first.

   Reference: Davis, C. (1998). *Patient practitioner interaction: An experiential manual for developing the art of health care* (3rd ed., p. 209). Thorofare, NJ: Slack, Inc.

8. Correct answer: (b)

   Rationale: The correct response in this situation is to provide the person modesty, and attempt to distract with other activities. If the activity did not cease, the assistant should leave the person's room.

   Reference: Navarra, T., et al. (1990). *Therapeutic communication, a guide to effective interpersonal skills for health care professionals* (p. 90). Thorofare, NJ: Slack.

9. Correct answer: (a)

   Rationale: The patient must achieve and demonstrate competence through physical practice.

   Reference: Davis, C. (1998). *Patient practitioner interaction: An experiential manual for developing the art of health care* (3rd ed., p. 210). Thorofare, NJ: Slack, Inc.

10. Correct answer: (b)

    Rationale: Body language portrays over half of the message to the listener, including eye contact, posture, and gestures.

    Reference: Davis, C. (1998). *Patient practitioner interaction: An experiential manual for developing the art of health care* (3rd ed., p. 144). Thorofare, NJ: Slack, Inc.

11. Correct answer: (b)

    Rationale: Clarification is an active listening technique that simplifies the perceived message in order to resolve any confusion.

    Reference: Davis, C. (1998). *Patient practitioner interaction: An experiential manual for developing the art of health care* (3rd ed., p. 106). Thorofare, NJ: Slack, Inc.

12. Correct answer: (a)

    Rationale: Reflection is a verbalization of the listener perception of the message.

    Reference: Davis, C. (1998). *Patient practitioner interaction: An experiential manual for developing the art of health care* (3rd ed., p. 106). Thorofare, NJ: Slack, Inc.

13. Correct answer: (d)

    Rationale: Restatement is an active listening technique that is used initially to demonstrate to the person that you are listening.

Reference: Davis, C. (1998). *Patient practitioner interaction: An experiential manual for developing the art of health care* (3rd ed., p. 106). Thorofare, NJ: Slack, Inc.

14. Correct answer: (c)

Rationale: Restatement is an active listening technique that is used initially to demonstrate to the person that you are listening.

Reference: Davis, C. (1998). *Patient practitioner interaction: An experiential manual for developing the art of health care* (3rd ed., p. 106). Thorofare, NJ: Slack, Inc.

PATIENT INSTRUCTION—CONSIDERING THE DEVELOPMENTAL LEVEL, CULTURAL BACKGROUND, SOCIAL HISTORY, HOME SITUATION, AND GEOGRAPHIC BARRIERS OF THE PATIENT

Nine Items

1. Correct answer: (c)

Rationale: The resident may not have easy access to an outpatient setting. The ultrasound intervention may be provided and monitored better than issuing a TENS unit. The ultrasound is also better suited for stiffness.

Reference: Anemaet, W., et al. (2000). *Home rehabilitation: Guide to clinical practice* (p. 16). St. Louis: Mosby.

2. Correct answer: (d)

Rationale: Paranoia is described as the persistence of perceived persecution by others.

Reference: Taber's cyclopedic medical dictionary (19th ed., p. 1578, 1579). Philadelphia: FA Davis.

3. Correct answer: (d)

Rationale: Grieving is normal after loss of function, specifically, denial, anger, bargaining, and sadness.

Reference: O'Sullivan. (2001). *Physical rehabilitation assessment and treatment* (4th ed., p. 32). Philadelphia: FA Davis.

4. Correct answer: (d)

Rationale: All of these choices are considered issues typically facing middle-aged adults, and should be considered as part of the patient's perspective.

Reference: Purtillo, R., & Haddad, A. (2002). *Health professional and patient interaction* (6th ed., pp. 274–277). Philadelphia: WB Saunders.

5. Correct answer: (c)

Rationale: Traditional Korean cultural values indicate that people should die at home.

Reference: Luckman, J. (2000). *Transcultural communication in health care* (p. 237). Albany: Delmar.

6. Correct answer: (c)

   Rationale: One-step, nonabstract, specific instructions are most appropriate in these situations.

   Reference: Navarra, T., et al. (1990). *Therapeutic communication, a guide to effective interpersonal skills for health care professionals* (p. 90). Thorofare, NJ: Slack, Inc.

7. Correct answer: (c)

   Rationale: The other three given cultures typically welcome close proximity during conversation.

   Reference: Luckman, J. (2000). *Transcultural communication in health care* (p. 54, 55). Albany: Delmar.

8. Correct answer: (a)

   Rationale: It is considered most appropriate to avoid distancing yourself from a Hispanic patient and their family.

   Reference: Salimbene, S. (2000). *What language does your patient hurt in? A practical guide to culturally competent patient care* (p. 31). St. Paul, MN: EMCParadigm.

9. Correct answer: (b)

   Rationale: In Arab culture the person who is suffering is expected to surrender their burdens, to be borne by their family. Some persons of this culture may not wish to act autonomously.

   Reference: Salimbene, S. (2000). *What language does your patient hurt in? A practical guide to culturally competent patient care* (p. 42). St. Paul, MN: EMCParadigm.

Procedural Interventions Group I: Exercise and Manual Therapy

OVERVIEW

This chapter includes questions covering procedural intervention questions included in the exam. There are 96 questions in this chapter that deal with exercise and manual therapy interventions.

KEY POINTS TO REVIEW

Exercise Interventions

- Aerobic exercise
- Cardiovascular exercise
- Strengthening
- Muscular endurance
- Stretching
- Range of motion
- Neuromuscular reeducation

- Perceptual training
- Balance
- Coordination
- Breathing exercise
- Aquatic exercise
- Postural exercise
- Developmental activity

Manual Therapy Interventions

- Peripheral joint mobilization
- Soft tissue mobilization

- Manual traction

EXERCISE—AEROBIC CAPACITY, AEROBIC TRAINING, AND CARDIOVASCULAR INTERVENTIONS

Eight Items

1. Which of the following statements is true about the physiologic development of aerobic and cardiovascular capacity?

    _____ a. between the ages of 5 and 15, body weight, lung volume, heart volume, and maximum oxygen uptake increase threefold

    _____ b. between the ages of 50 and 70, body weight, lung volume, heart volume, and maximum oxygen uptake decrease by half

    _____ c. between the ages of 5 and 15, body weight, lung volume, heart volume, and maximum oxygen uptake double

    _____ d. between the ages of 50 and 70, body weight, lung volume, heart volume, and maximum oxygen uptake decrease threefold

2. A person who performs well in long distance running may not perform well in weight lifting. Which term refers to this principle of exercise training?

    _____ a. overload principle

    _____ b. specificity principle

    _____ c. length-tension principle

    _____ d. sliding filament principle

3. A person is beginning outpatient cardiac rehabilitation after a mild myocardial infarction. Which statement is true about producing physiologic adaptation with cardiovascular training?

    _____ a. training effects will occur in a minimum of 1–3 weeks

    _____ b. training effects will occur in a minimum of 10–12 weeks

    _____ c. training effects will occur in a minimum of 5–8 weeks

    _____ d. training effects will occur in a minimum of 16–19 weeks

4. A person recently had a prolonged hospitalization, and is now very deconditioned. Which of the following is LEAST likely to occur with deconditioning?

    _____ a. decrease in total blood volume

    _____ b. decrease in plasma volume

    _____ c. increase in bone mineral density

    _____ d. increase in hypotension

5. During the early stage of cardiac rehabilitation, the treatment plan includes patient education, including teaching risk factors for future myocardial infarctions. Modifiable risk factors for myocardial infarction include which of the following?

    _____ a. gender

    _____ b. race

_____ c. age

_____ d. health

6. The physical therapist has instructed you to perform therapeutic exercise to improve aerobic conditioning, and increase endurance with a person in cardiac rehabilitation. Which of the following guidelines will BEST address the patient's goals?

_____ a. perform intense activity for 1–2 minutes, repeat after 4 minutes of rest or mild active exercise

_____ b. perform activity of submaximal intensity, lasting 30 seconds or more

_____ c. perform bursts of activity lasting 30 seconds or more, repeat daily

_____ d. perform activity with large muscles, submaximal intensity, for 3–5 minutes, repeated after rest or mild active exercise for a similar duration

7. Which of the following observations is LEAST appropriate at rating exercise intensity?

_____ a. metabolic equivalency table

_____ b. Berg scale

_____ c. Borg scale

_____ d. maximum heart rate

8. A physical therapist has requested you to perform cardiac rehabilitation with a person at 70–80% of their maximal heart rate. Which heart rate range would be MOST appropriate for a person 62 years of age?

_____ a. 100–110 beats per minute

_____ b. 120–135 beats per minute

_____ c. 130–155 beats per minute

_____ d. 110–125 beats per minute

EXERCISE—STRENGTHENING AND MUSCLE ENDURANCE INTERVENTIONS

Eight Items

1. A person in an outpatient physical therapy setting is performing therapeutic exercise interventions. Which statement is incorrect regarding the direct effects of repeated active muscle contraction?

_____ a. repeated muscle contraction causes vasodilatation to direct blood towards the active extremity

_____ b. repeated muscle contraction causes a decrease in peripheral resistance and stroke volume of the atria

_____ c. repeated muscle contraction causes vasodilatation to direct blood from nonworking muscles, kidneys, and the liver, to the active muscles

_____ d. repeated muscle contraction causes an increased hyperemia to the superficial skin tissue

2. Which of the following is the primary instruction that SHOULD be included in therapeutic strengthening for a person with potential heart problems or risk for stroke?

_____ a. always begin with submaximal isometrics and progress to eccentric contractions

_____ b. avoid overhead motions

_____ c. avoid delayed onset of muscle soreness by avoiding eccentric contractions

_____ d. don't hold your breath

3. When performing therapeutic exercise interventions, the activities are selected based upon the physical performance capabilities and needs of the patient. Exercise interventions also address the training of the needed muscle fiber types. Which muscle fiber type is solicited by performing anaerobic activities such as power lifting?

_____ a. type I

_____ b. type II

_____ c. type III

_____ d. type IV

4. You are performing therapeutic exercises with a person, 74 years of age, in an inpatient physical therapy setting. During today's session, the person complains of overall fatigue and asks for an extended rest period. Which of the following is the MOST probable cause for their symptoms?

_____ a. they are experiencing a depletion of potassium resources

_____ b. they are experiencing a depletion of calcium resources

_____ c. they are tired due to a lack of sleep in the hospital

_____ d. they are suffering from malaise

5. A person you have treated for several weeks has met their current long-term goals, will be returning to work next week, and will follow up with the physical therapist within the next 2 weeks if needed. Which of the following is a typical response of persons who have performed endurance training?

_____ a. lower resting heart rate

_____ b. lower stroke volume with exercise

_____ c. higher respiration rate with exercise

_____ d. higher cholesterol metabolism at rest

6. You have been performing therapeutic exercise interventions with a person recovering from a Bankart repair to the left upper extremity. The physical therapist has delegated a therapeutic strengthening progression within the person's tolerance. Varying the type of muscle work is one method of progressing therapeutic strengthening. Which statement is accurate about muscle work?

_____ a. concentric contractions should always be used before eccentric contractions

_____ b. isometric contractions produce more force than eccentric contractions

_____ c. maximal concentric contractions produce less force than maximal eccentric contraction

_____ d. eccentric contractions should follow isometric contractions

7. A person recently twisted their left knee while stepping off a loading dock. They were evaluated and determined to have injured their anterior cruciate ligament. The physical therapist has delegated the patient to you for closed-chain activities to strengthen their left knee. Which activity is MOST appropriate for this person?

_____ a. quad sets

_____ b. minisquats against a wall

_____ c. short-arc quads with emphasis on the vastus medialis oblique

_____ d. hamstring setting

8. A person is performing shoulder isometrics after a rotator cuff repair. Which statement is MOST accurate about isometric contractions?

_____ a. isometric contractions must be held for at LEAST 6 seconds against resistance to allow for peak tension and metabolic changes

_____ b. isometric contractions are the safest exercise intervention after an acute myocardial infarction

_____ c. isometric contractions must be performed in midrange to produce strength gains and physiologic adaptation

_____ d. isometric contractions must be held for at LEAST 10 seconds against resistance to allow for peak tension and metabolic changes

EXERCISE—STRETCHING AND RANGE OF MOTION INTERVENTIONS

Eight Items

1. A person has been performing therapeutic stretching for 3 weeks. Upon reevaluation, the physical therapist determines that they have not gained any range of motion. Therapeutic stretching without an increase in range of motion demonstrates which property of muscle?

_____ a. thixotrophy

_____ b. elasticity

_____ c. plasticity

_____ d. extensibility

2. When flexing the shoulder with the elbow extended at the same time, which muscle is mechanically insufficient?

_____ a. the biceps is passively insufficient

_____ b. the triceps is actively insufficient

_____ c. the biceps is actively insufficient

_____ d. the muscles are not insufficient in this position

3. A child is being treated by an interdisciplinary medical team to address cerebral palsy. Currently, the child is wearing a dynamic ankle-foot orthosis. When a muscle is held in a lengthened position via a prolonged stretching orthotic for several weeks, how does physiological lengthening occur?

_____ a. sarcomeres are added in series

_____ b. the muscle belly lengthens through series and parallel sarcomere addition

_____ c. sarcomeres are added in parallel

_____ d. physiological lengthening is not possible for a person with cerebral palsy

4. To achieve the desired physiological lengthening effects of therapeutic stretching, the stretch SHOULD be applied with which approach?

_____ a. short duration, high magnitude

_____ b. long duration, low magnitude

_____ c. short duration, low magnitude

_____ d. long duration, high magnitude

5. When applying a stretch to the pectoralis major muscle of a person with a recently healed clavicular fracture and cast removal, you apply a stretching force through their available length and hold the stretch. Which instruction would BEST compliment this therapeutic stretching intervention?

_____ a. hold their breath and contract the agonistic muscle

_____ b. inhale when the muscle is being lengthened and exhale when the stretch is being held

_____ c. hold their breath and contract the antagonistic muscle

_____ d. exhale when the muscle is being lengthened and inhale when the stretch is being held

6. An athlete, 27 years of age, is experiencing pain at the bottom of their heel. The treatment plan includes therapeutic stretching of the Achilles tendon. The stress placed upon the calcaneous by the Achilles tendon has caused bone spurring towards the plantar fascia. This is an anatomical example of which physical principle?

_____ a. Achilles' law

_____ b. McKenzie's law

_____ c. Wolff's law

_____ d. Storm's effect

7. When applying the hold-relax technique to a person lacking knee flexion, what SHOULD you instruct them to do?

_____ a. contract their quads, then contract their hamstrings

_____ b. contract their quads, then relax their quads

_____ c. contract their hamstrings, then contract their quads

_____ d. contract their hamstrings, then relax their hamstrings

8. A rapid stretching of a muscle is MOST likely to stimulate activation of which of the following neuromuscular structures?

_____ a. golgi tendon organ

_____ b. relaxation reflex

_____ c. moro ballistic reflex

_____ d. muscle spindle

EXERCISE—NEUROMUSCULAR REEDUCATION AND PERCEPTUAL INTERVENTIONS

Ten Items

1. You are using activities with a person in which they must reach and place objects in a specific position. Activities that challenge a person in controlling their range of active movement and the force of their muscular activity are MOST appropriate for which of the following conditions?

_____ a. dysmetria

_____ b. extinction

_____ c. dysphasia

_____ d. athetosis

2. A person is practicing functional tasks such as pulling intended objects out of a bag or purse. This technique is MOST appropriate for which of the following conditions?

_____ a. agnosia

_____ b. phonophoresis

_____ c. stereognosis

_____ d. dysmetria

3. A person is demonstrating synergistic movement while experiencing neurological impairment. A component of the flexor synergy for a patient who attempts to lift their arm up for an object would include which of the following component motions?

_____ a. scapular depression

_____ b. wrist extension

_____ c. scapular retraction

_____ d. forearm pronation

4. Which motion does NOT occur during D2 of proprioceptive neuromuscular facilitation for the upper extremity going into extension?

_____ a. wrist extension

_____ b. ulnar deviation

_____ c. pronation

_____ d. elbow flexion

5. With which neurological condition is a person MOST likely to exhibit "pusher's syndrome"?

_____ a. left hemiparesis

_____ b. Parkinson's disease

_____ c. right hemiparesis

_____ d. multiple sclerosis

6. A person who recently experienced a cerebral vascular accident is positioned on their left side, with their right shoulder flexed at a right angle. In addition, their right elbow is extended, and both the knees and the hip are flexed. This is the correct positioning for a person with hemiparesis affecting which half of the body?

_____ a. right

_____ b. left

_____ c. either half

_____ d. this is an inappropriate position for a person with a recent stroke

7. A person who was an unrestrained passenger in a motor vehicle crash suffered an upper motor neuron lesion. With an upper motor neuron lesion, which of the following signs would MOST likely be present?

_____ a. hypotonicity

_____ b. flaccidity

_____ c. hypertonicity

_____ d. impaired proprioception

8. A person is admitted to a rehabilitation unit after having a cerebral vascular accident primarily affecting the middle cerebral artery. Which clinical presentation is MOST likely for this person based upon the anatomical location of the lesion?

_____ a. expressive aphasia, if the person is right-hand dominant

_____ b. homonymous hemianopsia and contralateral hemiparesis

_____ c. contralateral hemiparesis, and perceptual deficits affecting the upper extremities more than the lower extremities

_____ d. contralateral hemiparesis, and perceptual deficits affecting the lower extremities more than the upper extremities

9. A physical therapist has delegated to you to provide neurodevelopmental interventions with a person who is recovering from a stroke. Which of the following strategies is LEAST consistent with neurodevelopmental interventions?

_____ a. facilitating controlled volition, avoiding synergistic patterns

_____ b. employing functional activities using the affected limbs

_____ c. facilitating early volition through synergistic patterns

_____ d. inhibiting spasticity and primitive reflexes through proper positioning

10. The BEST initial compensatory strategy with a person with significant motor and sensory impairment and left homonymous hemianopsia is which of the following?

_____ a. providing reminder signs on the left side of their room to decrease neglect

_____ b. positioning communication and feeding instruments on their right side

_____ c. positioning the person's bed so that the doorway is to their right

_____ d. instructing the person to turn their head to the left to facilitate vision

EXERCISE—BALANCE AND COORDINATION INTERVENTIONS

Seven Items

1. Which exercise protocol would be MOST appropriate for a person with coordination deficits?

_____ a. Frenkel's

_____ b. Codman's

_____ c. William's

_____ d. McKenzie's

2. A person is participating in interventions to address vestibular and balance deficits. Which activity BOTH challenges balance and stimulates the vestibular system?

_____ a. attempting to walk in straight line placing the feet heel to toe

_____ b. walking while moving the head side-to-side

_____ c. standing with feet shoulder-width apart with the eyes closed

_____ d. standing with feet shoulder-width apart and attempting to place feet closer together

3. Which therapeutic exercise activity is MOST appropriate to address a person's lack of balance?

_____ a. supine, short-arc quadriceps strengthening

_____ b. open-chain, long-arc motion of the lower extremities

_____ c. closed-chain, short-arc motion, progressing to long-arc motion of the lower extremities

_____ d. closed-chain, long-arc motion, progressing to short-arc motion of the lower extremities

4. A person is participating in interventions to address their lack of balance. Which balance activity is a direct progression towards a more challenging activity?

_____ a. stand with feet close together, progressing to standing with feet shoulder-width apart

_____ b. tandem walk upon a carpeted floor, progressing to walking on a noncarpeted surface placing their heel in front of their toes

_____ c. walk in circles and quick turns, progressing to smaller circles

_____ d. stand with feet close together, stepping forward heel to toe, then backward

5. The physical therapist has instructed you to perform preambulation activities to address a person with moderate balance impairment. Which of the following activities is a preambulatory technique to challenge a person's balance?

_____ a. stair-climbing

_____ b. short-sitting with perturbations

_____ c. marching in modified plantar grade

_____ d. standing from a seated position

6. When performing the Dix–Hallpike maneuver for a person with vertigo, which of the following signs will be exacerbated?

_____ a. vertigo

_____ b. ipsilateral paralysis

_____ c. nystagmus

_____ d. nausea

7. Balance interventions are MOST appropriate for a person with which of the following conditions?

_____ a. cranial nerve VII lesion

_____ b. lateral spinal cord lesion

_____ c. cranial verve VIII lesion

_____ d. peripheral neuropraxia

EXERCISE—BREATHING INTERVENTIONS

Eight Items

1. A person, 72 years of age, is being treated in an inpatient physical therapy setting. Their admitting diagnosis is chronic obstructive pulmonary disease. Which of the following breathing techniques will be MOST difficult?

_____ a. tidal volume strategies

_____ b. residual volume strategies

_____ c. expiratory volume strategies

_____ d. vital capacity strategies

2. A teenager with a history of asthma, referred to physical therapy to address tightness of the pectoral muscles, would also benefit from which of the following?

_____ a. chest mobility exercises

_____ b. instruction on shortness of breath positions

_____ c. postural drainage with percussion and vibration

_____ d. diaphragmatic breathing exercises with pursed-lip expiration

3. You are providing training in functional daily activities, and ambulation with a person who recently had a thoracotomy. Which technique is LEAST effective for improving chest expansion?

      _____ a. segmental breathing

      _____ b. incentive spirometer

      _____ c. chest mobility

      _____ d. pursed-lip breathing

4. Percussive interventions combined with postural drainage are MOST indicated for which of the following persons?

      _____ a. a person, 12 years of age, with cystic fibrosis

      _____ b. a person, 20 years of age, with tension pneumothorax

      _____ c. a person, 40 years of age, with atelectasis

      _____ d. a person, 40 years of age, with pneumonia

5. A person with bronchiectasis would NOT benefit from which intervention?

      _____ a. maintaining hydration through regular fluid intake

      _____ b. utilizing regular percussion and vibration especially several hours after the last meal

      _____ c. utilizing regular postural drainage especially in the morning

      _____ d. maintaining low levels of oxygenation during the early morning

6. A person who has poor mobility function and spends the majority of their time lying in a bed becomes more susceptible to pulmonary dysfunction. Which nosocomial infection is MOST likely to occur to someone with prolonged immobility?

      _____ a. emphysema

      _____ b. chronic bronchitis

      _____ c. pneumonia

      _____ d. respiratory alkalosis

7. A person, 15 years of age, had a motorcycle accident, which resulted in a complete injury to their spinal cord. Which level must they have at LEAST partially intact to breathe by means of their own diaphragm?

      _____ a. C2

      _____ b. C4

      _____ c. C6

      _____ d. T2

8. When teaching effective diaphragmatic breathing, you observe the person's respiration rate. If the person is an adult, what is the MOST appropriate respiration rate when using diaphragmatic breathing?

      _____ a. 6

      _____ b. 12

      _____ c. 24

      _____ d. 30

EXERCISE—AQUATIC INTERVENTIONS

Five Items

1. A person is performing therapeutic exercise and gait training in a therapeutic pool. What physical effect occurs during exercise in a therapeutic pool?
   ___ a. the center of gravity is shifted to the level of the lungs
   ___ b. drag forces acting upon the body are decreased
   ___ c. gravity acts upon the body to keep it afloat
   ___ d. hydrostatic pressure is decreased

2. A person who has weakness of many of their skeletal muscles would benefit from which aquatic therapy setting?
   ___ a. cooler water temperatures to decrease muscle viscosity
   ___ b. cooler water temperatures to increase muscle viscosity
   ___ c. warmer water temperatures to decrease viscosity
   ___ d. warmer water temperatures to increase viscosity

3. A person is participating in an aquatic exercise for the first time. They have had an open reduction and internal fixation of their right tibia. They are currently ambulating with bilateral axillary crutches and 30% weight bearing with their right lower extremity. The surgical incision is closed, and healing well. How much SHOULD their body be submerged during ambulation training in the pool?
   ___ a. to their fibular head
   ___ b. to their greater trochanter
   ___ c. to their iliac crests
   ___ d. to their xiphoid process

4. A person is participating in therapeutic activities during aquatic interventions. Which treatment position is NOT included during application of the Bad Ragaz technique?
   ___ a. plyometric
   ___ b. isotonic
   ___ c. isokinetic
   ___ d. isometric

5. Which physical effect of exercise in a therapeutic pool is correct?
   ___ a. being more submerged, buoyancy decreases
   ___ b. being less submerged, drag increases
   ___ c. being less submerged, buoyancy increases
   ___ d. being more submerged, drag decreases

EXERCISE—POSTURAL INTERVENTIONS

Eight Items

1. Which muscle is MOST commonly weak in a person who has been diagnosed with scoliosis?
   _____ a. ipsilateral erector spinae
   _____ b. contralateral erector spinae
   _____ c. iliopsoas
   _____ d. lower abdominals

2. A person is participating in physical therapy to address pain due to muscle imbalances, faulty movement patterns, and poor mechanical postures. When a person demonstrates a forward-head posture, which muscle would you MOST likely find to be short, and the person would benefit from which exercise?
   _____ a. sternocleidomastoid; cervical extension
   _____ b. splenius cervicus; cervical extension
   _____ c. sternocleidomastoid; chin tucks
   _____ d. splenius cervicus; chin tucks

3. A physical therapist evaluates a person with postural pain. The therapist describes the person as "resting on their ligaments," due to the reliance by the body's weight upon the iliofemoral ligaments. The therapist selects exercises to strengthen the gluteus maximus, and gait training to increase terminal stance duration. These interventions are MOST consistent with which posture?
   _____ a. lordosis
   _____ b. kyphosis
   _____ c. sway-back
   _____ d. flat low back

4. A person, 37 years of age, is employed as a full time truck driver. Currently, the person stands with their anterior superior iliac spine posterior to their pubis symphysis, when observed relative to the frontal plane. Which intervention is MOST appropriate to address this person's symptoms?
   _____ a. rectus abdominus strengthening
   _____ b. double knee-to-chest stretch
   _____ c. prone hip extension stretch
   _____ d. single knee-to-chest stretch

5. One of the benefits of good standing posture is the impact on energy expenditure. Which skeletal muscle SHOULD be activated to maintain knee extension for an optimal erect posture?
   _____ a. rectus femoris
   _____ b. vastus medialis
   _____ c. biceps femoris long head
   _____ d. gluteus maximus

6. A person stands with a right-hand dominant posture. Which muscle imbalance is considered typical with right-hand dominant posture?

_____ a. the right gluteus medius is weaker than the left

_____ b. the latissimus dorsi is longer on the right than the left

_____ c. the spine deviates to the right

_____ d. the right foot is more pronated than the left

7. When observing a person in static standing, you observe their scapula 3″ from the spine, the vertebral border aligned vertically, their olecranon facing laterally, and a slight posterior curve of the thoracic vertebrae. Based upon these observations, which postural intervention is MOST appropriate for this person?

_____ a. scapular retraction

_____ b. stretching into humeral external rotation and horizontal abduction

_____ c. prone extension assisted by the upper extremities

_____ d. stretching into humeral internal rotation

8. The posterior longitudinal ligament primarily serves which of the following functions?

_____ a. compress the lumbar vertebrae and protect the spinal cord

_____ b. limit vertebral extension

_____ c. limit vertebral flexion

_____ d. limit vertebral lateral flexion

EXERCISE—DEVELOPMENTAL INTERVENTIONS

Eight Items

1. An infant, 6 months of age, who is able to stand with weight bearing, can pass objects from hand to hand, and uses a radial-palmar grasp without adduction of the thumb has which of the following?

_____ a. acceptable development

_____ b. delayed grasp development

_____ c. delayed standing development

_____ d. lack of coordination development

2. A child experiencing normal growth pattern who is now able to pull themselves to standing, crawl, begin to creep, and able to assume quadruped from the pivot prone position, is probably about what age?

_____ a. 1 year of age

_____ b. 7–9 months of age

_____ c. 4–6 months of age

_____ d. 12–14 months of age

3. When working with children in physical therapy, the use of play or appropriately stimulating environments is necessary to achieve the desired outcomes. Which strategy is MOST appropriate for a child, 2 years of age?

    _____ a. use the body as a tool to climb on

    _____ b. use small toys

    _____ c. document progress on a chart using stars or stickers

    _____ d. initiate competition between the child and caregiver

4. A child in a pediatric physical therapy setting is throwing a beanbag at a target. Which of the following is not being addressed by this activity?

    _____ a. motor planning

    _____ b. eye-hand coordination

    _____ c. right-left discrimination

    _____ d. equilibrium

5. Which of the following treatment adaptations is LEAST appropriate for addressing the needs of a child with auditory impairment?

    _____ a. water play

    _____ b. toys with vibrating switches

    _____ c. gestures and signs

    _____ d. Simon-says

6. You are working in a pediatric setting, with a child and parent, on positional strategies. Which of the following goals is BEST addressed in supine than in prone?

    _____ a. improved gastric emptying

    _____ b. easier visual exploration

    _____ c. less reflux especially if head of the bed is 30° elevated

    _____ d. decreased risk of aspiration

7. In a pediatric physical therapy setting, some of the typical interventions include promoting controlled mobility through simple children's puzzles. Which of the following age ranges are MOST appropriate for the initial utilization of children's puzzles?

    _____ a. 6–9 months

    _____ b. 9–12 months

    _____ c. 12–18 months

    _____ d. 18–21 months

8. A child with Down syndrome is exhibiting a delay of postural tone. Which infant carrying position promotes head lifting and extensor tone?

    _____ a. holding both lower limbs with trunk leaning back upon the carrier

    _____ b. holding the child upon the hip of the carrier

    _____ c. using a backpack-style child carrier

    _____ d. the child is prone over the carrier's arm

MANUAL THERAPY—PERIPHERAL JOINT MOBILIZATION INTERVENTIONS

Eleven Items

1. A person being treated for left adhesive capsulitis of the glenohumeral joint with ultrasound for 8 minutes, passive range of motion, and joint mobilization. When the person's left shoulder is taken into the available range of motion, and large oscillations are applied at near end range, which grade of mobilization does this description MOST closely fit?
   _____ a. grade I
   _____ b. grade II
   _____ c. grade III
   _____ d. grade IV

2. Peripheral joint motion is BEST described by which of the following?
   _____ a. active joint motion within available range of movement
   _____ b. passive joint motion within available range of movement
   _____ c. oscillating the joint within the available range of movement
   _____ d. oscillating the joint to end range and beyond

3. A person is quite apprehensive during a passive range of motion intervention to their right shoulder. Which peripheral joint mobilization grades might the physical therapist recommend to facilitate their relaxation prior to passive range of motion?
   _____ a. grades I and II
   _____ b. grades II and III
   _____ c. grades III and IV
   _____ d. grades IV and V

4. During patellofemoral taping interventions, a pull in which direction is typically applied to the patella to facilitate normal tracking due to vastus medialis insufficiency?
   _____ a. superior
   _____ b. lateral
   _____ c. medial
   _____ d. inferior

5. A physical therapist has delegated peripheral joint mobilization of the glenohumeral joint to be performed upon a patient. The therapist has specified for the physical therapist assistant to apply a low grade oscillation with the patient's joint in the loose-packed position. Which of the following is the loose-packed position of the glenohumeral joint?
   _____ a. scapular plane, with 45° abduction
   _____ b. scapular plane, with 20° internal rotation

_____ c. scapular plane, with 55° abduction

_____ d. scapular plane, with 20° external rotation

6. Peripheral joint mobilization may be applied to joints in their loose-packed position. Which of the following is the closed-packed position of the glenohumeral joint?

_____ a. scapular plane, with 45° abduction

_____ b. sagittal plane, with 55° flexion

_____ c. maximal abduction and lateral rotation

_____ d. maximal extension and internal rotation

7. Peripheral joint mobilization may be applied to joints in their loose-packed position. Which of the following is the loose-packed position of the radiocarpal joint?

_____ a. slight flexion

_____ b. slight radial deviation

_____ c. slight ulnar deviation

_____ d. slight extension

8. Peripheral joint mobilization may be applied to joints in their loose-packed position. Which of the following is the loose-packed position of the tibiofemoral joint?

_____ a. full knee flexion

_____ b. 25°

_____ c. full knee extension

_____ d. 85°

9. Which of the following is an open-packed position of the tibiofemoral joint?

_____ a. full knee extension with tibial lateral rotation

_____ b. 85°

_____ c. 25°

_____ d. 20°

10. A person is participating in outpatient physical therapy to address hypomobility of the radiocarpal joint. One of the current indicated interventions is peripheral joint mobilization. Based upon the concave-convex rule, towards which direction are oscillations applied to increase radiocarpal flexion?

_____ a. volar

_____ b. dorsal

_____ c. medial

_____ d. lateral

11. Peripheral joint mobilization is MOST indicated for a person with which of the following conditions?

_____ a. lack of strength

_____ b. lack of muscle length

_____ c. capsular restriction

_____ d. stiff muscles

MANUAL THERAPY—SOFT TISSUE MOBILIZATION INTERVENTIONS

Nine Items

1. During a therapeutic massage intervention you are delivering a series of brisk blows in alternating fashion. Which stroke does this describe?
   - _____ a. tapotement
   - _____ b. effleurage
   - _____ c. kneading
   - _____ d. vibration

2. Prior to applying soft tissue interventions to a person on their first visit, you confirm the presence or absence of any precautions and contraindications. With the presence of which condition is it appropriate to perform therapeutic massage?
   - _____ a. area over hematomas
   - _____ b. area over herniated nucleus propulsus
   - _____ c. area over phlebitis
   - _____ d. area over pitting edema

3. A person, 34 years of age, is receiving treatment for right lateral epicondylitis. The plan states that they are to receive phonophoresis and massage to address pain. Which stroke would BEST assist in desensitizing the affected area while mobilizing deep tissue?
   - _____ a. superficial effleurage
   - _____ b. cross-fiber friction
   - _____ c. petrissage
   - _____ d. pincement

4. A person with a history of chronic and recurrent low back pain has been referred to physical therapy for treatment with electrical stimulation and therapeutic massage. When treating this person, it will be important to incorporate which parameters into each stroke of the massage intervention?
   - _____ a. speed, rhythm, and direction
   - _____ b. speed, rhythm, and pattern
   - _____ c. direction and pattern
   - _____ d. pattern and repetition

5. Massage in the direction of superficial muscle fibers with a soft stroke describes which of the following?
   - _____ a. tapotement
   - _____ b. deep friction
   - _____ c. petrissage
   - _____ d. effleurage

6. The supraspinatus is often a trigger point that elicits pain signals from which anatomical location?

____ a. the upper trapezius

____ b. the pectoral region

____ c. the brachioradialis

____ d. the deltoid

7. Trigger points are locations of hypersensitivity that produce reactions at other locations. Which anatomical location is LEAST likely a trigger point?

____ a. muscle belly of the sternocleidomastoid

____ b. superior medial border of the scapula

____ c. muscle belly of the middle trapezius

____ d. superior to the tibial tuberosity

8. Which of the following techniques of soft-tissue mobilization specifically seeks to reestablish the fascia to its gelatinous-like consistency?

____ a. Cyriax's deep friction

____ b. myofascial release

____ c. Trager method

____ d. Storms' technique of friction

9. Which of the following soft-tissue techniques is MOST appropriately used to lift and milk muscle tissue to release tension and waste products?

____ a. tapotement

____ b. deep friction

____ c. petrissage

____ d. effleurage

MANUAL THERAPY—MANUAL TRACTION INTERVENTIONS

Six Items

1. The physical therapist has requested that you apply manual joint traction to a person's right ankle prior to passive range of motion and stretching. Which of the following positions is MOST appropriate for applying a manual traction force?

____ a. person is prone with knee flexed to 90°

____ b. person is supine with ankle neutral

____ c. person is prone with ankle in 15° plantarflexion

____ d. person is supine with ankle in 5° dorsiflexion

2. Which of the following forces acting upon a joint is NOT reduced with the application of peripheral joint traction?

_____ a. shear

_____ b. tension

_____ c. compression

_____ d. torque

3. Which of the following indications is LEAST appropriate for the application of peripheral joint traction?

_____ a. to decrease pain

_____ b. to reduce hypomobility

_____ c. to facilitate the concurrent use of oscillations

_____ d. to increase joint mobility beyond anatomical limit

4. Which of the following Kaltenborn's grades of peripheral manual traction is sufficient in force to reduce compressive joint forces without separating articulating surfaces?

_____ a. grade I

_____ b. grade II

_____ c. grade III

_____ d. grade IV

5. Which of the following Kaltenborn's grade of traction is sufficient force to stretch soft tissue surrounding the joint in order to decrease hypomobility?

_____ a. grade I

_____ b. grade II

_____ c. grade III

_____ d. grade IV

6. Which peripheral joint mobilization technique is most effective for improving BOTH inversion and eversion of the subtalar joint?

_____ a. medial glide with contralateral rotation

_____ b. lateral glide with ipsilateral rotation

_____ c. medial glide with ipsilateral rotation

_____ d. distraction

ANSWERS AND RATIONALE

EXERCISE—AEROBIC CAPACITY, AEROBIC TRAINING, AND CARDIOVASCULAR INTERVENTIONS

Eight Items

1. Correct answer: (a)

   Rationale: This is the normal physiological development.

Reference: Kisner, C., & Colby, L. (2002). *Therapeutic exercise: Foundations and techniques* (4th ed., p. 137). Philadelphia: FA Davis.

2. Correct answer: (b)

   Rationale: Most beneficial effects of therapeutic exercise result in increased performance in the same types of activities as training. This is a result of the types of use of the body's organ systems, recruitment of muscle groups, and fiber types.

   Reference: Kisner, C., & Colby, L. (2002). *Therapeutic exercise: Foundations and techniques* (4th ed., p. 61). Philadelphia: FA Davis.

3. Correct answer: (b)

   Rationale: This is the minimum time period for cardiovascular training effects.

   Reference: Kisner, C., & Colby, L. (2002). *Therapeutic exercise: Foundations and techniques* (4th ed., p. 114). Philadelphia: FA Davis.

4. Correct answer: (c)

   Rationale: Bone density decreases with deconditioning.

   Reference: Kisner, C., & Colby, L. (2002). *Therapeutic exercise: Foundations and techniques* (4th ed., p. 115). Philadelphia: FA Davis.

5. Correct answer: (d)

   Rationale: The first three choices are nonmodifiable risk factors. Examples of other modifiable risk factors include smoking, weight, activity level, etc.

   Reference: Guccione, A. (2000). *Geriatric physical therapy* (2nd ed., p. 173). St. Louis: Mosby.

6. Correct answer: (d)

   Rationale: This is the safest and effective choice for increasing a person's endurance in cardiac rehabilitation.

   Reference: Kisner, C., & Colby, L. (2002). *Therapeutic exercise: Foundations and techniques* (4th ed., p. 160). Philadelphia: FA Davis.

7. Correct answer: (b)

   Rationale: The Berg scale is used to rate a person's balance.

   Reference: O'Sullivan. (2001). *Physical rehabilitation assessment and treatment* (4th ed., p. 208). Philadelphia: FA Davis.

8. Correct answer: (d)

   Rationale: Subtract the person's age from 220, and get 158. 70% and 80% of 158 equals 110 and 126 beats, respectively.

   Reference: Kisner, C., & Colby, L. (2002). *Therapeutic exercise: Foundations and techniques* (4th ed., p. 158). Philadelphia: FA Davis.

EXERCISE—STRENGTHENING AND MUSCLE ENDURANCE INTERVENTIONS

Eight Items

1. Correct answer: (b)

   Rationale: This effect occurs with repeated active muscle contractions.

   Reference: Kisner, C., & Colby, L. (2002). *Therapeutic exercise: Foundations and techniques* (4th ed., p. 119). Philadelphia: FA Davis.

2. Correct answer: (d)

   Rationale: Holding their breath produces a Valsalva maneuver, which increases their risk for stroke, aneurysm, or cardiac episode.

   Reference: Kisner, C., & Colby, L. (2002). *Therapeutic exercise: Foundations and techniques* (4th ed., p. 59). Philadelphia: FA Davis.

3. Correct answer: (b)

   Rationale: Type II fibers are fast-twitch, anaerobic fibers.

   Reference: Kisner, C., & Colby, L. (2002). *Therapeutic exercise: Foundations and techniques* (4th ed., p. 58, 116). Philadelphia: FA Davis.

4. Correct answer: (a)

   Rationale: Many older persons experience general muscle fatigue or total body fatigue due to depletion of potassium.

   Reference: Kisner, C., & Colby, L. (2002). *Therapeutic exercise: Foundations and techniques* (4th ed., p. 60). Philadelphia: FA Davis.

5. Correct answer: (a)

   Rationale: The second and third choices are the opposite of the actual benefits. The last choice is invalid.

   Reference: Kisner, C., & Colby, L. (2002). *Therapeutic exercise: Foundations and techniques* (4th ed., p. 165). Philadelphia: FA Davis.

6. Correct answer: (c)

   Rationale: This is the only valid choice. The first and last choices suggest absolutes, which are often poor choices.

   Reference: Kisner, C., & Colby, L. (2002). *Therapeutic exercise: Foundations and techniques* (4th ed., p. 67). Philadelphia: FA Davis.

7. Correct answer: (b)

   Rationale: The second choice is the only closed-chain activity.

   Reference: Kisner, C., & Colby, L. (2002). *Therapeutic exercise: Foundations and techniques* (4th ed., p. 68). Philadelphia: FA Davis.

8. Correct answer: (a)

   Rationale: Isometric exercises often facilitate the Valsalva maneuver, which is a risk for persons after acute myocardial infarction. The last two choices are false.

   Reference: Kisner, C., & Colby, L. (2002). *Therapeutic exercise: Foundations and techniques* (4th ed., p. 71). Philadelphia: FA Davis.

EXERCISE—STRETCHING AND RANGE OF MOTION INTERVENTIONS

Eight Items

1. Correct answer: (b)

   Rationale: Elasticity is the property of muscle that allows for it to resist deformation.

   Reference: Kisner, C., & Colby, L. (2002). *Therapeutic exercise: Foundations and techniques* (4th ed., p. 147). Philadelphia: FA Davis.

2. Correct answer: (d)

   Rationale: Of these muscles, the biceps is active and shortening over the shoulder joint, but for a given length over the extended elbow joint, therefore avoiding active insufficiency. The triceps is lengthened over the shoulder joint, but not over the elbow joint, therefore avoiding passive insufficiency. Shoulder flexion with the elbow extended avoids mechanical insufficiency.

   Reference: Lippert, L. (2000). *Clinical kinesiology for physical therapist assistants* (3rd ed., p. 38, 39). Philadelphia: FA Davis.

3. Correct answer: (a)

   Rationale: This is the physiological adaptation to prolonged therapeutic stretching interventions.

   Reference: Kisner, C., & Colby, L. (2002). *Therapeutic exercise: Foundations and techniques* (4th ed., p. 157). Philadelphia: FA Davis.

4. Correct answer: (b)

   Rationale: It takes almost 2 minutes to achieve silence of the muscle spindle.

   Reference: Kisner, C., & Colby, L. (2002). *Therapeutic exercise: Foundations and techniques* (4th ed., p. 160). Philadelphia: FA Davis.

5. Correct answer: (b)

   Rationale: This technique facilitates relaxation of the body.

   Reference: Kisner, C., & Colby, L. (2002). *Therapeutic exercise: Foundations and techniques* (4th ed., p. 368). Philadelphia: FA Davis.

6. Correct answer: (c)

   Rationale: The application of Wolff's law is that the body's structure responds to the forces placed upon it.

   Reference: Nordin, M., & Frankel, V. (2001). *Basic biomechanics of the musculoskeletal system* (3rd ed., p. 51). Philadelphia: Lippincott Williams & Wilkins.

7. Correct answer: (b)

   Rationale: This is the correct technique to improve lengthening of the quadriceps.

   Reference: O'Sullivan. (2001). *Physical rehabilitation assessment and treatment* (4th ed., p. 404). Philadelphia: FA Davis.

8. Correct answer: (d)

   Rationale: The spindle responds to rapid lengthening of the muscle.

   Reference: Norkin, C., & Levangie, P. (1992). *Joint structure and function: A comprehensive analysis* (2nd ed., p. 119). Philadelphia: FA Davis.

EXERCISE—NEUROMUSCULAR REEDUCATION AND PERCEPTUAL INTERVENTIONS

Ten Items

1. Correct answer: (a)

   Rationale: The term means difficulty in controlling the magnitude of volition, seen in cerebellar dysfunction.

   Reference: (1997). *Taber's Cyclopedic Medical Dictionary* (19th ed.). Philadelphia: FA Davis.

2. Correct answer: (c)

   Rationale: Stereognosis is the inability to recognize use and form of solid objects.

   Reference: (1997). *Taber's cyclopedic medical dictionary* (19th ed., p. 1872). Philadelphia: FA Davis.

3. Correct answer: (c)

   Rationale: During elevation of the upper extremity, scapular retraction, and scapular elevation, shoulder external rotation and abduction occur.

   Reference: Martin, S., & Kessler, M. (2000). *Neurologic intervention for physical therapist assistants* (p. 93). Philadelphia: WB Saunders.

4. Correct answer: (a)

   Rationale: The wrist flexes during the D2 pattern going into extension.

   Reference: Kisner, C., & Colby, L. (2002). *Therapeutic exercise: Foundations and techniques* (4th ed., p. 382). Philadelphia: FA Davis.

5. Correct answer: (a)

   Rationale: This condition may be the result of extensor tone with right cerebral hemisphere lesions.

   Reference: Martin, S., & Kessler, M. (2000). *Neurologic intervention for physical therapist assistants* (p. 137). Philadelphia: WB Saunders.

6. Correct answer: (a)

   Rationale: This is a pressure strategy for promoting proprioceptive feedback from the right side of the body.

Reference: O'Sullivan. (2001). *Physical rehabilitation assessment and treatment* (4th ed., p. 550). Philadelphia: FA Davis.

7. Correct answer: (c)

   Rationale: This is most consistent with upper motor neuron injuries.

   Reference: Lippert, L. (2000). *Clinical kinesiology for physical therapist assistants* (3rd ed., p. 67). Philadelphia: FA Davis.

8. Correct answer: (c)

   Rationale: The middle cerebral artery supplies the motor and sensory cortices where these somatic functions occur.

   Reference: O'Sullivan. (2001). *Physical rehabilitation assessment and treatment* (4th ed., p. 526). Philadelphia: FA Davis.

9. Correct answer: (c)

   Rationale: Neurodevelopmental techniques are directed at inhibiting synergistic patterns to achieve skilled volition.

   Reference: Martin, S., & Kessler, M. (2000). *Neurologic intervention for physical therapist assistants* (p. 111). Philadelphia: WB Saunders.

10. Correct answer: (d)

    Rationale: This is the only compensatory strategy of the choices; the others challenge the person's deficit.

    Reference: Martin, S., & Kessler, M. (2000). *Neurologic intervention for physical therapist assistants* (p. 90). Philadelphia: WB Saunders.

EXERCISE—BALANCE AND COORDINATION INTERVENTIONS

Seven Items

1. Correct answer: (a)

   Rationale: Frenkel's is a protocol of exercises to address dysmetria.

   Reference: O'Sullivan. (2001). *Physical rehabilitation assessment and treatment* (4th ed., p. 730, 731). Philadelphia: FA Davis.

2. Correct answer: (b)

   Rationale: Walking while moving the head side-to-side challenges a person's balance and both vestibular systems.

   Reference: O'Sullivan. (2001). *Physical rehabilitation assessment and treatment* (4th ed., p. 837). Philadelphia: FA Davis.

3. Correct answer: (c)

   Rationale: Closed-chain activities are more functional for balance training than open-chain. Balance activities are progressed from short-arc to long-arc.

Reference: Kisner, C., & Colby, L. (2002). *Therapeutic exercise: Foundations and techniques* (4th ed., p. 94). Philadelphia: FA Davis.

4. Correct answer: (c)

Rationale: The first two activities are the reverse of the progression sequence. The last choice lacks progression. More narrow bases of support, closing the eyes, sharper direction changes, and accommodating surfaces provide more challenges to balance.

Reference: O'Sullivan. (2001). *Physical rehabilitation assessment and treatment* (4th ed., p. 837). Philadelphia: FA Davis.

5. Correct answer: (a)

Rationale: Stair-climbing is not a preambulation activity.

Reference: Kisner, C., & Colby, L. (2002). *Therapeutic exercise: Foundations and techniques* (4th ed., p. 556). Philadelphia: FA Davis.

6. Correct answer: (c)

Rationale: The Dix–Hallpike maneuver is performed in supine, and may exacerbate nystagmus.

Reference: Goodman, C., & Snyder, T. (2000). *Differential diagnosis in physical therapy* (3rd ed., p. 1135). Philadelphia: WB Saunders.

7. Correct answer: (c)

Rationale: Cranial nerve VIII is the vestibulococchlear nerve which innervates the vestibular system. Balance will be most directly impaired with this condition.

Reference: O'Sullivan. (2001). *Physical rehabilitation assessment and treatment* (4th ed., p. 839). Philadelphia: FA Davis.

EXERCISE—BREATHING INTERVENTIONS

Eight Items

1. Correct answer: (c)

Rationale: Persons with COPD develop decreases in expiratory volumes.

Reference: Hillegass, E., & Sadowsky, H. (2001). *Essentials of cardiopulmonary physical therapy* (2nd ed., p. 280). Philadelphia: WB Saunders.

2. Correct answer: (a)

Rationale: Chest mobility will maximize expansion and ventilation capacity of the lungs.

Reference: Kisner, C., & Colby, L. (2002). *Therapeutic exercise: Foundations and techniques* (4th ed., p. 756). Philadelphia: FA Davis.

3. Correct answer: (d)

Rationale: Pursed-lip breathing can decrease respiratory rate and increase tidal volume, but does not improve chest expansion.

Reference: Kisner, C., & Colby, L. (2002). *Therapeutic exercise: Foundations and techniques* (4th ed., p. 754). Philadelphia: FA Davis.

4. Correct answer: (a)

   Rationale: Postural drainage and percussion are interventions to mobilize lung secretions. The other three choices are contraindications for the combination of percussive interventions with postural drainage.

   Reference: Campbell, S., et al. (2000). *Physical therapy for children* (2nd ed., p. 749). Philadelphia: WB Saunders.

5. Correct answer: (d)

   Rationale: Physical therapy interventions are directed towards thinning secretions and maintaining pulmonary hygiene. Persons with bronchiectasis may develop low ventilation resulting in hypoxia, which is addressed with supplemental oxygen.

   Reference: Hillegass, E., & Sadowsky, H. (2001). *Essentials of cardiopulmonary physical therapy* (2nd ed., p. 274). Philadelphia: WB Saunders.

6. Correct answer: (c)

   Rationale: Pneumonia infections occur more easily to a person with limited mobility, renal lesions, and diabetes.

   Reference: Goodman, C., & Snyder, T. (2000). *Differential diagnosis in physical therapy* (3rd ed., p. 157). Philadelphia: WB Saunders.

7. Correct answer: (b)

   Rationale: The innervation for the diaphragm is the third to fifth cervical neurological level.

   Reference: Lippert, L. (2000). *Clinical kinesiology for physical therapist assistants* (3rd ed., p. 296). Philadelphia: FA Davis.

8. Correct answer: (b)

   Rationale: Normal respiration for adults is 12–18 per minute, with or without the diaphragmatic technique.

   Reference: Pierson, F. (2002). *Principles and techniques of patient care* (3rd ed., p. 60). Philadelphia: WB Saunders.

EXERCISE—AQUATIC INTERVENTIONS

Five Items

1. Correct answer: (a)

   Rationale: In a pool environment, buoyancy keeps the body afloat; hydrostatic pressure and drag forces upon the body are increased.

   Reference: Bates, A., & Hanson, N. (1996). *Aquatic physical therapy* (p. 24). Philadelphia: WB Saunders.

2. Correct answer: (b)

   Rationale: Viscosity is a resistance to movement through a fluid medium. The greater the viscosity, the greater the resistance to movement. A person who is weaker would benefit from decreased viscosity.

   Reference: Bates, A., & Hanson, N. (1996). *Aquatic physical therapy* (p. 24, 25). Philadelphia: WB Saunders.

3. Correct answer: (d)

   Rationale: At the level of their xiphoid process, up to 70% of their body weight is being supported by buoyancy.

   Reference: Bates, A., & Hanson, N. (1996). *Aquatic physical therapy* (p. 25). Philadelphia: WB Saunders.

4. Correct answer: (a)

   Rationale: Bad Ragaz consists of three positions: isotonic, isokinetic, and isometric.

   Reference: Prentice, W., & Voight, M. (2001). *Techniques in musculoskeletal rehabilitation* (p. 202). New York: McGraw-Hill.

5. Correct answer: (d)

   Rationale: When the body is more submerged, buoyancy and drag increase.

   Reference: Behrens, B., & Michlovitz, S. (1996). *Physical agents: Theory and practice for the physical therapist assistant* (p. 137). Philadelphia: FA Davis.

EXERCISE—POSTURAL INTERVENTIONS

Eight Items

1. Correct answer: (d)

   Rationale: The lower abdominals have been shown to be more directly linked to scoliosis.

   Reference: Kendall, F., et al. (1993). *Muscles: Testing and function* (4th ed., p. 124, 125). Baltimore: Williams & Wilkins.

2. Correct answer: (c)

   Rationale: The forward-head posture is an extension posture. The primary intervention is chin tucks or cervical retraction.

   Reference: Kendall, F., et al. (1993). *Muscles: Testing and function* (4th ed., p. 74). Baltimore: Williams & Wilkins.

3. Correct answer: (c)

   Rationale: Sway-back posture is characterized by a slouching and pelvic sway-forward. There is a general lack of acceleration during gait.

   Reference: Kisner, C., & Colby, L. (2002). *Therapeutic exercise: Foundations and techniques* (4th ed., p. 600). Philadelphia: FA Davis.

4. Correct answer: (d)

   Rationale: The posture described is a posterior pelvic tilt. A person with posterior tilted pelvis is indicated for hamstring and gluteus maximus stretching, with paraspinal and hip flexor strengthening. The double knee-to-chest stretch emphasizes a stretch force upon the paraspinals, whereas the single knee-to-chest stretch addresses the gluteus maximus.
   Reference: Kisner, C., & Colby, L. (2002). *Therapeutic exercise: Foundations and techniques* (4th ed., p. 601). Philadelphia: FA Davis.

5. Correct answer: (d)

   Rationale: No muscle activity at the knee is required to maintain knee extension during optimal stance posture. A lack of hip extension by the gluteals may result in a lack of knee extension.
   Reference: Norkin, C., & Levangie, P. (1992). *Joint structure and function: A comprehensive analysis* (2nd ed., p. 429). Philadelphia: FA Davis.

6. Correct answer: (a)

   Rationale: Right-hand dominant posture occurs with depression of the right shoulder girdle, with elevation of the right pelvic girdle. The elevation of the right side of the pelvis leads to an adducted position, and is consistent with ipsilateral gluteus medius weakness.
   Reference: Kendall, F., et al. (1993). *Muscles: Testing and function* (4th ed., p. 81). Baltimore: Williams & Wilkins.

7. Correct answer: (b)

   Rationale: Each of these is normal postural alignment with the exception of the humerus. The olecranon should face posteriorly. Shortness or stiffness of the pectoral major muscles is indicated and addressed with horizontal abduction with external rotation.
   Reference: Sahrmann, S. (2002). *Diagnosis and treatment of movement impairment syndromes* (p. 199). St. Louis: Mosby.

8. Correct answer: (c)

   Rationale: The posterior longitudinal ligament limits vertebral flexion.
   Reference: Norkin, C., & Levangie, P. (1992). *Joint structure and function: A comprehensive analysis* (2nd ed., p. 136). Philadelphia: FA Davis.

EXERCISE—DEVELOPMENTAL INTERVENTIONS

Eight Items

1. Correct answer: (a)

   Rationale: These are typical motor milestones in normal development. Adduction of the thumb is not typical until the 7 month.

Reference: Martin, S., & Kessler, M. (2000). *Neurologic intervention for physical therapist assistants* (p. 60). Philadelphia: WB Saunders.

2. Correct answer: (b)

   Rationale: These milestones are typical in the 8–9 months of age.

   Reference: Martin, S., & Kessler, M. (2000). *Neurologic intervention for physical therapist assistants* (p. 58). Philadelphia: WB Saunders.

3. Correct answer: (a)

   Rationale: This is done by using familiarity, repetition, interest, and exploration of themselves and their environments.

   Reference: Anemaet, W., et al. (2000). *Home rehabilitation: Guide to clinical practice* (p. 72). St. Louis: Mosby.

4. Correct answer: (d)

   Rationale: Equilibrium is better addressed through dynamic displacement and adjustment of the trunk.

   Reference: Anemaet, W., et al. (2000). *Home rehabilitation: Guide to clinical practice* (p. 80). St. Louis: Mosby.

5. Correct answer: (d)

   Rationale: Each of other treatment adaptations is appropriate to address the needs of a child with auditory impairment. Simon-says is primarily a verbal treatment strategy.

   Reference: Anemaet, W., et al. (2000). *Home rehabilitation: Guide to clinical practice* (p. 70). St. Louis: Mosby.

6. Correct answer: (b)

   Rationale: The other choices are advantages of using the prone position. Visual exploration is better achieved in the supine position.

   Reference: Anemaet, W., et al. (2000). *Home rehabilitation: Guide to clinical practice* (p. 92, 93). St. Louis: Mosby.

7. Correct answer: (c)

   Rationale: This is the appropriate age range for simple puzzles.

   Reference: Anemaet, W., et al. (2000). *Home rehabilitation: Guide to clinical practice* (p. 76). St. Louis: Mosby.

8. Correct answer: (d)

   Rationale: In the prone position, the extensor is stimulated by the forces of gravity.

   Reference: Martin, S., & Kessler, M. (2000). *Neurologic intervention for physical therapist assistants* (p. 355). Philadelphia: WB Saunders.

MANUAL THERAPY—PERIPHERAL JOINT MOBILIZATION INTERVENTIONS

Eleven Items

1. Correct answer: (c)

   Rationale: Large oscillations applied up to the limit of available motion are classified as grade III.

   Reference: Kisner, C., & Colby, L. (2002). *Therapeutic exercise: Foundations and techniques* (4th ed., p. 224). Philadelphia: FA Davis.

2. Correct answer: (c)

   Rationale: Joint mobilization are oscillations applied with the anatomical range of motion.

   Reference: Kisner, C., & Colby, L. (2002). *Therapeutic exercise: Foundations and techniques* (4th ed., p. 216). Philadelphia: FA Davis.

3. Correct answer: (a)

   Rationale: Grades I and II are used primarily to relieve pain and improve relaxation.

   Reference: Kisner, C., & Colby, L. (2002). *Therapeutic exercise: Foundations and techniques* (4th ed., p. 224). Philadelphia: FA Davis.

4. Correct answer: (c)

   Rationale: The vastus medialis muscle is credited with exerting some medial directed force upon the patella.

   Reference: Kisner, C., & Colby, L. (2002). *Therapeutic exercise: Foundations and techniques* (4th ed., p. 249). Philadelphia: FA Davis.

5. Correct answer: (c)

   Rationale: The loose-packed position for the glenohumeral joint is 55° of scaption.

   Reference: Rothstein, J., et al. (1998). *The rehabilitation specialist's handbook* (2nd ed., p. 108). Philadelphia: FA Davis.

6. Correct answer: (c)

   Rationale: When the head of the humerus is fully elevated and laterally rotated, it is in the maximal closed-packed position.

   Reference: Rothstein, J., et al. (1998). *The rehabilitation specialist's handbook* (2nd ed., p. 108). Philadelphia: FA Davis.

7. Correct answer: (c)

   Rationale: With the wrist in anatomical position, the slightly ulnar deviation, the wrist is in loose-packed position.

   Reference: Rothstein, J., et al. (1998). *The rehabilitation specialist's handbook* (2nd ed., p. 109). Philadelphia: FA Davis.

8. Correct answer: (b)

   Rationale: The knee is in the loose-packed position between 20° and 30°.

   Reference: Rothstein, J., et al. (1998). *The rehabilitation specialist's handbook* (2nd ed., p. 109). Philadelphia: FA Davis.

9. Correct answer: (b)

   Rationale: The open-packed position is any position other than the maximum closed-packed or loose-packed position of a joint.

   Reference: Rothstein, J., et al. (1998). *The rehabilitation specialist's handbook* (2nd ed., p. 108, 109). Philadelphia: FA Davis.

10. Correct answer: (b)

    Rationale: The scaphoid has a convex proximal surface moving on a concave distal surface of the radius. When a convex surface moves upon a concave surface, arthrokinematics occurs in the opposite direction of osteokinematic motion. During wrist flexion the carpals should be mobilized dorsally.

    Reference: Kisner, C., & Colby, L. (2002). *Therapeutic exercise: Foundations and techniques* (4th ed., p. 240). Philadelphia: FA Davis.

11. Correct answer: (c)

    Rationale: Peripheral joint mobilization is indicated to address capsular hypomobility.

    Reference: Kisner, C., & Colby, L. (2002). *Therapeutic exercise: Foundations and techniques* (4th ed., p. 216). Philadelphia: FA Davis.

MANUAL THERAPY—SOFT TISSUE MOBILIZATION INTERVENTIONS

Nine Items

1. Correct answer: (a)

   Rationale: Tapotement is described as brisk alternating blows, also referred to as tapping.

   Reference: Rothstein, J., et al. (1998). *The rehabilitation specialist's handbook* (2nd ed., p. 930). Philadelphia: FA Davis.

2. Correct answer: (b)

   Rationale: A herniated disk may be cause for caution, but it is not contraindicated for therapeutic massage.

   Reference: Loving, J. (1999). *Massage therapy theory and practice* (p. 37). Stamford, CT: Appleton & Lange.

3. Correct answer: (b)

   Rationale: Cross-fiber friction is used as a counterirritant intervention.

   Reference: Loving, J. (1999). *Massage therapy theory and practice* (p. 102). Stamford, CT: Appleton & Lange.

4. Correct answer: (b)

   Rationale: Direction is necessary only for lymphatic drainage.

   Reference: Tappan, F. (1998). *Healing massage techniques: Holistic, classic, and emerging methods* (2nd ed., p. 77). Norwalk, CT: Appleton & Lange.

5. Correct answer: (d)

   Rationale: Effleurage typically progresses from superficial as described here, to deep.

   Reference: Rothstein, J., et al. (1998). *The rehabilitation specialist's handbook* (2nd ed., p. 930). Philadelphia: FA Davis.

6. Correct answer: (d)

   Rationale: The supraspinatus trigger has proximate sensory innervation to the deltoid muscle.

   Reference: Rothstein, J., et al. (1998). *The rehabilitation specialist's handbook* (2nd ed., p. 941). Philadelphia: FA Davis.

7. Correct answer: (d)

   Rationale: Each of these are anatomical trigger points, except the patellar tendon.

   Reference: Rothstein, J., et al. (1998). *The rehabilitation specialist's handbook* (2nd ed., p. 935, 936). Philadelphia: FA Davis.

8. Correct answer: (b)

   Rationale: Myofascial release is directly targeted at altering the collagenous properties of fascia.

   Reference: Tappan, F. (1988). *Healing massage techniques: Holistic, classic, and emerging methods* (2nd ed., p. 300). Norwalk, CT: Appleton & Lange.

9. Correct answer: (c)

   Rationale: Petrissage is the kneading of soft tissues to release tension and potential wastes of the soft tissue.

   Reference: Tappan, F. (1988). *Healing massage techniques: Holistic, classic, and emerging methods* (2nd ed., p. 77). Norwalk, CT: Appleton & Lange.

MANUAL THERAPY—MANUAL TRACTION INTERVENTIONS

Six Items

1. Correct answer: (b)

   Rationale: Manual joint traction is applied with the ankle in neutral.

   Reference: Kisner, C., & Colby, L. (2002). *Therapeutic exercise: Foundations and techniques* (4th ed., p. 253). Philadelphia: FA Davis.

2. Correct answer: (b)

Rationale: Peripheral manual traction increases the distraction force upon the joint.

Reference: Prentice, W., & Voight, M. (2001). *Techniques in musculoskeletal rehabilitation* (p. 241). New York: McGraw-Hill.

3. Correct answer: (d)

Rationale: Peripheral joint traction is not used to manipulate the joint beyond anatomical limits.

Reference: Prentice, W., & Voight, M. (2001). *Techniques in musculoskeletal rehabilitation* (p. 241). New York: McGraw-Hill.

4. Correct answer: (a)

Rationale: Grade I traction force only reduces joint compression. Grade II is required to achieve separation of joint surfaces.

Reference: Prentice, W., & Voight, M. (2001). *Techniques in musculoskeletal rehabilitation* (p. 241). New York: McGraw-Hill.

5. Correct answer: (c)

Rationale: Grade III stretch force is required beyond the point of limitation to achieve surrounding soft tissue stretching.

Reference: Prentice, W., & Voight, M. (2001). *Techniques in musculoskeletal rehabilitation* (p. 241). New York: McGraw-Hill.

6. Correct answer: (d)

Rationale: Distraction affects all planes of the subtalar joint.

Reference: Kisner, C., & Colby, L. (2002). *Therapeutic exercise: Foundations and techniques* (4th ed., p. 253). Philadelphia: FA Davis.

CHAPTER 6

Procedural Interventions Group II: Transfers, Functional Activities, Gait Training, Assistive Devices, Adaptive Devices, and Environment Modification

OVERVIEW

This chapter includes questions covering procedural intervention questions included in the exam. There are 102 questions in this chapter that deal with transfers, functional activities, gait training, equipment training, and environment modification interventions.

KEY POINTS FOR REVIEW

Performing Transfers

- Devices

- Weight-bearing statuses

- Transfer techniques

- Levels of assistance

- Patient instruction

- Body mechanics

- Medical considerations

Performing Functional Activities and Training

- Prehension
- Patient/family training
- Activities of daily living
- Equipment training
- Medical considerations
- Functional mobility

Gait Training

- Assistive devices
- Weight-bearing statuses
- Gait deviations
- Balance deficits
- Normal gait cycle
- Preambulation activities

Applying, Adjusting, and Equipment Training

- Adaptive equipment
- Assistive equipment
- Orthotic equipment
- Prosthetic equipment
- Protective equipment
- Supportive equipment

Modification of Environment

- Work
- Home
- Leisure

PERFORMING TRANSFERS

Nineteen Items

1. A person recently underwent bilateral transtibial amputations. When performing sliding board transfer training, which patient instruction is MOST incorrect?
   - _____ a. lean to the left to place the board under the right lower extremity
   - _____ b. grip the distal end of the board before sliding to prevent displacement of the board
   - _____ c. use a wheelchair with removable armrests
   - _____ d. lean slightly forward and scoot in several short movements

2. A person who recently had a hip arthroplasty is now toe-touch weight bearing on their left lower extremity and having difficulty with ambulation. Today you are working with the person on transfers between the bed and the wheelchair. Which is MOST functional to accomplish transfer training from the bed to the wheelchair?

    ____ a. position the wheelchair to the left and use a standard walker

    ____ b. position the wheelchair to the right and use a standard walker

    ____ c. position the wheelchair to the right, stand, and pivot the person

    ____ d. position the wheelchair to the left, stand, and pivot the person

3. Which single-caregiver transfer technique from wheelchair to mat table is SAFEST when transferring a person without spinal precautions, who requires maximal assistance?

    ____ a. platform wheeled walker

    ____ b. slideboard

    ____ c. stand-pivot

    ____ d. scoot-pivot

4. A person with a spinal cord injury, diagnosed as C4 complete, has been delegated to you for a session in the standing frame. Which transfer technique is MOST appropriate to get the person from a wheelchair to a standing frame?

    ____ a. slideboard

    ____ b. two-person lift

    ____ c. stand-pivot

    ____ d. single-person lift

5. Which of the following instructions to a person will reduce the resistive forces of friction upon their body during bed mobility?

    ____ a. flex hips and knees, and lift buttocks prior to scooting up in bed

    ____ b. elevate head of bed prior to scooting down in bed

    ____ c. use the handrail on the side towards which they are rolling

    ____ d. lift head when scooting left or right

6. You are about to perform a transfer with a person from an adjustable treatment mat table to a manual wheelchair. They are currently being treated for a left cerebral vascular accident and hemiparesis. They will stand and ambulate approximately 5′ using a hemiwalker, and then sit in the wheelchair. Which is the correct side for you to stand during this transfer?

    ____ a. directly in front of the person during sit-to-stand

    ____ b. to the person's left throughout

    ____ c. to the person's right throughout

    ____ d. directly in front of the person during sit-to-stand, then to the correct side during ambulation

7. A person being treated in a bariatric medicine setting is being transferred using a mechanical hydraulic lift. When using a mechanical hydraulic lift for transferring a person from a wheelchair to the mat table, you SHOULD do which of the following?

   _____ a. place the lifting device directly in front of the wheelchair and increase the width of the base

   _____ b. place the lifting device directly in front of the wheelchair, secure the person in the sling, and open the valve prior to lifting the person

   _____ c. attach the shorter segments of the chain to the lower portion of the sling

   _____ d. instruct the person to hold onto the support bar when moving the lifting device

8. A person has arrived in the physical therapy treatment area in a wheelchair. Which of the following steps is accurate regarding transferring this person to a higher, nonadjustable treatment table?

   _____ a. transfer the person towards their affected side, have them stand, and then place their foot upon a step stool

   _____ b. transfer the person to standing, then have them place their affected lower extremity upon a step stool

   _____ c. transfer the person towards then unaffected side, with their foot prepositioned upon a step stool

   _____ d. transfer the person to standing, and then have them step up to a step stool with their unaffected lower extremity

9. Which is MOST accurate about placement of a gait belt?

   _____ a. the belt should be placed on a person in supine prior to ambulation

   _____ b. the belt should be placed on a person just above the iliac crests

   _____ c. the belt should be placed away from the axilla, when a person has an ostomy bag

   _____ d. the belt should be placed tight enough, not to allow the thickness of a hand under it

10. When teaching a person to perform a stand-pivot transfer from the bed to the wheelchair, where should they initially place their hands to stand? Assume the person is already sitting on the edge of the bed.

    _____ a. around your neck or waist

    _____ b. on the edge of the bed or handrails if available

    _____ c. upon the armrests of the wheelchair

    _____ d. on the handles of the assistive device

11. A person is participating in motor reeducation to improve their ability to stand from a seated position. To facilitate contribution from the lower trunk, which motor component MUST occur?

    _____ a. anterior pelvic tilt with spinal flexion

    _____ b. posterior pelvic tilt with spinal flexion

    _____ c. anterior pelvic tilt with spinal extension

    _____ d. posterior pelvic tilt with spinal extension

12. A person, 58 years of age, had a total hip arthroplasty (posterior approach) yesterday. Today is their first attempt to transfer from supine to sitting, and transfer from bed to the wheelchair. During

transfer training, the person requires assistance for more than half of the effort to complete the task. Which level of assistance term is MOST accurate about these observations?

_____ a. the person requires minimal assistance

_____ b. the person requires moderate assistance

_____ c. the person requires maximal assistance

_____ d. the person requires contact guard assistance

13. After a prolonged illness, a person is profoundly deconditioned, and is dependent in bed mobility, positioning, and transfers. When treating this person on a mat table, by yourself, you need to position the person closer to the foot of the table. Which technique is the MOST correct to accomplish this task?

_____ a. from the supine position, place the hips and knees in flexion, swing feet off the table, while assisting trunk and head into sitting position, perform low bottom squat-pivots towards foot of table, and then return to supine

_____ b. flex the person's hips and knees, roll their hips and shoulders squarely toward you, extend lower extremities, slide the person towards foot of table, and return to supine or repeat previous steps until in correct position

_____ c. from the supine position, position the person into hook-lying, position yourself at the person's head, lift shoulder, and support alignment of cervical spine, and push the person towards the foot of the table in repeated movements as tolerated by the patient

_____ d. flex the person's hips, position yourself at the person's feet, cradle, and lift pelvis, and pull the person in repeated movements of 6"–10" towards the foot of the table

14. A person who recently had a cerebral vascular accident is MORE likely to be challenged by participating in transfer training using which technique?

_____ a. transfer towards their weaker side

_____ b. transfer towards their stronger side

_____ c. transfer using a sliding board

_____ d. transfer into the wheelchair using a mechanical lift

15. Which of the following is MOST appropriate for a person after a hip replacement?

_____ a. from supine, the person moves their legs towards edge of bed while maintaining upper extremity support posterior to hips, and then scoots forward until feet are placed securely on the floor

_____ b. from supine, the person raises onto their elbows, slides alternating legs towards edge of bed while maintaining upper extremity support lateral to hips, and then scoots forward until feet are placed securely on the floor

_____ c. from supine, the person raises onto their elbows, slides alternating legs towards edge of bed while maintaining upper extremity support anterior to hips, and then scoots forward until feet are placed securely on the floor

_____ d. from supine, the person flexes hips and knees, and rolls hips and shoulders simultaneously into sidelying, eases legs off edge of bed, and pushes up into sitting

16. A person who is demonstrating a sliding board transfer, removes the right armrest, leans to the left, and places the board approximately at midthigh under their right lower extremity. Next, they attempt transfers in two to three scoots to the right. Based upon this information, which of the following cues should be given to them?

    _____ a. they need to reposition the sliding board closer to the popliteal crease

    _____ b. they need to perform the transfer in seven to eight scoots

    _____ c. they need to perform the transfer in one single scoot

    _____ d. they are performing the transfer correctly

17. Which intervention would be considered MOST appropriate when treating a person who underwent a left transtibial amputation one week ago?

    _____ a. stand-pivot transfer, mat to wheelchair, with the wheelchair on the left

    _____ b. slideboard transfer, mat to wheelchair, with the wheelchair on the left

    _____ c. slideboard transfer, wheelchair to mat, with the mat to the right

    _____ d. ambulate with a small-base quad cane in the right hand, non-weight-bearing on the left lower extremity

18. Upon achieving a full upright standing posture from sitting, a person experiences orthostatic hypotension. Which of the following descriptions is LEAST accurate regarding orthostatic hypotension?

    _____ a. it is more pronounced in standing

    _____ b. blood pressure tends to decrease with standing activities

    _____ c. prolonged inactivity exacerbates this condition

    _____ d. this condition can only be addressed through prescribed medication

19. You are preparing to perform a three-person carry of a person who is of moderate size and dependent for all forms of mobility. Which of the following is correct regarding a three-person transfer?

    _____ a. the lifter closest to the head verbalizes the instructions

    _____ b. the middle lifter faces the other two lifters to prevent rotation and controls the person's pelvis

    _____ c. the person is carried facing away from the lifters when on respiratory isolation

    _____ d. the third person is the person being lifted

PERFORMING FUNCTIONAL ACTIVITIES AND FUNCTIONAL TRAINING

Twenty Items

1. Which of the following is the LEAST important consideration for a person's safety with toilet transfer training?

    _____ a. the person's diagnosis

    _____ b. the person's cognition

_____ c. the person's surgical precautions

_____ d. the person's age

2. When performing transfer training in and out of a car, which of the following is considered MOST critical to the type of instructions given to the person?

_____ a. the person is 72 years of age

_____ b. the person has a three week status of postthoracic spine fracture

_____ c. the person had a left total hip arthroplasty three years ago

_____ d. the person complains of vertigo and nausea with prolonged automobile rides

3. A person ambulates with a standard walker, 250′ to and from the therapy area, requires supervision only for transfers and gait training, and walks up and down 16 stair steps in both directions, using a right-side handrail. Which activity needs to be further addressed?

_____ a. the person lives in a two-level home

_____ b. the person's front yard is an uneven terrain

_____ c. the person does not own a bedside commode

_____ d. the person has a large dog in their home

4. As you are observing a person's first attempt to compression wrap themselves after a below-the-knee amputation, what do you look for in an effective wrap?

_____ a. constrict proximally

_____ b. bandage loosely wrapped, to prevent cutting off circulation

_____ c. greatest pressure distally

_____ d. wrinkles only on medial aspect of leg

5. Which position-stretch should be avoided by a person after a transfemoral amputation?

_____ a. iliofemoral adduction

_____ b. iliofemoral abduction

_____ c. iliofemoral neutral

_____ d. iliofemoral extension

6. A person with paresis of the upper extremities is having difficulty with precision hand movements. Which prehension pattern is the LEAST precise of these grasp patterns?

_____ a. pad-to-tip

_____ b. tip-to-tip

_____ c. pad-to-side

_____ d. two-jaw chuck

7. You are treating a person in a subacute rehabilitation setting, addressing activities of daily living. Which of the following are classified as instrumental activities of daily living?

_____ a. bed mobility

_____ b. performing sit-to-stand

_____ c. ambulation

_____ d. making a phone call

8. You are treating a person who has difficulty performing sit-to-stand from a standard toilet. They ambulate 75' with a standard walker without supervision. Which of the following BEST addresses this person's function?

_____ a. adult incontinence pad and bedpan

_____ b. raised toilet seat

_____ c. bathroom stall bars

_____ d. bedside commode

9. Which tasks are directly related to instrumental activities of daily living?

_____ a. velocity of gait and chair rise time

_____ b. chair rise time and grip strength

_____ c. grip strength and velocity of gait

_____ d. grip strength, velocity of gait, and chair rise time

10. A person who is recovering from a spinal cord injury has function at the tenth thoracic level. Which activity would be MOST difficult with this level of impairment?

_____ a. use of hip flexors during midswing

_____ b. independent manual wheelchair mobility

_____ c. vital capacity of 100%

_____ d. upper body dressing

11. A person with function at which neurological level should AVOID functional tenodesis of the finger flexors?

_____ a. C4

_____ b. C6

_____ c. C7

_____ d. L1

12. A person who has a spinal cord injury and full function at the seventh cervical neurological level would be LEAST appropriate for which activity?

_____ a. dependent bed mobility

_____ b. independent use of wheelchair

_____ c. functional grip

_____ d. modified independent transfers

13. A person with a spinal cord injury underwent surgical fusion of the fifth to seventh cervical vertebrae four weeks ago. Now they are beginning to regain function of the sixth cervical neurological level. The physical therapist sets a goal for compensatory grasp utilizing tenodesis. Which stretching technique should be avoided?

_____ a. keeping interphalangeal joints flexed during upper extremity weight bearing

_____ b. stretching into wrist and finger flexion, holding for 30 seconds or more

_____ c. providing passive range of motion into finger flexion, abduction, and extension to neutral

_____ d. stretching into wrist extension and finger extension, holding for 30 seconds or more

14. A person who has a spinal cord injury and neurological impairment is currently rehabilitating at an inpatient facility. One of the interventions in the person's plan of care is to establish tenodesis. Which of the following is a common functional example of tenodesis?

_____ a. allowing contracture of the extrinsic finger flexors to facilitate grip for a person with quadriplegia and some preserved function of extensor carpi radialis

_____ b. allowing contracture of the anterior tibialis to decrease the occurrence of foot drop for a person with paraplegia and some preserved function of the hip flexors

_____ c. allowing contracture of the hamstrings to facilitate wheelchair positioning for a person with paraplegia and some preserved function of iliopsoas

_____ d. allowing contracture of the pectoral muscles to maintain optimal forward positioning in sitting

15. When instructing a person in daily functional skills, you find that a person is concerned about their ability to cross the street. Which velocity must be achieved for crossing through a marked pedestrian crosswalk?

_____ a. 1.22 meters per second

_____ b. 2.11 meters per second

_____ c. .5 meters per second

_____ d. 5 meters per second

16. A person requires moderate assistance to transfer from a wheelchair into a hospital bed. Which technique will provide the BEST lower extremity support?

_____ a. having the person participate with their upper extremity

_____ b. block their uninvolved leg

_____ c. block their involved leg

_____ d. having the person place their feet upon a stool while sitting in the wheelchair

17. A person is rehabilitating from a spinal cord injury. The person has a goal to gain full use of their intercostals, have a functional gait with the assistance of hip-knee-ankle-foot orthosis and a platform walker, and be independent with floor transfers. What is the highest possible neurological level of function that would enable the person to accomplish this goal?

_____ a. T8

_____ b. T12

_____ c. L4

_____ d. S1

18. A physical therapist assistant is training a person with bed mobility. Which technique is LEAST appropriate for a person with spinal precautions?

_____ a. to have the person flatten the bed

_____ b. to have the person flex their knees

_____ c. to utilize a draw sheet placed from the occiput to the popliteal crease when assisting with two persons

_____ d. to utilize a mechanical lift for persons over 300 pounds who require maximal assistance

19. A person who had a crushing injury to their lower back three weeks ago, continues to experience intermittent urinary incontinence. Which active intervention would BEST benefit the person in managing their urinary incontinence?

_____ a. direct current electrical stimulation

_____ b. consume more orange juice

_____ c. pelvic muscle contraction

_____ d. increase clear water intake

20. When preparing a person for discharge to home, you are comparing the benefits of using a walker or a cane, since they function at level of minimal contact assistance during morning treatment sessions. Which statement is true regarding the use of standard canes?

_____ a. canes are safer when used bilaterally

_____ b. canes can support only up to 25% of an individual's weight

_____ c. canes can support only up to 10% of an individual's weight

_____ d. canes are not as safe as walkers on stairs

GAIT TRAINING: USE OF ASSISTIVE DEVICES, CONSIDERATION OF PROPER WEIGHT-BEARING STATUSES, GAIT DEVIATIONS, BALANCE DEFICITS, COMPONENTS OF THE GAIT CYCLE, AND PREGAIT ACTIVITIES

Thirty-three Items

1. When observing normal gait and deviations, it is important to know the sequence of phases in the gait cycle, and to which task of gait they are directed. Which of the following choices is the MOST correct sequence of gait phases?

_____ a. initial contact, terminal swing, midswing, and midstance

_____ b. midswing, terminal swing, initial contact, and loading response

_____ c. initial contact, midstance, and terminal swing loading response

_____ d. midstance, terminal stance, initial swing, and preswing

2. Peak activity of the quadriceps femoris muscle group is observed at which phase of normal gait?

_____ a. midstance

_____ b. loading response

_____ c. initial contact

_____ d. terminal stance

3. Which pregait activity would be the MOST immediate progression after practicing kneeling activity?

_____ a. standing

_____ b. short-sitting

_____ c. long-sitting

_____ d. modified plantar-grade

4. Which pregait activity has the least base of support with the highest center of gravity?

_____ a. prone on elbows

_____ b. half-kneeling

_____ c. modified plantar-grade

_____ d. hook-lying

5. A person ambulates lacking differentiation of the trunk, shoulders, and hips. During the swing period, they rely heavily upon their hip flexors, and lack counterrotation between the shoulder and hip girdles. Which pregait activity is MOST appropriate to address this movement deficit?

_____ a. bridging

_____ b. segmental rolling, sidelying to supine, and upper extremity initiating

_____ c. quadruped creeping

_____ d. log rolling

6. A physical therapist has requested that you to teach a four-point gait pattern to a patient. Which of the following describes that pattern?

_____ a. left crutch, right foot, right crutch, left foot, . . .

_____ b. left crutch, right crutch, swing through, right foot, . . .

_____ c. left crutch, right foot, left foot, right crutch, . . .

_____ d. right crutch, right foot, left crutch, left foot, . . .

7. A person has a left trimalleolar fracture, and has orders for ambulation training, using an assistive device, with a non-weight-bearing status. Which progression is MOST appropriate during the second ambulation session with a person who is non-weight-bearing using a standard walker for 10'?

_____ a. stand the person in the parallel bars, close standby, and follow with the wheelchair

_____ b. apply safety belt, use a standard walker, and attempt to increase ambulation distance while maintaining correct weight-bearing status

_____ c. attempt ambulation using a wheeled walker, using a safety belt, maintain correct weight-bearing status, and attempt to increase ambulation distance

_____ d. apply safety belt and begin stair step training using one rail and a cane

8. Which statement is MOST accurate about the normal gait cycle?
   _____ a. equal time should be spent in stance and swing periods of the ipsilateral lower extremity
   _____ b. equal time should be spent in stance and swing periods of the contralateral lower extremity
   _____ c. more time should be spent in the stance period than the swing period of the ipsilateral lower extremity
   _____ d. less time should be spent in the stance period than the swing period of the contralateral lower extremity

9. A person who is lifting their foot excessively from the floor during the acceleration period of gait is demonstrating which of the following gait deviations?
   _____ a. calcaneous gait
   _____ b. hemiparetic gait
   _____ c. steppage gait
   _____ d. vaulting gait

10. A person who has decreased weight-bearing on an injured lower extremity is demonstrating which of the following gait deviations?
    _____ a. tabetic
    _____ b. antalgic
    _____ c. steppage
    _____ d. cadence

11. When ambulating someone who is demonstrating a Trendelenburg gait pattern, you are MOST likely to observe which of the following deviations?
    _____ a. increased hip abduction during ipsilateral midswing
    _____ b. increased hip abduction during ipsilateral midstance
    _____ c. decreased hip abduction during ipsilateral midswing
    _____ d. decreased hip abduction during ipsilateral midstance

12. While ambulating with a person using a wheeled walker, you observe that their weight shifting is not evenly distributed. Upon closer observation, you observe that the person demonstrates an increased lateral protrusion of the hip during ipsilateral stance. Based upon this observation, which gait deviation should be recorded?
    _____ a. hemiparetic gait
    _____ b. Trendelenberg gait
    _____ c. gluteus medius gait
    _____ d. scissors gait

13. You are performing gait training with a person who has a peroneal nerve palsy. Which gait deviation will MOST likely be observed?
    _____ a. Trendelenburg
    _____ b. vaulting

_____ c. foot drop

_____ d. ataxic

14. Which audible gait deviation occurs when performing gait training with a person who has paresis of the ankle dorsiflexors?

    _____ a. drop foot during swing phase

    _____ b. medial whip during swing phase

    _____ c. Trendelenburg gait during stance phase

    _____ d. foot slap during loading response phase

15. Which clinical gait observation is consistent with a lack of ipsilateral knee and hip flexion throughout the gait cycle?

    _____ a. tabetic

    _____ b. steppage

    _____ c. contralateral vaulting

    _____ d. lurch

16. What is the FIRST thing you should do upon standing a person from a standard wheelchair, to adjust a pair of axillary crutches?

    _____ a. cue the person to hold one of the devices and drop their other upper extremity to check the position of the axillary pad and hand grip

    _____ b. cue the person to place the devices 6" anteriorly and laterally

    _____ c. cue the person to stand erect

    _____ d. cue the person to avoid leaning excessively onto the devices

17. You are observing a person's gait pattern, specifically including their step length. Which of the following step length parameters is accurate?

    _____ a. normal step length for a female adult is 1.28 meters

    _____ b. normal step length for a child is 1.28 meters

    _____ c. normal step length for a toddler is 1.25 meters

    _____ d. normal step length for a person with a middle cerebral artery lesion is typically less than 1.28 meters

18. While observing a person ambulating, you note that they excessively lean their trunk left during left midstance. Which condition would MOST likely result in that gait deviation?

    _____ a. left greater than right leg length

    _____ b. right gluteus medius weakness

    _____ c. left iliotibial band contracture

    _____ d. left dyskinesia syndrome

19. You are preparing to perform gait training with a person who is partial-weight-bearing upon their left lower extremity. Which condition is a direct contraindication for applying a gait belt upon this person?

_____ a. recent diagnosis of an abdominal aortic aneurysm

_____ b. recent ostomy placement

_____ c. recent multiple rib fractures

_____ d. recent thoracis spinal surgery

20. A person has two steps to enter their two-story home without handrails, and a rail on their right-hand side when ascending 16 steps to the second floor. The person is currently ambulating with supervision only, for a distance of 200′, using a short-based quad cane, and right lower extremity weight-bearing as tolerated. Which of the following techniques is MOST appropriate when performing stair training with this person for descending their stair steps from the second floor?

_____ a. grabbing the handrail with the left upper extremity and using the assistive device in the right hand

_____ b. using the assistive device in the right hand, without using the handrail

_____ c. using the assistive device in the left hand, without using the handrail

_____ d. grabbing the handrail with the right upper extremity and using the assistive device in the left hand

21. A person who has achieved ambulation using a standard walker for 200′ with supervision only, and can maintain non-weight-bearing with their right lower extremity, is now ready for training with curb walking. What is the correct training technique for this person to practice ambulating off of a curb using an assistive device?

_____ a. placing the assistive device and then stepping down with their left lower extremity

_____ b. backing up to the curb, placing the assistive device down, and then stepping down with their left lower extremity

_____ c. placing their left lower extremity down, and then the assistive device

_____ d. backing up to the curb, stepping down with their left lower extremity, and then placing the assistive device down

22. A person diagnosed with Parkinson's disease six years ago would be least likely to demonstrate which of the following?

_____ a. festinating gait with decreased base of support

_____ b. increased counterrotation between the shoulder and hip girdles

_____ c. decreased occurrence of heel-off

_____ d. flexed postures at hip and knee

23. A person with diabetes and a history of chronic pressure sores with delayed healing has recently undergone a left transtibial amputation. Physical therapy for this person will focus on preprosthetic training, mobility training, and upper extremity conditioning. Which of the following interventions would be MOST appropriate?

_____ a. figure-eight wrapping

_____ b. patellofemoral taping

_____ c. medium frequency electrical stimulation

_____ d. straight-leg raises

24. Which of the following is MOST accurate about closed-loop skills?

_____ a. playing softball is a closed-loop skill

_____ b. a closed-loop skill requires that the distal segment of the extremity remains relatively stationary

_____ c. closed-loop skills require more perceptual information

_____ d. closed-loop skills maintain set parameters

25. Which function is compromised with an injury to the eighth cranial nerve?

_____ a. swallowing

_____ b. vision

_____ c. smell

_____ d. balance

26. A person who was an unrestrained passenger in a motor vehicle crash sustained a spinal cord injury. A lesion that affects the corticospinal tracts will MOST often result in which of the following?

_____ a. loss of light touch perception

_____ b. motor deficits

_____ c. proprioceptive deficits

_____ d. loss of temperature sensation in the extremities

27. Someone who has remained in a primarily horizontal position for a prolonged period of time often experiences orthostatic hypotension during treatment sessions. Which of the following is LEAST accurate about orthostatic hypotension?

_____ a. it can occur as a result of a patient assuming an upright position

_____ b. it is common after long periods of bed rest

_____ c. it is common in elderly persons

_____ d. it only lasts for 24 hours

28. While performing gait training with a person who has right hemiparesis, you observe a plantarflexed posture, consistently, during the midswing and terminal swing phases of gait. Which of the following is the MOST likely explanation for this observation?

_____ a. the person lacks contraction of the anterior tibialis and extensor hallicus longus

_____ b. the person has a decreased kinesthesia function in the right lower extremity

_____ c. the person has an exaggerated flexor synergy of the right lower extremity

_____ d. the person lacks distal segment proprioception and kinesthesia

29. A person with left hemiparesis having difficulty with foot clearance during the swing phase of gait would BEST benefit from which intervention?

_____ a. active bridging in supine

_____ b. sit-to-stand without upper extremity support

_____ c. active plantarflexion while seated on therapeutic exercise ball

_____ d. forward step-ups onto a step stool

30. The physical therapist has delegated crutch training to you with a person who is partial-weight-bearing on the left lower extremity for the next three weeks. Which adjustment would be MOST accurate for a pair of forearm crutches?

_____ a. forearm cuff should cover distal third of forearm

_____ b. forearm cuff should be placed at proximal third of forearm

_____ c. forearm cuff should be placed $1''$–$1^{1}/_{2}''$ proximal to the olecranon

_____ d. forearm cuff should be placed $1''$–$1^{1}/_{2}''$ distal to the olecranon

31. A person is performing preprosthetic training after recent amputation of their bilateral lower extremities. Which of the following is the MOST common nontraumatic reason for lower extremity amputation?

_____ a. pregnancy

_____ b. sports injury

_____ c. chronic obstructive pulmonary disease

_____ d. peripheral vascular disease

32. A person who recently had a cerebral vascular accident affecting the left hemisphere of their brain has weak right dorsiflexors graded 2/5 during manual muscle testing. Which type of gait deviation would you MOST likely observe them doing?

_____ a. flat-footed

_____ b. hip hiking

_____ c. antalgic

_____ d. steppage

33. A person, 44 years of age, sustained a left hip injury while falling off a ladder, four weeks ago. The rehabilitation is progressing, but the person continues to have weakness in the gluteus medius muscle. Which type of gait pattern is LEAST likely to occur as a compensation for gluteus medius weakness?

_____ a. abductor gait

_____ b. extensor gait

_____ c. Trendelenberg gait

_____ d. both (a) and (c)

APPLICATION, ADJUSTMENT, AND TRAINING IN THE USE OF ADAPTIVE EQUIPMENT

Four Items

1. A person with a three-year history of Parkinson's disease demonstrates a festinating gait. Which shoe adaptation would BEST address this gait deviation?

_____ a. medial foot wedge

_____ b. lateral foot wedge

_____ c. anterior foot wedge

_____ d. posterior foot wedge

2. A person with a true leg length discrepancy of $1^3/_4$ inches, who complains of acute low back pain, is being treated with ultrasound and therapeutic exercises to decrease spasms and promote mobility. Which device would also benefit the person, and potentially decrease the occurrence of low back pain?

_____ a. contralateral longitudinal arch support

_____ b. ipsilateral shoe lift

_____ c. contralateral shoe lift

_____ d. ipsilateral longitudinal arch support

3. A person with severe spasticity, who MOST often assumes a posture of hip adduction and scissoring during attempted ambulation, also has limited head control. Which device would meet the needs of this person for stability positioning?

_____ a. posterior thorax and abduction wedges

_____ b. head support and knee spica

_____ c. head support and posterior thorax wedges

_____ d. abduction wedge and head support

4. A person has a spinal cord injury, requires respiratory assistance, is dependent in bed mobility, has no motor recruitment in the upper extremities, and can use a chin control on a power wheelchair. These functions and adaptations are MOST appropriate for a person with at LEAST partial function at which spinal level?

_____ a. C4

_____ b. C5

_____ c. C6

_____ d. C7

APPLICATION, ADJUSTMENT, AND TRAINING IN THE USE OF ASSISTIVE EQUIPMENT

Five Items

1. When measuring crutches for a person that is non-weight-bearing on their left lower extremity after a knee arthroscopy, at least how many fingers should fit between the axilla and axillary pad of the crutches?

_____ a. 4

_____ b. 1

_____ c. 2

_____ d. 0

2. When measuring crutches for a person who is partial-weight-bearing upon their left lower extremity, where should the handgrips be positioned?

_____ a. place the grips where the person feels most comfortable

_____ b. at midrange of the triceps excursion, for greatest strength

_____ c. at full elbow extension

_____ d. at 20° of elbow flexion

3. A person who plays high school basketball recently fractured their right distal fibula. The physician has ordered the person to maintain non-weight-bearing with the involved lower extremity. Which assistive device pattern is MOST appropriate for this person?

_____ a. four-point alternating with crutches

_____ b. swing-through with crutches

_____ c. two-point alternating with wheeled walker

_____ d. two-point alternating with bilateral canes

4. Which of the following sequences is an accurate progression of ambulating assistive devices?

_____ a. axillary crutches, wheeled walker, quad cane, and standard cane

_____ b. wheeled-walker, small-base quad cane, large-base quad cane, and axillary crutches

_____ c. standard walker, large-base quad cane, small-base quad cane, and standard cane

_____ d. parallel bars, standard cane, wheeled walker, and axillary crutches

5. When planning discharge transition from a rehabilitation setting, wheelchair options are being addressed with a person as their primary means of locomotion. The person will need to ascend and descend 12'-wide concrete steps to enter and exit their place of employment. Which wheelchair option is LEAST necessary?

_____ a. folding frame

_____ b. antitipping bars

_____ c. removable armrests

_____ d. treaded tires

APPLICATION, ADJUSTMENT, AND TRAINING IN THE USE OF ORTHOTIC EQUIPMENT

Four Items

1. After donning a lower extremity orthotic, and ambulating, the orthotic is removed and the skin is inspected. Which time limit is used as the threshold criteria for the disappearance of skin blemishes?

_____ a. 1–3 seconds

_____ b. 5 seconds

_____ c. 30 seconds

_____ d. 10 seconds

2. A person who repeatedly demonstrates a right foot drop during the swing phase of gait would benefit MOST from which ankle orthotic feature?

_____ a. neutral dorsiflexion stop

_____ b. controlled ankle motion setting of 15°-0°-40°

_____ c. neutral plantarflexion stop

_____ d. plantarflexion assist

3. A person who recently suffered fractures to the anterior surfaces of their cervical vertebrae has shown significant skeletal instability at the fourth and fifth cervical vertebrae. The person has also demonstrated increasing neurological impairment at the fifth cervical nerve root distribution and below. Maximal stabilization of these segments in this situation would BEST be achieved through which orthotic?

_____ a. halo

_____ b. soft collar

_____ c. Milwaukee brace

_____ d. Philadelphia collar

4. A young child who has been diagnosed with myelodysplasia affecting the fifth lumbar neurological level, would BEST be provided with which of the following orthotics?

_____ a. parapodium

_____ b. hip-knee-ankle-foot orthosis

_____ c. knee-ankle-foot orthosis

_____ d. ankle-foot orthosis

APPLICATION, ADJUSTMENT, AND TRAINING IN THE USE OF PROSTHETIC EQUIPMENT

Four Items

1. A person who is participating in lower extremity prosthetic training demonstrates an abducted gait pattern. What would explain this observation?

_____ a. prosthesis is too long

_____ b. prosthetic does not provide enough knee friction

_____ c. prosthetic lateral wall is too high

_____ d. prosthesis is positioned in adduction

2. Which gait deviation typically occurs with a prosthesis that is too short?

_____ a. abducted gait

_____ b. cirumducted gait

_____ c. lateral trunk bending

_____ d. vaulting

3. Which strategy is used to facilitate knee extension for persons using prosthetic limbs after an above the knee amputations?

_____ a. activate hip flexors

_____ b. activate hip extensors

_____ c. activate quadriceps

_____ d. activate rectus femoris

4. A person using a transtibial prosthesis demonstrates a lack of knee flexion during early stance. Which condition would facilitate this deviation?

_____ a. low heeled shoe

_____ b. socket too posterior

_____ c. weak quadriceps

_____ d. all of the above

APPLICATION, ADJUSTMENT, AND TRAINING IN THE USE OF PROTECTIVE EQUIPMENT

Five Items

1. A person has hemiplegia and decreased sensory perception of the left lower extremity. Which device would prevent breakdown of the skin over the posterior calcaneus?

_____ a. ankle-foot orthosis

_____ b. multipodus boot

_____ c. ankle air splint

_____ d. bed tent

2. Having a person perform isometrics and avoiding hyperextension are interventions consistent with which of the following?

_____ a. capsular mobilization

_____ b. joint protection

_____ c. myotendonous stretching

_____ d. strengthening for a poor minus muscle

3. A person with an acute ankle sprain is being educated regarding the use of an air splint for the ankle. Which of the following wear guidelines is MOST appropriate for acute-phase wear of protective devices?

_____ a. wear up to 12 hours after injury

_____ b. wear up to 24 hours after injury

_____ c. wear up to 36 hours after injury

_____ d. wear up to 48 hours after injury

4. Which joint dysfunction is correctly addressed through the application of a Swedish knee cage?

_____ a. tibial torsion

_____ b. genu varum

_____ c. genu valgum

_____ d. genu recurvatum

5. A person is having an acute exacerbation of their rheumatoid arthritis. The physical therapist has applied a protective device to the person and requested that you reinforce joint protection education with the person today. Which intervention is also appropriate for this person?

_____ a. minisquats if the lower extremities are not involved

_____ b. isometrics at end range

_____ c. gentle eccentric use of the involved musculature

_____ d. tendon gliding exercises

APPLICATION, ADJUSTMENT, AND TRAINING IN THE USE OF SUPPORTIVE EQUIPMENT

Five Items

1. Which statement is LEAST accurate about the use of an upper extremity sling?

_____ a. they maintain the protective position of glenohumeral internal rotation and adduction

_____ b. they decrease the distraction forces through the glenohumeral joint

_____ c. they can be used for neurogenic subluxation of the glenohumeral joint

_____ d. they are contraindicated after surgical repair of the rotator cuff

2. A person is wearing a sling for strict precautions to prevent glenohumeral subluxation. Which supportive device is MOST complimentary to an upper extremity sling?

_____ a. upper extremity air splint

_____ b. abduction splint

_____ c. swathe

_____ d. universal cuff

3. A person has severe lymphedema and requires daily wear of a compression garment. What is the minimal pressure range necessary for safe and effective compression of severe lymphedema?

_____ a. up to 30 mm Hg

_____ b. up to 50 mm Hg

_____ c. more than 30 mm Hg

_____ d. more than 50 mm Hg

4. A person participating in physical therapy interventions to address functional mobility and physical endurance requires the use of low concentration supplemental oxygen. Which application is MOST appropriate for this person during the physical therapy treatment session?

_____ a. apply the oxygen using a nasal cannula

_____ b. apply the oxygen using an oronasal mask

_____ c. apply the oxygen using an oxygen tent

_____ d. apply the oxygen using a manual respiratory bag

5. A physical therapist assistant is working one-on-one with a person performing physical endurance interventions. The person is on supplemental oxygen delivered via nasal cannula. Which physical sign is the FIRST warning that the person is not adequately tolerating the physical activity?

_____ a. muscle soreness

_____ b. dyspnea

_____ c. cyanosis

_____ d. calf cramping

MODIFICATION OF THE ENVIRONMENT FOR HOME, WORK, OR LEISURE

Three Items

1. A person is returning to their employment setting. The employer is addressing several reasonable modifications to facilitate entry and exit safety. Which is the minimal slope requirement for an outdoor ramp?

_____ a. 1:6

_____ b. 1:12

_____ c. 1:20

_____ d. 1:24

2. A person is preparing for transition from a rehabilitative setting to a home setting. The person will require the long-term use of a wheelchair as their primary mode of mobility. Which modification is required to facilitate mobility around their home environment?

_____ a. insulation of hot water pipes under sinks

_____ b. at least 32″ doorway openings

_____ c. at least 32″ countertops

_____ d. padding of handrails

3. Which environmental modification is MOST applicable for a person with impaired grasp function?

_____ a. surface grading

_____ b. surface beveling

_____ c. surface nosing

_____ d. surface knurling

ANSWERS AND RATIONALE

PERFORMING TRANSFERS

Nineteen Items

1. Correct answer: (b)

   Rationale: Avoid gripping the end of the board as it can cause injury to the fingers

   Reference: Pierson, F. (2002). *Principles and techniques of patient care* (3rd ed., p. 146). Philadelphia: WB Saunders.

2. Correct answer: (b)

   Rationale: Use of an assistive device is more functional and appropriate for a person to maintain toe-touch weight bearing. Moving the person to their right or uninvolved side is easier.

   Reference: Pierson, F. (2002). *Principles and techniques of patient care* (3rd ed., p. 161). Philadelphia: WB Saunders.

3. Correct answer: (d)

   Rationale: A scoot-pivot transfer allows the lowest center of gravity with the least amount of lifting. This transfer may be contraindicated for persons with spinal precautions.

   Reference: Nixon, V., & Schneider, F. (1985). *Spinal cord injury: A guide to functional outcomes in physical therapy management* (p. 104, 105). Maryland: Aspen.

4. Correct answer: (b)

   Rationale: A two-person lift is most appropriate; a second-best choice would be slideboard, but not a stand-pivot.

   Reference: Pierson, F. (2002). *Principles and techniques of patient care* (3rd ed., p. 151). Philadelphia: WB Saunders.

5. Correct answer: (a)

   Rationale: Beginning in this position, the person has significantly less surface contact, and therefore reduces friction forces. When elevating the head of the bed, greater friction occurs in the lower portions of the body. There is not enough information in the second or third choices to serve as a valid option for reducing friction.

   Reference: Pierson, F. (2002). *Principles and techniques of patient care* (3rd ed., p. 133). Philadelphia: WB Saunders.

6. Correct answer: (c)

    Rationale: You should only stand in front of the person, when they are not using an assistive device. A person with a left cerebral vascular accident will most likely have impairments on the right side of their body. You should stand on the person's affected side during ambulation.

    Reference: Minor, M., & Minor, S. (1999). *Patient care skills* (p. 406).

7. Correct answer: (a)

    Rationale: The base of support can be widened to increase stability or position around wheelchairs. The shorter chains should be attached to the upper portion of the sling, the person should not hold onto the support bar, and the hydraulic valve must be closed to lift the person.

    Reference: Pierson, F. (2002). *Principles and techniques of patient care* (3rd ed., p. 156). Philadelphia: WB Saunders.

8. Correct answer: (d)

    Rationale: Difficult transfers should first be attempted towards the uninvolved side. The person should achieve standing before stepping upon the step stool.

    Reference: Minor, M., & Minor, S. (1999). *Patient care skills* (p. 262).

9. Correct answer: (b)

    Rationale: A gait belt should be placed on a person in sitting, towards the axilla when they have an ostomy bag, and you should have enough space to place your hand around the belt.

    Reference: Pierson, F. (2002). *Principles and techniques of patient care* (3rd ed., p. 224). Philadelphia: WB Saunders.

10. Correct answer: (b)

    Rationale: The person should be taught to push up from the surfaces they are sitting on.

    Reference: Minor, M., & Minor, S. (1999). *Patient care skills* (p. 259).

11. Correct answer: (c)

    Rationale: Tilting the pelvis anteriorly and extending the spine prepares the trunk component to initiate standing.

    Reference: O'Sullivan. (2001). *Physical rehabilitation assessment and treatment* (4th ed., p. 422, 423). Philadelphia: FA Davis.

12. Correct answer: (c)

    Rationale: Maximal assistance is defined as participation in the task, with 50–75% to complete the task.

    Reference: Pierson, F. (2002). *Principles and techniques of patient care* (3rd ed., p. 128). Philadelphia: WB Saunders.

13. Correct answer: (d)

    Rationale: This is the correct body-mechanics advantage for moving a person towards the foot of a treatment table or bed.

    Reference: Pierson, F. (2002). *Principles and techniques of patient care* (3rd ed., p. 133). Philadelphia: WB Saunders.

14. Correct answer: (a)

Rationale: Initially it is more challenging to transfer towards their weaker side, but eventually it is desired that the person can transfer towards either direction.

Reference: Pierson, F. (2002). *Principles and techniques of patient care* (3rd ed., p. 140). Philadelphia: WB Saunders.

15. Correct answer: (a)

Rationale: By maintaining their hands behind their hips, they reduce their hip flexion posture and their chance of dislocation.

Reference: Pierson, F. (2002). *Principles and techniques of patient care* (3rd ed., p. 139). Philadelphia: WB Saunders.

16. Correct answer: (d)

Rationale: All of the steps are correct for a sliding board transfer.

Reference: Nixon, V., & Schneider, F. (1985). *Spinal cord injury: A guide to functional outcomes in physical therapy management* (p. 80, 81). Maryland: Aspen.

17. Correct answer: (c)

Rationale: Transfers will initially be easier toward the uninvolved side.

Reference: O'Sullivan. (2001). *Physical rehabilitation assessment and treatment* (4th ed., p. 634). Philadelphia: FA Davis.

18. Correct answer: (b)

Rationale: Orthostatic hypotension can be addressed through use of short-duration standing, or upright activities in sitting, the parallel bars, standing frames, or tilt tables.

Reference: O'Sullivan. (2001). *Physical rehabilitation assessment and treatment* (4th ed., p. 423). Philadelphia: FA Davis.

19. Correct answer: (a)

Rationale: All three lifters face the same direction, and the person being lifted is faced towards them.

Reference: Minor, M., & Minor, S. (1999). *Patient care skills* (p. 230).

PERFORMING FUNCTIONAL ACTIVITIES AND FUNCTIONAL TRAINING

Twenty Items

1. Correct answer: (d)

Rationale: Each of these is an important consideration with transfer training. Age is the least relevant of these choices.

Reference: Pierson, F. (2002). *Principles and techniques of patient care* (3rd ed., p. 129). Philadelphia: WB Saunders.

2. Correct answer: (b)

Rationale: Age and automobile tolerance are not considered as critical as precautions following spinal injury. A person, 3 years after a total hip replacement no longer has surgical precautions.

Reference: Pierson, F. (2002). *Principles and techniques of patient care* (3rd ed., p. 130). Philadelphia: WB Saunders.

3. Correct answer: (b)

Rationale: The person is ambulating on indoor level surfaces, and may not be safe on uneven terrain. A bedside commode is not specifically indicated for a person who can ambulate up to 250'.

Reference: Pierson, F. (2002). *Principles and techniques of patient care* (3rd ed., p. 251). Philadelphia: WB Saunders.

4. Correct answer: (c)

Rationale: Greater pressure distally facilitates passive movement of fluids towards the thorax.

Reference: Pierson, F. (2002). *Principles and techniques of patient care* (3rd ed., p. 310). Philadelphia: WB Saunders.

5. Correct answer: (b)

Rationale: This position increases risk of contracture.

Reference: O'Sullivan. (2001). *Physical rehabilitation assessment and treatment* (4th ed., p. 632, 633). Philadelphia: FA Davis.

6. Correct answer: (c)

Rationale: This prehensile pattern can actually be performed by individuals with paralysis of all hand muscles.

Reference: Norkin, C., & Levangie, P. (1992). *Joint structure and function: A comprehensive analysis* (2nd ed., p. 295). Philadelphia: FA Davis.

7. Correct answer: (d)

Rationale: The other activities are considered basic activities of daily living.

Reference: O'Sullivan. (2001). *Physical rehabilitation assessment and treatment* (4th ed., p. 725). Philadelphia: FA Davis.

8. Correct answer: (b)

Rationale: If the person is ambulatory and safe, raising the height of the seat will facilitate the sit-to-stand transfer.

Reference: O'Sullivan. (2001). *Physical rehabilitation assessment and treatment* (4th ed., p. 340). Philadelphia: FA Davis.

9. Correct answer: (d)

Rationale: Each of these tasks and balance are directly related to instrumental activities of daily living.

Reference: Guccione, A. (2000). *Geriatric physical therapy* (2nd ed., p. 211). St. Louis: Mosby.

10. Correct answer (a)

    Rationale: The lungs should not be impaired, the upper extremities are not affected, but the hip flexors required lumbar cord function.

    Reference: Martin, S., & Kessler, M. (2000). *Neurologic intervention for physical therapist assistants* (p. 193). Philadelphia: WB Saunders.

11. Correct answer: (d)

    Rationale: The use of tenodesis can be used for persons with C6-C7 function to facilitate grasp. Persons with function above that can benefit from the use of the tenodesis hand posture as a hook. A person with function at L1 is not indicated for tenodesis compensation at the wrist.

    Reference: Somers, M. (2001). *Spinal cord injury: Functional rehabilitation* (2nd ed., p. 178). New Jersey: Prentice Hall.

12. Correct answer: (a)

    Rationale: A person with full function of the seventh cervical neurological level should be addressing modified independence with bed mobility.

    Reference: Nixon, V., & Schneider, F. (1985). *Spinal cord injury: A guide to functional outcomes in physical therapy management* (p. 65). Maryland: Aspen.

13. Correct answer: (d)

    Rationale: If a stretch is applied to the long finger flexors concurrently across the wrist and finger joints, the flexor tendons may lose the required tendon tension for a tenodesis grasp.

    Reference: Somers, M. (2001). *Spinal cord injury: Functional rehabilitation* (2nd ed., p. 178). New Jersey: Prentice Hall.

14. Correct answer: (a)

    Rationale: Tenodesis is typically used for producing a functional grip. Contracture of the anterior tibialis is rare and unlikely. Contracture of the hamstrings will prevent safe and effective positioning and pressure distribution in sitting and lying.

    Reference: Somers, M. (2001). *Spinal cord injury: Functional rehabilitation* (2nd ed., p. 178). New Jersey: Prentice Hall.

15. Correct answer: (a)

    Rationale: This is the standard for pedestrian velocity crosswalk design.

    Reference: Guccione, A. (2000). *Geriatric physical therapy* (2nd ed., p. 215). St. Louis: Mosby.

16. Correct answer: (c)

    Rationale: Block the leg that is most likely to buckle.

    Reference: Minor, M., & Minor, S. (1999). *Patient care skills* (p. 260).

17. Correct answer: (b)

Rationale: A person with function at T12 can support themselves upright and have full control of their intercostals. They would still require HKAFO and a walker to ambulate.

Reference: Somers, M. (2001). *Spinal cord injury: Functional rehabilitation* (2nd ed., p. 359). New Jersey: Prentice Hall.

18. Correct answer: (b)

Rationale: Lumbar spinal precautions do not allow for flexion of the knees.

Reference: (2000). *Physical therapist's clinical companion* (p. 339). Springhouse, PA: Springhouse Corporation.

19. Correct answer: (c)

Rationale: The first choice is not an active intervention for the patient. Choices (b) and (d) may potentially increase occurrence of incontinence. Pelvic muscle strengthening will increase their chances of controlling their urinary incontinence.

Reference: Guccione, A. (2000). *Geriatric physical therapy* (2nd ed., p. 345). St. Louis: Mosby.

20. Correct answer: (b)

Rationale: The other statements are false regarding canes.

Reference: Guccione, A. (2000). *Geriatric physical therapy* (2nd ed., p. 215). St. Louis: Mosby.

GAIT TRAINING: USE OF ASSISTIVE DEVICES, CONSIDERATION OF PROPER WEIGHT-BEARING STATUSES, GAIT DEVIATIONS, BALANCE DEFICITS, COMPONENTS OF THE GAIT CYCLE, AND PREGAIT ACTIVITIES

Thirty-three Items

1. Correct answer: (b)

Rationale: These are the seventh, eighth, first, and second phases of the normal gait cycle.

Reference: Perry, J. (1992). *Gait analysis: Normal and pathological function* (p. 10). Thorofare, NJ: Slack.

2. Correct answer: (b)

Rationale: Loading response is a peak phase for accepting weight onto the forward limb.

Reference: Perry, J. (1992). *Gait analysis: Normal and pathological function* (p. 159). Thorofare, NJ: Slack.

3. Correct answer: (d)

Rationale: Modified plantar-grade raises the center of gravity and decreases the base of support.

Reference: O'Sullivan. (2001). *Physical rehabilitation assessment and treatment* (4th ed., p. 420). Philadelphia: FA Davis.

4. Correct answer: (c)

Rationale: Modified plantar-grade is the highest progression of these pregait activities.

Reference: O'Sullivan. (2001). *Physical rehabilitation assessment and treatment* (4th ed., p. 420). Philadelphia: FA Davis.

5. Correct answer: (c)

Rationale: This activity facilitates counterrotation of the shoulder and hips.

Reference: O'Sullivan. (2001). *Physical rehabilitation assessment and treatment* (4th ed., p. 417). Philadelphia: FA Davis.

6. Correct answer: (a)

Rationale: The device leads the contralateral limb.

Reference: Pierson, F. (2002). *Principles and techniques of patient care* (3rd ed., p. 110). Philadelphia: WB Saunders.

7. Correct answer: (b)

Rationale: The first and third choices are not progressions, and the fourth is not appropriate for a standard walker.

Reference: Pierson, F. (2002). *Principles and techniques of patient care* (3rd ed., p. 248). Philadelphia: WB Saunders.

8. Correct answer: (c)

Rationale: During normal gait, more time is spent in the stance period than swing.

Reference: Perry, J. (1992). *Gait analysis: Normal and pathological function* (p. 4). Thorofare, NJ: Slack.

9. Correct answer: (c)

Rationale: The foot is lifted excessively to compensate for foot drop.

Reference: Rothstein, J., et al. (1998). *The rehabilitation specialist's handbook* (2nd ed., p. 817). Philadelphia: FA Davis.

10. Correct answer: (b)

Rationale: An antalgic gait occurs during attempts to weight-bear on a painful extremity.

Reference: Rothstein, J., et al. (1998). *The rehabilitation specialist's handbook* (2nd ed., p. 816). Philadelphia: FA Davis.

11. Correct answer: (d)

Rationale: A Trendelenburg gait deviation is observed with weakness of the gluteus medius muscle. Weakness of the gluteus medius muscle often manifests in the inability to maintain a near abducted posture of the lower extremity during midstance.

Reference: Rothstein, J., et al. (1998). *The rehabilitation specialist's handbook* (2nd ed., p. 817). Philadelphia: FA Davis.

12. Correct answer: (c)

   Rationale: The lateral protrusion of the weight-bearing hip is consistent with an increase in hip adduction due to lack of gluteus medius effort on the stance leg.

   Reference: Rothstein, J., et al. (1998). *The rehabilitation specialist's handbook* (2nd ed., p. 817). Philadelphia: FA Davis.

13. Correct answer: (c)

   Rationale: The peroneal nerve innervates the anterior tibialis.

   Reference: Lippert, L. (2000). *Clinical kinesiology for physical therapist assistants* (3rd ed., p. 392). Philadelphia: FA Davis.

14. Correct answer: (d)

   Rationale: A foot slap is the only audible gait deviation of the given choices.

   Reference: Rothstein, J., et al. (1998). *The rehabilitation specialist's handbook* (2nd ed., p. 817). Philadelphia: FA Davis.

15. Correct answer: (c)

   Rationale: The lack of limb shortening would most likely produce the deviation of vaulting on the contralateral side.

   Reference: Rothstein, J., et al. (1998). *The rehabilitation specialist's handbook* (2nd ed., p. 854). Philadelphia: FA Davis.

16. Correct answer: (c)

   Rationale: The person must stand erect in order to achieve the correct personal and device posture, prior to checking for proper fit.

   Reference: Pierson, F. (2002). *Principles and techniques of patient care* (3rd ed., p. 222). Philadelphia: WB Saunders.

17. Correct answer: (a)

   Rationale: Normal step length for a female adult is 1.28 meters, while for children and toddlers it is shorter, and there is no standard length for a person with a middle cerebral artery lesion.

   Reference: Perry, J. (1992). *Gait analysis: Normal and pathological function* (p. 432). Thorofare, NJ: Slack.

18. Correct answer: (c)

   Rationale: A greater length of the left lower extremity would result in leaning the trunk to right during right midstance. Gluteus medius weakness is seen in ipsilateral stance. A short ITB would result in the center of gravity moving closer to the area of support (left hip).

   Reference: Perry, J. (1992). *Gait analysis: Normal and pathological function* (p. 276). Thorofare, NJ: Slack.

19. Correct answer: (c)

Rationale: The aneurysm is stated as diagnosed, not incised. The presence of an ostomy bag would indicate a high (axillary) belt placement. Multiple rib fractures and pregnancy are contraindications for placing a gait belt on a person.

Reference: Pierson, F. (2002). *Principles and techniques of patient care* (3rd ed., p. 128). Philadelphia: WB Saunders.

20. Correct answer: (a)

Rationale: The assistive device typically belongs to the contralateral (left upper extremity) one, but the use of the descending handrail on the left side combined with the use of the assistive device provide for greater stability.

Reference: Pierson, F. (2002). *Principles and techniques of patient care* (3rd ed., p. 250). Philadelphia: WB Saunders.

21. Correct answer: (a)

Rationale: A person only needs to back to a curb when ascending. When descending, place the assistive device first, and then the weight-bearing extremity.

Reference: Pierson, F. (2002). *Principles and techniques of patient care* (3rd ed., p. 259). Philadelphia: WB Saunders.

22. Correct answer: (b)

Rationale: A festinating gait, bilateral decreased heel-off, a flexed posture, and decreased counterrotation of the shoulder and hip girdles are consistent with prolonged Parkinson's disease.

Reference: O'Sullivan. (2001). *Physical rehabilitation assessment and treatment* (4th ed., p. 754). Philadelphia: FA Davis.

23. Correct answer: (a)

Rationale: Figure-eight wrapping addresses prosthetic preparation. The other choices do not address mobility, prosthetic preparation, or upper extremity conditioning.

Reference: O'Sullivan. (2001). *Physical rehabilitation assessment and treatment* (4th ed., p. 630, 631). Philadelphia: FA Davis.

24. Correct answer: (d)

Rationale: Closed-loop skills occur in reliable environments, with minimal variation.

Reference: Martin, S., & Kessler, M. (2000). *Neurologic intervention for physical therapist assistants* (p. 41). Philadelphia: WB Saunders.

25. Correct answer: (d)

Rationale: The eighth cranial nerve is the vestibulocochlear nerve.

Reference: O'Sullivan. (2001). *Physical rehabilitation assessment and treatment* (4th ed., p. 189). Philadelphia: FA Davis.

26. Correct answer: (b)

   Rationale: The corticospinal tracts are the primary motor tracts of the spinal cord.

   Reference: Martin, S., & Kessler, M. (2000). *Neurologic intervention for physical therapist assistants* (p. 187). Philadelphia: WB Saunders.

27. Correct answer: (d)

   Rationale: The first three choices are true regarding orthostatic hypotension. The condition may persist for a variable period of time, until physiologic tolerance to upright positions is achieved.

   Reference: Pierson, F. (2002). *Principles and techniques of patient care* (3rd ed., p. 325). Philadelphia: WB Saunders.

28. Correct answer: (a)

   Rationale: These muscles dorsiflex the ankle during the swing phases of gait.

   Reference: Perry, J. (1992). *Gait analysis: Normal and pathological function* (p. 163, 164). Thorofare, NJ: Slack.

29. Correct answer: (d)

   Rationale: This activity challenges a person's ability to dorsiflex and achieve adequate limb clearance.

   Reference: O'Sullivan. (2001). *Physical rehabilitation assessment and treatment* (4th ed., p. 261). Philadelphia: FA Davis.

30. Correct answer: (d)

   Rationale: This is the correct placement for support and mobility of the humeroulnar joint.

   Reference: Pierson, F. (2002). *Principles and techniques of patient care* (3rd ed., p. 220). Philadelphia: WB Saunders.

31. Correct answer: (d)

   Rationale: Peripheral vascular disease is the most common cause of lower extremity amputations.

   Reference: O'Sullivan. (2001). *Physical rehabilitation assessment and treatment* (4th ed., p. 620). Philadelphia: FA Davis.

32. Correct answer: (d)

   Rationale: Excessive step height may occur to compensate for foot clearance.

   Reference: Lippert, L. (2000). *Clinical kinesiology for physical therapist assistants* (3rd ed., p. 427). Philadelphia: FA Davis.

33. Correct answer: (b)

   Rationale: Either the abductor lurch or Trendelenberg deviations may occur with weakness of the gluteus medius muscle during the stance period of gait.

   Reference: O'Sullivan. (2001). *Physical rehabilitation assessment and treatment* (4th ed., p. 270). Philadelphia: FA Davis.

APPLICATION, ADJUSTMENT, AND TRAINING IN THE USE OF ADAPTIVE EQUIPMENT

Four Items

1. Correct answer: (c)

   Rationale: A person with a festinating gait pattern has an anterior shift in their center of gravity. An anterior foot wedge would direct their center of gravity more posterior and decrease the mechanical instability.
   Reference: O'Sullivan. (2001). *Physical rehabilitation assessment and treatment* (4th ed., p. 754). Philadelphia: FA Davis.

2. Correct answer: (b)

   Rationale: An ipsilateral shoe lift may compensate for some of the true leg length discrepancy.
   Reference: Kendall, F., et al. (1993). *Muscles: Testing and function* (4th ed., p. 100). Baltimore: Williams & Wilkins.

3. Correct answer: (d)

   Rationale: The mobility of the pelvic girdle, spine, and head must be accomplished through tone inhibition to achieve sitting stability.
   Reference: Martin, S., & Kessler, M. (2000). *Neurologic intervention for physical therapist assistants* (pp. 118–199). Philadelphia: WB Saunders.

4. Correct answer: (a)

   Rationale: Persons with C5 or below function will elicit motor recruitment in the upper extremities. Respiratory assistance and chin control are consistent with partial function at C4.
   Reference: Nixon, V., & Schneider, F. (1985). *Spinal cord injury: A guide to functional outcomes in physical therapy management* (p. 48). Maryland: Aspen.

APPLICATION, ADJUSTMENT, AND TRAINING IN THE USE OF ASSISTIVE EQUIPMENT

Five Items

1. Correct answer: (c)

   Rationale: The axillary pad should be approximately two to four finger widths below the axilla.
   Reference: Pierson, F. (2002). *Principles and techniques of patient care* (3rd ed., p. 222). Philadelphia: WB Saunders.

2. Correct answer: (d)

   Rationale: This position allows for sufficient contraction of the triceps muscle group.
   Reference: Pierson, F. (2002). *Principles and techniques of patient care* (3rd ed., p. 222). Philadelphia: WB Saunders.

3. Correct answer: (b)

   Rationale: Teenagers tend to prefer crutches over walkers. Swing through pattern of crutch walking is the preferred gait pattern. The use of the other patterns is inappropriate.

   Reference: Minor, M., & Minor, S. (1999). *Patient care skills* (p. 299, 300).

4. Correct answer: (c)

   Rationale: This is a progression from devices of greater bases of support to lesser.

   Reference: Minor, M., & Minor, S. *Patient care skills* (p. 290).

5. Correct answer: (b)

   Rationale: Antitipping bars would inhibit stair locomotion.

   Reference: Pierson, F. (2002). *Principles and techniques of patient care* (3rd ed., p. 189). Philadelphia: WB Saunders.

APPLICATION, ADJUSTMENT, AND TRAINING IN THE USE OF ORTHOTIC EQUIPMENT

Four Items

1. Correct answer: (d)

   Rationale: Skin blemishes should disappear within 10 seconds.

   Reference: Rothstein, J., et al. (1998). *The rehabilitation specialist's handbook* (2nd ed., p. 857). Philadelphia: FA Davis.

2. Correct answer: (c)

   Rationale: The neutral plantarflexion stop will improve limb clearance during swing phase.

   Reference: Prentice, W., & Voight, M. (2001). *Techniques in musculoskeletal rehabilitation* (p. 332). New York: McGraw-Hill.

3. Correct answer: (a)

   Rationale: The halo or Minerva device provides the maximal spinal stabilization.

   Reference: O'Sullivan. (2001). *Physical rehabilitation assessment and treatment* (4th ed., p. 1041). Philadelphia: FA Davis.

4. Correct answer: (d)

   Rationale: The child has function above the fifth lumbar neurological level, and only requires stabilization distal to the knee.

   Reference: Nixon, V., & Schneider, F. (1985). *Spinal cord injury: A guide to functional outcomes in physical therapy management* (p. 164). Maryland: Aspen.

APPLICATION, ADJUSTMENT, AND TRAINING IN THE USE OF PROSTHETIC EQUIPMENT

Four Items

1. Correct answer: (a)

   Rationale: The abducted gait pattern compensates for decreased floor clearance.

   Reference: Rothstein, J., et al. (1998). *The rehabilitation specialist's handbook* (2nd ed., p. 837). Philadelphia: FA Davis.

2. Correct answer: (c)

   Rationale: Lateral trunk bending tends to occur with a prosthetic that is too short.

   Reference: Rothstein, J., et al. (1998). *The rehabilitation specialist's handbook* (2nd ed., pp. 836–838). Philadelphia: FA Davis.

3. Correct answer: (b)

   Rationale: Activation of the hip extensors brings the proximal segment of the prosthesis posterior creating an extension moment at the knee.

   Reference: O'Sullivan. (2001). *Physical rehabilitation assessment and treatment* (4th ed., p. 654). Philadelphia: FA Davis.

4. Correct answer: (d)

   Rationale: Each of these choices can contribute to early stance lack of knee flexion.

   Reference: O'Sullivan. (2001). *Physical rehabilitation assessment and treatment* (4th ed., p. 665). Philadelphia: FA Davis.

APPLICATION, ADJUSTMENT, AND TRAINING IN THE USE OF PROTECTIVE EQUIPMENT

Five Items

1. Correct answer: (b)

   Rationale: An ankle-foot orthosis or ankle air splints are not pressure relieving devices. The bed tent prevents pressure and friction upon the anterior foot and toes.

   Reference: Seymour, R. (2002). *Prosthetics and orthotics: Lower limb and spinal* (p. 359). Philadelphia: Lippincott Williams & Wilkins.

2. Correct answer: (b)

   Rationale: Joint protection programs include isometric stabilization in a protected range of motion.

   Reference: Kisner, C., & Colby, L. (2002). *Therapeutic exercise: Foundations and techniques* (4th ed., p. 425). Philadelphia: FA Davis.

3. Correct answer: (d)

   Rationale: The use of protective devices after acute injury is typically indicated for up to 48 hours after injury.

   Reference: Kisner, C., & Colby, L. (2002). *Therapeutic exercise: Foundations and techniques* (4th ed., p. 288, 289). Philadelphia: FA Davis.

4. Correct answer: (d)

   Rationale: The Swedish knee cage prevents hyperextension of the knee joint during gait and weight-bearing.

   Reference: O'Sullivan. (2001). *Physical rehabilitation assessment and treatment* (4th ed., p. 379). Philadelphia: FA Davis.

5. Correct answer: (d)

   Rationale: Tendon gliding exercises are typically included with joint protection programs.

   Reference: Kisner, C., & Colby, L. (2002). *Therapeutic exercise: Foundations and techniques* (4th ed., p. 425). Philadelphia: FA Davis.

APPLICATION, ADJUSTMENT, AND TRAINING IN THE USE OF SUPPORTIVE EQUIPMENT

Five Items

1. Correct answer: (d)

   Rationale: Slings are typically indicated after rotator cuff repair.

   Reference: Kisner, C., & Colby, L. (2002). *Therapeutic exercise: Foundations and techniques* (4th ed., p. 348). Philadelphia: FA Davis.

2. Correct answer: (c)

   Rationale: A swathe is the wrapping material to stabilize the sling against the person's abdomen.

   Reference: Kisner, C., & Colby, L. (2002). *Therapeutic exercise: Foundations and techniques* (4th ed., p. 348). Philadelphia: FA Davis.

3. Correct answer: (d)

   Rationale: More than 50 mm Hg of pressure is required for interventions to address severe lymphedema.

   Reference: O'Sullivan. (2001). *Physical rehabilitation assessment and treatment* (4th ed., p. 599). Philadelphia: FA Davis.

4. Correct answer: (a)

   Rationale: The nasal cannula is most appropriate for low to moderate levels of supplemental oxygen delivery.

   Reference: Pierson, F. (2002). *Principles and techniques of patient care* (3rd ed., p. 290). Philadelphia: WB Saunders.

5. Correct answer: (b)

Rationale: Any or all of these should be considered signs that a person is not properly tolerating the physical activity in any situation. The first to occur is difficulty breathing.

Reference: Pierson, F. (2002). *Principles and techniques of patient care* (3rd ed., p. 290). Philadelphia: WB Saunders.

MODIFICATION OF THE ENVIRONMENT FOR HOME, WORK, OR LEISURE

Three Items

1. Correct answer: (c)

Rationale: A 1:20 slope is appropriate for an outdoor ramp.

Reference: O'Sullivan. (2001). *Physical rehabilitation assessment and treatment* (4th ed., p. 337). Philadelphia: FA Davis.

2. Correct answer: (b)

Rationale: Hot water pipes are insulated for safety, not mobility. Countertops should be no higher than 31", and doorways should be at least 32".

Reference: O'Sullivan. (2001). *Physical rehabilitation assessment and treatment* (4th ed., p. 340, 341). Philadelphia: FA Davis.

3. Correct answer: (d)

Rationale: A knurled surface is roughened to facilitate grip upon the object.

Reference: O'Sullivan. (2001). *Physical rehabilitation assessment and treatment* (4th ed., p. 357). Philadelphia: FA Davis.

Procedural Interventions Group III: Physical Agents and Modalities

OVERVIEW

This chapter includes questions covering procedural interventions included in the exam. There are 120 questions in this chapter that deal with physical agents and modalities.

KEY POINTS FOR REVIEW

Intermittent Compression

- Recommended pressures
- Girth measurement
- Medical considerations

- Skin observations
- Equipment setup
- Physiological effects

Superficial Thermal Modalities

- Moist heat packs
- Cryotherapies
- Ultraviolet therapy
- Infrared
- Types of heating

- Physiological effects
- Equipment setup
- Skin observations
- Medical considerations
- Temperature ranges

Ultrasound and Phonophoresis

- Medical considerations
- Physiological considerations
- Equipment setup
- Mediums

Electrical Stimulation and Iontophoresis

- Electrode placement and number
- Medical considerations
- Electrical stimulation parameters
- Physiological effects

Biofeedback

- Equipment setup
- Treatment parameters

Mechanical Modalities

- Spinal traction
- Tilt table
- Standing frame
- Continuous passive motion devices
- Medical conditions
- Equipment setup
- Physiological effects

Whirlpool and Hubbard Tank

- Temperature ranges
- Equipment setup
- Physiological effects
- Medical considerations

INTERMITTENT COMPRESSION

Eleven Items

1. A person is referred to physical therapy to address lymphedema in the upper extremity after a mastectomy procedure. Which intermittent initial compression pressure setting would be MOST appropriate for a person with postmastectomy lymphedema?

    _____ a. 20 mm Hg

    _____ b. 60 mm Hg

    _____ c. 80 mm Hg

    _____ d. 120 mm Hg

2. Which of the following intermittent compression settings is the minimum pressure required for effective application to address lower extremity edema?

_____ a. 30 mm Hg

_____ b. 60 mm Hg

_____ c. 90 mm Hg

_____ d. 130 mm Hg

3. Prior to applying a mechanical compression unit to a person, the physical therapist assistant checks for the presence of contraindications. Which of the following is a contraindication for intermittent compression therapy?

_____ a. traumatic edema in the extremity

_____ b. venous insufficiency in the extremity

_____ c. stasis ulcers in the extremity

_____ d. recent fracture in the extremity

4. Which statement is MOST accurate concerning mechanical compression to address edema?

_____ a. use of compressive garment between treatments is necessary to maintain progress gained at each treatment session

_____ b. use of compressive garments is contraindicated between mechanical compression treatment sessions

_____ c. custom compressive garments should not be used between mechanical compression treatment sessions, secondary to the cost of each garment

_____ d. girth measurements should be performed by the patient at home

5. Before performing intermittent compression therapy with a person having left lower extremity edema, you check for contraindications. Which of the following conditions would MOST require you to consult with the physical therapist prior to applying intermittent compression?

_____ a. venous insufficiency

_____ b. blood pressure reading 140/70

_____ c. deep vein thrombosis

_____ d. chronic obstructive pulmonary disease

6. A person has been referred to physical therapy to address bilateral lower extremity edema. The physical therapist has selected intermittent compression therapy to address the goal of reducing lymphedema in the lower extremities. Which intervention is the MOST complimentary intervention to intermittent compression to reduce lymphedema?

_____ a. interferential stimulation at 120 pulses per second

_____ b. Russian stimulation at 50 pulses per second

_____ c. high-voltage stimulation at 15 pulses per second

_____ d. moist heat pack

7. You are preparing to apply mechanical compression therapy to a person to address edema in their left upper extremity. Which clinical observation SHOULD be made prior to applying mechanical compression therapy for the patient's safety?

_____ a. heart rate

_____ b. girth measurement

_____ c. extremity length

_____ d. blood pressure

8. Before performing intermittent compression therapy with a person having right lower extremity edema, you check for contraindications. Which condition would MOST require you to consult with the physical therapist prior to applying intermittent compression?

_____ a. congestive heart failure

_____ b. lymphedema

_____ c. diabetes

_____ d. chronic obstructive pulmonary disease

9. A person has experienced prolonged edema in their right lower extremity. Currently, they have been evaluated by a physical therapist who delegated to you to perform sequential chamber intermittent compression. Which treatment parameters are MOST appropriate for applying this intervention?

_____ a. set the chambers to pressures differing by at LEAST 5 mm Hg, all less than systolic and diastolic blood pressure

_____ b. set the proximal chamber to a pressure less than diastolic pressure, reduce the middle cell by 20 mm Hg, and reduce the distal cell by another 20 mm Hg

_____ c. set all chambers to a pressure less than systolic blood pressure

_____ d. set the distal chamber to a pressure less than diastolic pressure, reduce the middle cell by 20 mm Hg, and reduce the proximal cell by another 20 mm Hg

10. Use of mechanical compressive devices facilitates the reduction of peripheral edema. MOST of the body's lymphatic circulation is carried into the thoracic duct. Which lymphatic vessel does the right upper extremity empty into?

_____ a. right thoracic duct

_____ b. right lymphatic duct

_____ c. superior vena cava

_____ d. inferior vena cava

11. Prior to the application of mechanical intermittent compression, the physical therapist assistant checks the skin to observe the severity of pitting edema. Upon depression into the skin with an index finger, a 4 millimeter impression occurs. Based upon this information, which of the following grades is documented for pretreatment edema?

_____ a. 1+

_____ b. 2+

_____ c. 3+

_____ d. 4+

SUPERFICIAL THERMAL MODALITIES—PARAFFIN, MOIST HEAT PACKS, CRYOTHERAPY, AND INFRARED

Twenty-two Items

1. A person is participating in a paraffin intervention, using the dip and wrap technique. Which of the following means of heat exchange is being demonstrated by this intervention?

   _____ a. conversion

   _____ b. conduction

   _____ c. convection

   _____ d. radiation

2. A moist heat pack is applied to a person in supine, using a commercial hot pack cover and several layers of toweling for insulation. Given this application, which method of heat exchange occurs with the application of moist heat packs?

   _____ a. conversion

   _____ b. conduction

   _____ c. convection

   _____ d. radiation

3. A person evaluated by the physical therapist is found to have left elbow tendonitis. The treatment plan includes friction massage, phonophoresis, and stretching, followed by an ice massage. Which physiological responses generally occur from therapeutic cold interventions?

   _____ a. vasodilation, increased elasticity of tissue, and decreased phagocytosis

   _____ b. increased phagocytosis, decreased nerve conduction velocity, and vasodilation

   _____ c. vasoconstriction, increased nerve conduction velocity, and decreased phagocytosis

   _____ d. decreased nerve conduction velocity, decreased phagocytosis, and vasoconstriction

4. Which of the following precautions is LEAST necessary with the application of ultraviolet light interventions?

   _____ a. certain prescription medications cause an increase in sensitivity

   _____ b. eye protection should be worn during all applications

   _____ c. MED tests are required for the initial treatment

   _____ d. monitor pre-, peak-, and postperipheral pulse rate

5. A person is scheduled to receive a paraffin treatment today to address arthralgia at the first metacarpal-phalangeal joint. Prior to the person arriving at the facility, you check the temperature on

the paraffin unit. Which of the following Fahrenheit temperature settings is MOST appropriate for the paraffin unit?

_____ a. 104°

_____ b. 115°

_____ c. 126°

_____ d. 155°

6. A person has just arrived to an outpatient physical therapy setting for a treatment plan, which includes paraffin. Which of the following steps must be performed prior to every paraffin intervention?

_____ a. wash the body part

_____ b. check vital signs

_____ c. measure girth of body part

_____ d. apply protective nonlatex disposable glove or layer of plastic to body part

7. Ultraviolet therapy is used in a variety of dermatologic conditions. Prior to performing any intervention, the patient would be screened for contraindications relevant to ultraviolet therapy. Which of the following conditions would be contraindicated?

_____ a. acne vulgaris

_____ b. lupus erythematosis

_____ c. aseptic open wound

_____ d. psoriasis

8. Prior to selecting a moist heat pack from a hydrocollator unit, you observe the current temperature. Which of the following Fahrenheit readings is the correct operating temperature for the application of moist heat packs?

_____ a. 175°

_____ b. 160°

_____ c. 125°

_____ d. 104°

9. Which of the following thermal modalities has the LEAST depth of penetration and tissue temperature change?

_____ a. moist heat pack

_____ b. infrared

_____ c. pulsed ultrasound

_____ d. short-wave diathermy

10. A person is experiencing a lack of superficial peripheral circulation for which the physical therapist has selected a heat intervention to address. Which statement is MOST accurate regarding radiant heat?

_____ a. long infrared waves are absorbed primarily in the stratum corneum of the epidermis

_____ b. short infrared waves are reflected in all layers of the epidermis and dermis

_____ c. heat is reduced where the infrared waves are absorbed

_____ d. medium infrared waves have the greatest depth of penetration

11. Prior to applying a cryotherapy intervention to a person to address a localized tendonitis following therapeutic exercise, you check for the presence of contraindications. After doing so, you explain to the person the expected stages of perception experienced during a cryotherapy intervention. What is the correct sequence of the stages of cold perception?

_____ a. cold, numbness, burning, and aching

_____ b. burning, cold, aching, and numbness

_____ c. cold and numbness only

_____ d. cold, burning, aching, and numbness

12. A person is being treated in an outpatient physical therapy setting to address lumbar dysfunction. The physical therapist has requested that you perform mechanical lumbar traction with the person in supine with a standard moist heat pack over their lumbar region. Which of the following steps will be MOST important to the person's safety during these interventions?

_____ a. adding extra layers of towels between the person and the moist heat pack

_____ b. using a conservative progression of traction

_____ c. checking the person's vital signs before and after treatment

_____ d. setting the angle of pull to 0°

13. A person is performing interventions to address medial epicondylitis. The physical therapist has requested that you apply a cold pack during today's therapy session. Which guideline is MOST accurate about cold pack applications?

_____ a. the cervical sized cold packs are applied for up to 12 minutes

_____ b. the standard sized cold packs are applied for up to 20 minutes

_____ c. cold packs are applied up to the point of numbness

_____ d. cold packs are applied up to the point of reduced edema or inflammation

14. Which of the following statements is true regarding radiant heat?

_____ a. short infrared waves penetrate more deeply than long waves

_____ b. long infrared waves affect nerve endings and vascular beds in the dermis

_____ c. long infrared waves stimulate more perspiration than shorter waves

_____ d. short infrared waves penetrate up to 2 millimeters

15. A person has a superficial open wound with an infection. Which superficial thermal heat intervention is MOST appropriate to decrease the presence of bacteria and the wound's resistance to infection?

_____ a. hyperbaric oxygen

_____ b. ultraviolet B waves

_____ c. ultraviolet C waves

_____ d. infrared waves

16. You are preparing a moist heat pack to apply to a person's lumbar region. Based upon this information, how many layers are required for safe application of this intervention?
    _____ a. the lumbar region typically requires eight to ten layers of toweling
    _____ b. the lumbar region typically requires four to six layers of toweling
    _____ c. two to six layers of toweling is appropriate
    _____ d. six to eight layers of toweling is appropriate

17. Which of the following paraffin intervention techniques is the MOST safe to increase superficial tissue temperature?
    _____ a. immersion
    _____ b. dip immersion
    _____ c. glove
    _____ d. painting

18. A person who is experiencing an acute right postural torticollis has been delegated to you for therapeutic exercise instructions. The physical therapist requested that you apply a vapocoolant spray to reduce the pain perception while instructing the person in use of gentle active range of motion activities and postural awareness. Which application is MOST appropriate for this person?
    _____ a. gently stretch towards right lateral rotation, and left lateral flexion, and apply in one direction along right sternocleidomastoid and upper trapezius while stretching
    _____ b. gently stretch left sternocleidomastoid and right upper trapezius and apply in one direction
    _____ c. apply in bidirectional sweeping motions along left sternocleidomastoid and upper trapezius
    _____ d. apply in one direction, along right sternocleidomastoid and upper trapezius

19. Which of the following is the safest and MOST effective temperature setting for fluidotherapy?
    _____ a. 95°–105°
    _____ b. 100°–110°
    _____ c. 155°–165°
    _____ d. 110°–125°

20. A person has been evaluated by the physical therapist and has consented to receiving paraffin treatments to address their right foot symptoms. Which contraindication is MOST critical regarding the application of this intervention?
    _____ a. breaks in the skin
    _____ b. history of heart disease
    _____ c. rheumatoid arthritis in remission
    _____ d. normal sensation

21. Which condition is NOT a contraindication common to all superficial heat interventions?
    _____ a. vascular insufficiency
    _____ b. infected wound
    _____ c. acute injury
    _____ d. metal implants

22. A person is a long distance runner with recurrent injuries involving the hamstrings. The person typically experiences a low tolerance to hamstring stretching during periods of exacerbation. Which superficial thermal intervention BEST compliments therapeutic stretching of the hamstrings for this person?

____ a. phonophoresis

____ b. moist heat pack

____ c. ice massage

____ d. vapocoolant spray

ULTRASOUND AND PHONOPHORESIS

Twenty Items

1. When therapeutic ultrasonic waves pass through human tissue, the sound waves change from mechanical to thermal energy. This event describes which of the following therapeutic means of heat exchange?

____ a. conduction

____ b. conversion

____ c. radiation

____ d. convection

2. The physical therapist has asked you to perform an intervention with a person who has a left hamstring strain. The intervention includes the application of ultrasound with a 10% hydrocortisone cream application, on a continuous setting at 1.0 watts per squared centimeter. Which type of heat intervention has been described?

____ a. iontophoresis

____ b. diaphoresis

____ c. phonophoresis

____ d. diathermy

3. Ultrasound interventions are typically applied with an ultrasound gel or submerged in water. What is the primary purpose of the gel or water?

____ a. the gel or water acts as a coupling agent

____ b. the gel or water acts as a comforting agent for the patient, and has typically a warm temperature

____ c. the gel or water provides the clinician a visual guide for where the sound head is being placed

____ d. the gel or water provides a stimulus to the superficial nerve endings

4. Which of the following effects is LEAST likely to occur with a pulsed ultrasound application?

____ a. stable cavitation

____ b. microstreaming

_____ c. mechanical vibration

_____ d. vigorous heating

5. A person is being treated at your facility with the goal of decreasing low back pain. Their current plan of care includes the application of moist heat, followed by ultrasound and soft tissue mobilization. What physiological response is generally expected to occur with these interventions?

_____ a. vasoconstriction of the skin, increased tidal volume, and lower respiratory rate

_____ b. increased cardiac output and increased basal metabolic rate

_____ c. increased intestinal blood flow and raised cardiac output

_____ d. increased cardiac output and decreased basal metabolic rate

6. Which condition is an absolute contraindication for continuous therapeutic ultrasound?

_____ a. closed epiphyseal plates

_____ b. pregnancy

_____ c. in the area of a thrombus

_____ d. a person with benign cancer

7. Which treatment adjustment is LEAST appropriate when applying therapeutic ultrasound using the indirect method?

_____ a. use the 1 megahertz frequency

_____ b. conductive gel is not needed

_____ c. increase the intensity by .5 watts per centimeter squared

_____ d. avoid use over irregular surfaces of the extremity

8. A physical therapy facility regularly has preventative maintenance checks performed on each of their physical modality machines. Which of the following findings would pose the greatest safety hazard for patient care?

_____ a. oil and trapped micropockets of air on the ultrasound applicator

_____ b. a severed electrical cord

_____ c. beam nonuniformity ratio greater than 6.0

_____ d. a broken fuse

9. How does the application of a moist heat pack immediately before applying therapeutic ultrasound affect the penetration of the ultrasound?

_____ a. attenuation is increased with prior application of moist heat packs

_____ b. attenuation is decreased with prior application of moist heat packs

_____ c. attenuation does not change with prior application of moist heat packs

_____ d. ultrasound penetrates deeper with prior application of moist heat packs

10. Which of the following is LEAST contraindicated for therapeutic ultrasound applications?

_____ a. application to the skin over the spinal cord

_____ b. application to an area of metastasized cancer

_____ c. application to areas of arterial insufficiency

_____ d. application to an area of bleeding

11. A physical therapist has requested that you apply therapeutic ultrasound to a person. For which condition is the indirect method of application MOST indicated?

_____ a. Peyronie's disease

_____ b. De Quervains

_____ c. carpal tunnel

_____ d. Osgood–Schlatters

12. Which term is associated with the surface area of the ultrasound applicator that actually produces sound waves?

_____ a. piezoelectric effect

_____ b. beam nonuniformity ratio

_____ c. effective radiating area

_____ d. treatment area

13. Which therapeutic ultrasound setting is MOST appropriate for treating superficial areas of the body?

_____ a. 1.5 watts per centimeter squared

_____ b. .75 watts per centimeter squared

_____ c. 1 megahertz

_____ d. 3 megahertz

14. What treatment parameters are documented to represent the intensity setting during an ultrasound treatment?

_____ a. watts per centimeter squared

_____ b. megahertz

_____ c. duty cycle

_____ d. pulsed

15. Which statement is most accurate regarding metallic implants and the application of ultrasound?

_____ a. ultrasound may be applied to areas over metal implants

_____ b. ultrasound can only be safely applied near metallic implants that are beyond the effective radiating area

_____ c. ultrasound is safe over methylmethacrylate cement, but not screws and plates

_____ d. ultrasound can be used safely over methylmethacrylate cement or metallic implants

16. Which statement about the depth of effective heating is true regarding 1 megahertz therapeutic ultrasound application to the gluteus maximus?

_____ a. more than half of the ultrasound energy is absorbed by the skin

_____ b. more than half of the ultrasound energy is absorbed before entering the muscle

_____ c. more than half of the ultrasound energy is absorbed by the muscle

_____ d. less than half of the ultrasound energy is absorbed before reaching bone

17. A physical therapist has directed you to perform therapeutic ultrasound to a person with subacromial bursitis. Which ultrasound setting is MOST appropriate for addressing subacromial bursitis?

_____ a. no more than 1.5 watts per squared centimeter

_____ b. no more than .5 watts per squared centimeter

_____ c. no more than 2.5 watts per squared centimeter

_____ d. no more than 2.0 watts per squared centimeter

18. A person is receiving therapeutic ultrasound at 1 megahertz. Which structure typically absorbs more of the ultrasound energy at this frequency?

_____ a. skin

_____ b. tendon

_____ c. muscle

_____ d. fat

19. Which ultrasound treatment parameter is MOST appropriate for addressing a person with left temporomandibular joint pain?

_____ a. indirect, pulsed

_____ b. moving, continuous

_____ c. stationary, pulsed

_____ d. moving, pulsed

20. A physical therapist has delegated a therapeutic ultrasound intervention to an area of a person's body to you. During palpation, you estimate their treatment area to be approximately 2 centimeters in thickness. Which ultrasound frequency setting is MOST appropriate for an area of this thickness?

_____ a. 1 megahertz

_____ b. 2 megahertz

_____ c. 3 megahertz

_____ d. 5 megahertz

ELECTRICAL STIMULATION AND IONTOPHORESIS

Twenty-two Items

1. Which type of therapeutic electrical current is considered more appropriate to address a person with acute pain?

_____ a. interferential stimulation and high frequency

_____ b. high-voltage pulsed stimulation and positive current

_____ c. low-voltage, positive current, and low frequency

_____ d. biphasic and negative current

2. A person with a stage four decubitus ulcer at the left calcaneus is receiving therapeutic electrical stimulation to retard wound infection. Which electrical stimulation parameter is MOST appropriate to inhibit wound infection?

    _____ a. high-voltage, negative current, 100 pulses per second, and low intensity

    _____ b. high-voltage, positive current, 60 pulses per second, and low intensity

    _____ c. low-voltage, alternating current, 35 pulses per second, and low intensity

    _____ d. premodulated current, 3 pulses per second, and high intensity

3. Which electrical stimulation intervention provides a medium-frequency alternating current ?

    _____ a. low-voltage transcutaneous electrical nerve stimulation unit

    _____ b. high-voltage stimulation unit

    _____ c. Russian stimulation unit

    _____ d. interferential stimulation unit

4. There are several types of electrical stimulation current that can address the reducing of a person's pain level. Which device would provide the person more independence towards accomplishing this goal?

    _____ a. recurrent stimulation unit

    _____ b. low-voltage stimulation unit

    _____ c. Russian stimulation unit

    _____ d. transcutaneous electrical nerve stimulation unit

5. Which statement is LEAST accurate regarding therapeutic microcurrent applications?

    _____ a. the intensity setting is at a subsensory level

    _____ b. the intensity setting is less than 1 milliamp

    _____ c. the frequency setting is less than 50 hertz

    _____ d. the interpulse duration is greater than 50 microseconds

6. You are preparing a treatment area for a person who is attending physical therapy for high-voltage stimulation to the paraspinal muscles. High-voltage stimulators are identifiable by which of the following characteristics?

    _____ a. high-voltage stimulation devices have an output meter up to 150 milliamps

    _____ b. high-voltage stimulation devices do not offer the choice of the polarity setting

    _____ c. high-voltage stimulation devices require at LEAST two sets of active leads

    _____ d. high-voltage stimulation devices have a dedicated dispersive pad

7. Which electrical stimulation intervention would be MOST indicated for a person with right foot drop?

    _____ a. low-voltage alternating current, 10–50 pulses per second, at 150 microsecond pulse duration

    _____ b. high-voltage direct current, positive, 5–30 pulses per second, at 150 microsecond pulse duration

    _____ c. interferential stimulation, 8–20 pulses per second, at 150 microsecond pulse duration

    _____ d. Russian stimulation, 30–50 pulses per second, at 150 microsecond pulse duration

8. A person 39 years of age, with a prolonged history of low back pain, is currently being treated with transcutaneous electrical nerve stimulation and postural exercises. A transcutaneous electrical nerve stimulation unit may be used to accomplish which of the following?

_____ a. reduction of myalgia

_____ b. reduction of edema

_____ c. reduction of vasoconstriction

_____ d. muscle reeducation

9. A physical therapist assistant is applying a low-voltage direct current to a person with right ankle edema, in supine with the lower extremity elevated. Which of the following electrode placements is MOST effective in reducing edema?

_____ a. place the cathode at the site of edema

_____ b. place the dispersive electrode at the ankle

_____ c. place the cathode at the calf muscle

_____ d. place the anodes at the ankle

10. When applying neuromuscular electrical stimulation to solicit a motor response, which treatment parameters are MOST effective?

_____ a. a pulse duration of 200 microseconds and a frequency of 35 pulses per second

_____ b. a pulse rate of 200 pulses per second and a pulse duration of 300 microseconds

_____ c. a pulse width of 100 microseconds and a 35 hertz frequency

_____ d. a beat frequency of 35 hertz and a pulse width of 50 microseconds

11. When preparing to apply electrical stimulation electrodes to a person, the physical therapist assistant cleans the area to be treated. Which of the following is MOST appropriate for preparing a person with dry skin for an electrical stimulation intervention?

_____ a. apply a moist heat pack to increase perspiration

_____ b. clean the skin with an alcohol swab

_____ c. shave the skin to remove any hair

_____ d. apply a thin layer of moisturizer when the skin is excessively dry

12. Which intervention is MOST appropriate for regarding interferential stimulation?

_____ a. interferential currents to provide sensory level stimulation

_____ b. interferential currents applied using two electrodes

_____ c. interferential currents to produce a motor level response

_____ d. interferential currents used concurrent to ultrasound therapy

13. Which therapeutic electrical current would be MOST indicated for a person with denervation of a peripheral nerve?

_____ a. low-voltage direct current, positive

_____ b. high-voltage direct current, positive

_____ c. low-voltage direct current, negative

_____ d. high-voltage alternating current

14. A physical therapist assistant is preparing to apply iontophoresis to a person with lateral epicondylitis. Which statement is true regarding the application of the electrodes?

_____ a. the negative electrode should be twice the size of the positive electrode

_____ b. the active electrode should be the opposite polarity of the medication

_____ c. the electrodes should be positioned in a criss-cross pattern.

_____ d. the anode should be used to apply positively charged medications

15. A physical therapist requests that you provide a medium-frequency biphasic current to a person's quadriceps muscle to facilitate voluntary contraction during an exercise intervention. Russian stimulation is MOST effective at what parameters?

_____ a. using a 10 seconds on, and 50 seconds off, duty cycle

_____ b. using a 35–50 hertz frequency

_____ c. using a pulse duration of less than 100 microseconds

_____ d. using an interpulse duration of greater than 200 microseconds

16. A physical therapist and a physical therapist assistant are discussing interventions for a person with potential electrical sensitivities. When are therapeutic electrical stimulation descriptions MOST accurate?

_____ a. direct currents cannot produce twitch motor responses

_____ b. 1 milliamp is sufficient to produce sensory responses

_____ c. alternating currents cannot produce tetanic motor responses

_____ d. 3 milliamps is sufficient to produce motor responses

17. Which condition is LEAST indicated for neuromuscular electrical stimulation?

_____ a. decrease in edema

_____ b. improvement in acute pain

_____ c. decrease in spasticity

_____ d. improvement in endurance of type II muscle fibers

18. A person is receiving therapeutic electrical stimulation intervention to address myogenic pain in the lumbar paraspinal region. Which statement is MOST accurate about electrode placement with interferential applications?

_____ a. the best method of targeting the location of pain is trial and error

_____ b. the best method of targeting the location of pain is to place electrodes of the same channel on either side of the area

_____ c. the best method of targeting the location of pain is to surround the target area

_____ d. the best method of targeting the location of pain is to place each channel diagonally crossing through the area

19. Which of the following is NOT considered a precaution or contraindication for transcutaneous electrical nerve stimulation?

_____ a. inhibition of pain during operation of heavy equipment

_____ b. inhibition of pain in the presence of myocardial arrythmia

_____ c. inhibition of pain over a herniated nucleus propulsus

_____ d. inhibition of pain over the area of the carotid sinus

20. Which condition is MOST indicated for the given electrical stimulation intervention?

_____ a. muscle weakness, interferential stimulation

_____ b. drop foot, transcutaneous electrical nerve stimulation

_____ c. myalgia, Russian stimulation

_____ d. spasticity, neuromuscular stimulation

21. A physical therapist's documented goals include that the patient should increase their right middle deltoid strength from poor to poor plus and right shoulder active range of motion from 40° to 50° in 2 weeks. Which intervention would BEST address these goals?

_____ a. short-wave diathermy

_____ b. neuromuscular electrical stimulation

_____ c. transcutaneous electrical nerve stimulation

_____ d. fluidotherapy

22. Prior to applying an electrical stimulation intervention, a physical therapist questions the person regarding other existing medical conditions. Which of the following is NOT considered a general contraindication for therapeutic electrical stimulation intervention?

_____ a. a person who suspects they are pregnant

_____ b. a person who has an implanted pacemaker

_____ c. a person who is deconditioned

_____ d. a person who is diagnosed with stage two cancer

BIOFEEDBACK

Six Items

1. What is the purpose of skin preparation before applying biofeedback electrodes?

_____ a. improve cross-talk detection

_____ b. decrease motor unit action potential detection

_____ c. decrease skin impedance

_____ d. improve nerve conduction velocity

2. Which intervention would be MOST effective in providing feedback to a person with a median nerve injury?

_____ a. neuromuscular stimulation to the triceps

_____ b. neuromuscular stimulation to the pronator

_____ c. surface electromyography placed over the triceps

_____ d. surface electromyography placed over the pronator

3. When applying biofeedback for motor recruitment, where should the initial threshold setting begin?

_____ a. just above the baseline

_____ b. just below the baseline

_____ c. at the level of the third volitional contraction

_____ d. at zero

4. Which application of biofeedback is LEAST appropriate for facilitating motor practice?

_____ a. open practice

_____ b. electrical myography

_____ c. mirror

_____ d. verbal cueing

5. Which placement of electrodes results in detection of fewer motor unit action potentials?

_____ a. 1–2 centimeter spacing

_____ b. 2–5 centimeter spacing

_____ c. placing the ground electrode between the active electrodes

_____ d. 5–8 centimeter spacing

6. When applying biofeedback for muscle inhibition, which electrode placement is MOST effective?

_____ a. monitoring the agonistic muscle

_____ b. monitoring the antagonistic muscle

_____ c. monitoring the immediately proximal muscle

_____ d. monitoring the synergistic muscle

MECHANICAL MODALITIES—SPINAL TRACTION, TILT TABLE, STANDING FRAMES, AND CONTINUOUS PASSIVE MOTION DEVICES

Twenty-two Items

1. You have a person in a standing frame to address bone density and tolerance to upright posture. The person is recovering from a spinal cord injury. Which level is autonomic dysreflexia of primary concern?

_____ a. injuries affecting the sixth thoracic level and above

_____ b. injuries affecting the eighth thoracic level and above

_____ c. injuries resulting in paraplegia

_____ d. injuries affecting the third thoracic level and above

2. A person who has been diagnosed with discogenic neuropathy would BEST respond to which mechanical traction settings?

     ____ a. prone static for 10 minutes

     ____ b. prone intermittent for 10 minutes

     ____ c. supine static for 15 minutes

     ____ d. supine intermittent for 15 minutes

3. A person, who had a total knee replacement three days ago, is being placed upon a continuous passive motion device several times a day. Which setting is MOST appropriate in promoting pain relief?

     ____ a. 4 cycles per minute

     ____ b. 45 seconds per cycle

     ____ c. 3 cycles per minute

     ____ d. 25 seconds per cycle

4. A person recently experienced a spine twisting injury when sliding into second base during a softball tournament. The current plan of care includes static pelvic traction for 10 minutes, beginning with 40% of their total body weight. Which of the following would be precautions for applying this intervention?

     ____ a. herniated vertebral disk

     ____ b. chronic muscle spasm

     ____ c. osteoporosis

     ____ d. subacute muscle spasm

5. When applying mechanical spinal traction, which statement is true about the duration of force applied?

     ____ a. on time must be equal to or greater than off time

     ____ b. on time must be less than off time

     ____ c. at least 7 seconds is required to maximize vertebral separation

     ____ d. at least 12 seconds is required to maximize vertebral separation

6. The standing frame is used for individuals who are unable to achieve and maintain full erect standing. Which statement is LEAST accurate about the physiological effects of standing interventions?

     ____ a. standing programs facilitate extensor tone of the upper extremity muscles

     ____ b. standing programs can increase bone mineral density

     ____ c. standing programs can deepen the acetabulum in children

     ____ d. standing programs facilitate tolerance to upright postures

7. A person recently had a total knee replacement, and is participating in exercise and mobility interventions. In addition, the surgeon has ordered that the person have a continuous passive motion device applied three times a day. Desired physiological effects of continuous passive motion (CPM) devices do NOT include which of the following?

     ____ a. increasing the rate of collagen formation

     ____ b. improving the orientation of collagen fibers

     ____ c. improved tissue extensibility

     ____ d. limit contracture formation

8. Which intervention is MOST challenging for a person who is participating in physical therapy to address orthostatic hypotension?

    _____ a. standing frame

    _____ b. tilt table

    _____ c. parallel bars

    _____ d. elevating the head of a hospital bed

9. A physical therapist assistant is placing a person, recovering from a spinal injury, in a standing frame and elevating their body towards standing. Which of the following is MOST important during this intervention?

    _____ a. monitor vital signs throughout elevation

    _____ b. inform the patient that achieving full standing may not correlate to improved function

    _____ c. inform the patient that a full upright posture may exacerbate orthostatic hypotension

    _____ d. monitor amount of weight borne through their extremities

10. Which condition is an indication for mechanical spinal traction?

    _____ a. vertebral hypermobility

    _____ b. medial disk protrusion

    _____ c. paraspinal muscle spasm

    _____ d. posterior spinal fusion

11. A person is receiving mechanical cervical traction to address discogenic symptoms at the midcervical region. Which angle of pull produces the optimum increases in the intervertebral spaces?

    _____ a. 0°

    _____ b. 12°

    _____ c. 15°

    _____ d. 25°

12. Which condition is of MOST concern when applying mechanical spinal traction?

    _____ a. pregnancy

    _____ b. recent vertebral fracture

    _____ c. spinal stenosis

    _____ d. respiratory insufficiency

13. A person who is experiencing poor tolerance to full upright postures has been evaluated, and is beginning a treatment session on the tilt table today. Large straps are used to secure the person prior to elevating the tilt table. Which of the following is NOT a primary location for applying the stabilizing belts when using the tilt table?

    _____ a. chest

    _____ b. knees

    _____ c. pelvis

    _____ d. cervical spine

14. A person with moderate lumbar nerve root dysfunction and severe pain received their first mechanical traction session 2 days ago. Since that session, they have been completely pain free. Which of the following actions is most appropriate when they inform you of this at their next visit?

_____ a. decrease the pull and duration of traction in this visit

_____ b. recommend discontinuing the intervention to the physical therapist

_____ c. increase pull and duration of traction in this visit

_____ d. increase the angle and decrease the pull of traction in this visit

15. A person with vertebral artery pathology is considered to have a condition MOST contraindicated for which mechanical interventions?

_____ a. intermittent mechanical compression therapy

_____ b. standing frame and tilt table

_____ c. mechanical cervical traction

_____ d. mechanical pelvic traction

16. A person with an injury to their spinal cord has a current preambulation goal of tolerating a standing frame, fully upright, with stable vitals signs, for 30 minutes. The trunk stabilizing attachment is used for persons who lack adequate postural control. Which of the following neurological levels of function is typically necessary for adequate stabilization of the trunk and pelvis?

_____ a. second thoracic

_____ b. fifth thoracic

_____ c. ninth thoracic

_____ d. first lumbar

17. A person has recently battled a chronic illness resulting in a prolonged hospitalization and extensive bed rest. A physical therapist has requested that you perform tilt table interventions with this person. Which body system is LEAST likely affected with elevation of a person on a tilt table?

_____ a. integumentary

_____ b. respiratory

_____ c. endocrine

_____ d. cardiovascular

18. A person with subacute lumbar paraspinal spasms finds relief of symptoms in extension postures. The physical therapist requests that you apply mechanical traction interventions to this person. Which application of lumbar traction is MOST appropriate for this person?

_____ a. prone

_____ b. supine

_____ c. sitting

_____ d. semirecumbent

19. The physical therapist requests that you instruct a person in self-traction techniques to facilitate relief of symptoms when they are at work. Which technique is MOST effective in addressing a person with

subacute cervical discogenic pain?

_____ a. self-traction performed by a push-up from an arm chair, holding for 10–15 seconds

_____ b. mechanical traction in sidelying, with the head slightly elevated, holding for 20 minutes

_____ c. mechanical traction in supine, with the head slightly elevated, holding for 60 seconds

_____ d. self-traction performed by gripping an overhead bar, and partially squatting, for 3–5 seconds

20. A physical therapist assistant is performing a tilt table intervention with a person for the first time today. Which physiological observation is an indication to a person's poor response to a tilt table intervention?

_____ a. change in consciousness

_____ b. excessive perspiration

_____ c. increased pedal pulse

_____ d. paresthesia of the distal extremities

21. A physical therapist requests that you instruct a person in use of a home, over-the-door cervical traction unit. Which of the following adjustments will appropriately promote the application of the intervention in the position of flexion?

_____ a. have the person lay supine

_____ b. have the person face away from the door

_____ c. have the person face towards the door

_____ d. have the person lean sideways toward the door

22. A person is evaluated by a physical therapist regarding recurrent low back pain. Which condition is LEAST appropriate to address with mechanical spinal traction?

_____ a. presence of disk protrusion

_____ b. presence of lateral spinal stenosis

_____ c. presence of upper extremity radiculopathy

_____ d. presence of pressure on the spinal cord

WHIRLPOOLS AND HUBBARD TANKS

Seventeen Items

1. A person is referred to physical therapy, and is evaluated by the physical therapist. Which condition is considered LEAST appropriate for whirlpool interventions?

_____ a. the presence of venous insufficiency

_____ b. the presence of lymphatic insufficiency

_____ c. the presence of active wound bleeding

_____ d. the presence of localized infection

2. A physical therapist requests that you prepare a Hubbard tank with very warm water for a person. What is the maximum Fahrenheit temperature for Hubbard tank interventions?

_____ a. 110°

_____ b. 102°

_____ c. 106°

_____ d. 100°

3. While preparing the hydrotherapy for a whirlpool intervention to a person with a decubitus wound to the sacrum, you begin filling the whirlpool tank. Which of the following Fahrenheit temperature settings is MOST appropriate for this person?

_____ a. 90°–94°

_____ b. 94°–98°

_____ c. 98°–104°

_____ d. 106°–108°

4. Which dilution ratio is MOST appropriate for chloramine-T?

_____ a. 1 gram per gallon

_____ b. 10 grams per gallon

_____ c. 50 grams per sixty gallons

_____ d. 500 grams per Hubbard tank

5. After completing a whirlpool treatment and sending a person back to their room, you prepare to disinfect the whirlpool tank. Which of the following materials is MOST appropriate for effective disinfection of a whirlpool tank?

_____ a. 1:20 dilution of sodium hypochlorite

_____ b. antimicrobial soap

_____ c. isopropyl alcohol

_____ d. phenolic germicidal detergent

6. Whirlpools can be used as a thermal agent for the human body. Submersion in a whirlpool tank establishes heat exchange by which of the following means?

_____ a. conduction

_____ b. conversion

_____ c. convection

_____ d. radiation

7. Which electrical device must be properly grounded to allow a person to operate the equipment while submerged in the tank?

_____ a. the electrical plug in ground-fault interrupter outlet can be operated if properly grounded

_____ b. no electrical equipment can be operated by the person inside the tank

_____ c. the ceiling mounted on electrical overhead lift can be operated if properly grounded

_____ d. only the on/off switch of the agitator can be operated if properly grounded

8. A physical therapist assistant is scheduling the use of whirlpool therapy equipment. Which physical requirement is necessary for placing a person in a highboy tank?

_____ a. full extension of the lower extremity

_____ b. lateral flexion of the thoracic spine

_____ c. hip and knee flexion

_____ d. independent in wheelchair transfers

9. When other whirlpool additives for cleansing are not available, sodium hypochlorite can be substituted. Which dilution ratio is MOST appropriate for adding sodium hypochlorite to a whirlpool tank?

_____ a. 1:10

_____ b. 1:200

_____ c. 1:20

_____ d. 1:100

10. Which of the following skin ulcer conditions is LEAST effectively managed with whirlpool intervention?

_____ a. tunneling wounds

_____ b. granulizing wounds

_____ c. reepithelializing wounds

_____ d. primarily closed wounds

11. A person is having difficulty with wound healing due to impaired peripheral circulation. Which of the following is a desired effect of using an extremity tank for providing whirlpool interventions?

_____ a. effects of gravity-dependent positioning

_____ b. effects of compression upon the edge of the tank

_____ c. effects of warm water

_____ d. effects of removing granulous tissue

12. Whirlpools can be used as a thermal agent for the human body. After submersion in a whirlpool tank, and with the agitator activated, heat exchange primarily occurs by which of the following means?

_____ a. conduction

_____ b. conversion

_____ c. convection

_____ d. radiation

13. A person has progressed in their wound healing, and the physical therapist has determined that standard whirlpool intervention is too excessive in pressure. Which medical device provides the LEAST irrigation pressure per square inch?

_____ a. bulb syringe

_____ b. spray bottle

_____ c. saline squeeze bottle

_____ d. half-intensity pulsed lavage

14. Application of a whirlpool intervention accomplishes which desired method of wound debridement?

_____ a. manual debridement

_____ b. enzymatic debridement

_____ c. nonselective debridement

_____ d. autolytic debridement

15. Which tissue condition SHOULD be considered inappropriate for debridement by means of whirlpool intervention?

_____ a. necrotic tissue

_____ b. devitalized tissue

_____ c. exudate wastes

_____ d. cellulitis

16. Which observation is not necessary for documenting the status of an open wound being addressed with whirlpool intervention?

_____ a. peripheral blood pressure

_____ b. color, shape, and size

_____ c. odor

_____ d. pulses, sensation, and depth

17. Which open wound conditions are MOST indicated for hydrotherapy intervention?

_____ a. wounds with granulation

_____ b. wounds with malodorous exudate

_____ c. wounds with cellulitis

_____ d. wounds covered with adherent eschar up to 60%

ANSWERS AND RATIONALE

INTERMITTENT COMPRESSION

Eleven Items

1. Correct answer: (a)

   Rationale: Recommended intermittent compression pressure settings for the upper extremities are 20–50 mm Hg.

   Reference: Behrens, B., & Michlovitz, S. (1996). *Physical agents: Theory and practice for the physical therapist assistant* (p. 219). Philadelphia: FA Davis.

2. Correct answer: (a)

   Rationale: The minimum recommended pressure for the lower extremities is 30 mm Hg of pressure. Higher pressures can be applied as long as they are less than the diastolic blood pressure.

Reference: Behrens, B., & Michlovitz, S. (1996). *Physical agents: Theory and practice for the physical therapist assistant* (p. 219). Philadelphia: FA Davis.

3. Correct answer: (d)

   Rationale: Each of these is an indication for intermittent compression, except the recent injury, which is contraindicated.

   Reference: Hayes, K. (2002). *Manual for physical agents* (5th ed., p. 84). New York: Prentice.

4. Correct answer: (a)

   Rationale: Mechanical compression intervention is followed by application of a compressive garment.

   Reference: Behrens, B., & Michlovitz, S. (1996). *Physical agents: Theory and practice for the physical therapist assistant* (p. 219). Philadelphia: FA Davis.

5. Correct answer: (c)

   Rationale: Blood clots are a contraindication for intermittent compression therapy.

   Reference: Hayes, K. (2002). *Manual for physical agents* (5th ed., p. 85). New York: Prentice.

6. Correct answer: (c)

   Rationale: High-voltage stimulation at a low pulse rate produces a muscle "pumping" action to increase venous return from an extremity. Interferential stimulation best addresses pain, and Russian stimulation is used to facilitate motor responses. Moist heat may exacerbate lymphedema.

   Reference: Prentice, W. (2002). *Therapeutic modalities for physical therapists* (2nd ed., p. 404, 405). New York: McGraw-Hill.

7. Correct answer: (d)

   Rationale: Blood pressure must be checked prior to, during, and after mechanical compression therapy to avoid exceeding diastolic pressure with machine settings.

   Reference: Behrens, B., & Michlovitz, S. (1996). *Physical agents: Theory and practice for the physical therapist assistant* (p. 219). Philadelphia: FA Davis.

8. Correct answer: (a)

   Rationale: With congestive heart failure, the increase of peripheral circulation return may dangerously strain the heart.

   Reference: Prentice, W. (2002). *Therapeutic modalities for physical therapists* (2nd ed., p. 406). New York: McGraw-Hill.

9. Correct answer: (d)

   Rationale: The greatest pressure should be located most distal on the extremity, to facilitate venous return.

   Reference: Prentice, W. (2002). *Therapeutic modalities for physical therapists* (2nd ed., p. 405). New York: McGraw-Hill.

10. Correct answer: (b)

    Rationale: The right upper extremity and thoracic region empty into the right lymphatic duct.

Reference: Goodman, C., & Snyder, T. (2002). *Differential diagnosis in physical therapy* (3rd ed., p. 483). Philadelphia: WB Saunders.

11. Correct answer: (b)

Rationale: The other choices are used for 2, 6, and 8 millimeters impressions, respectively.

Reference: Anemaet, W., et al. (2000). *Home rehabilitation: Guide to clinical practice* (p. 509). St. Louis: Mosby.

SUPERFICIAL THERMAL MODALITIES— PARAFFIN, MOIST HEAT PACKS, CRYOTHERAPY, AND INFRARED

Twenty-two Items

1. Correct answer: (b)

Rationale: The paraffin conducts directly onto the skin, and any movement of the paraffin medium is negligible.

Reference: Behrens, B., & Michlovitz, S. (1996). *Physical agents: Theory and practice for the physical therapist assistant* (p. 61). Philadelphia: FA Davis.

2. Correct answer: (b)

Rationale: The heat conducts through the layers, by reducing thermal resistance through moisture, and conducts heat to the skin.

Reference: Behrens, B., & Michlovitz, S. (1996). *Physical agents: Theory and practice for the physical therapist assistant* (p. 59). Philadelphia: FA Davis.

3. Correct answer: (d)

Rationale: These are the desired physiological responses to cryotherapy.

Reference: Prentice, W. (2002). *Therapeutic modalities for physical therapists* (2nd ed., p. 208, 209). New York: McGraw-Hill.

4. Correct answer: (d)

Rationale: Ultraviolet therapy is superficial mild thermal agent, which has little effect upon peripheral pulse rate.

Reference: Behrens, B., & Michlovitz, S. (1996). *Physical agents: Theory and practice for the physical therapist assistant* (p. 124, 125). Philadelphia: FA Davis.

5. Correct answer: (c)

Rationale: This is the standard operating temperature for paraffin equipment.

Reference: Behrens, B., & Michlovitz, S. (1996). *Physical agents: Theory and practice for the physical therapist assistant* (p. 61). Philadelphia: FA Davis.

6. Correct answer: (a)

Rationale: The other choices may be necessary in some cases, but the hands must be washed for infection control every time.

Reference: Hayes, K. (2002). *Manual for physical agents* (5th ed., p. 13). New York: Prentice.

7. Correct answer: (b)

Rationale: Ultraviolet energy may exacerbate lupus erythematosis. The other conditions are typical indications for ultraviolet intervention.

Reference: Hayes, K. (2002). *Manual for physical agents* (5th ed., p. 74). New York: Prentice.

8. Correct answer: (b)

Rationale: The standard recommended temperature settings vary from 155° to 170°. This particular reference used 160°.

Reference: Michlovitz, S. (1990). *Thermal agents in rehabilitation* (2nd ed., p. 94). Philadelphia: FA Davis.

9. Correct answer: (b)

Rationale: Infrared energy typically penetrates less than 1 millimeter, and less than moist heat packs. Ultrasound and short-wave diathermies heat at least 3–5 centimeters of depth.

Reference: Prentice, W. (2002). *Therapeutic modalities for physical therapists* (2nd ed., p. 232). New York: McGraw-Hill.

10. Correct answer: (a)

Rationale: Long infrared waves are absorbed primarily in the stratum corneum of the epidermis.

Reference: Hayes, K. (2002). *Manual for physical agents* (5th ed., p. 5). New York: Prentice.

11. Correct answer: (d)

Rationale: These are the typical stages of cold perception. These have also been published in the sequence of cold, aching, burning, and then numbness.

Reference: Hayes, K. (2002). *Manual for physical agents* (5th ed., p. 66). New York: Prentice.

12. Correct answer: (a)

Rationale: A person lying upon the moist heat packs prevents the typical dissipation of heat, and therefore will receive a greater heating at a quicker rate.

Reference: Hayes, K. (2002). *Manual for physical agents* (5th ed., p. 10). New York: Prentice.

13. Correct answer: (d)

Rationale: Cryotherapy interventions should not exceed the point of anesthesia.

Reference: Prentice, W. (2002). *Therapeutic modalities for physical therapists* (2nd ed., p. 215). New York: McGraw-Hill.

14. Correct answer: (a)

Rationale: Short infrared waves penetrate more deeply than long waves, up to 10 millimeters, affecting free nerve endings and vascular beds in the dermis.

Reference: Hayes, K. (2002). *Manual for physical agents* (5th ed., p. 5). New York: Prentice.

15. Correct answer: (c)

    Rationale: Hyperbaric oxygen can produce the same effects, but is not a thermal modality. UV-B produces erythema and pigmentation. Infrared is not considered bactericidal.

    Reference: Hayes, K. (2002). *Manual for physical agents* (5th ed., p. 72, 73). New York: Prentice.

16. Correct answer: (d)

    Rationale: The lumbar region has little influence on the number of required layers of toweling, six to eight is typically appropriate.

    Reference: Behrens, B., & Michlovitz, S. (1996). *Physical agents: Theory and practice for the physical therapist assistant* (p. 59). Philadelphia: FA Davis.

17. Correct answer: (c)

    Rationale: This produces the least amount of temperature increase, but is the most easily tolerated and commonly used paraffin technique.

    Reference: Hayes, K. (2002). *Manual for physical agents* (5th ed., p. 13). New York: Prentice.

18. Correct answer: (a)

    Rationale: This is the correct position to lengthen and treat the typically involved musculature.

    Reference: Hayes, K. (2002). *Manual for physical agents* (5th ed., p. 64). New York: Prentice.

19. Correct answer: (d)

    Rationale: This is the correct temperature setting for fluidotherapy, also known as the dry whirlpool.

    Reference: Prentice, W. (2002). *Therapeutic modalities for physical therapists* (2nd ed., p. 235). New York: McGraw-Hill.

20. Correct answer: (a)

    Rationale: Skin integrity is the primary concern of these choices. Paraffin is a much localized thermal modality. The last two choices are not contraindications.

    Reference: Hayes, K. (2002). *Manual for physical agents* (5th ed., p. 13). New York: Prentice.

21. Correct answer: (d)

    Rationale: Metal implants are not contraindicated for superficial heat interventions.

    Reference: Prentice, W. (2002). *Therapeutic modalities for physical therapists* (2nd ed., p. 225). New York: McGraw-Hill.

22. Correct answer: (d)

    Rationale: This is the only effective intervention that would address the large muscles of the hamstrings resulting in decreased sensory input, and improved tolerance to stretching.

    Reference: Cameron, M. (1999). *Physical agents in rehabilitation: From research to practice* (p. 145). Philadelphia: WB Saunders.

ULTRASOUND AND PHONOPHORESIS

Twenty Items

1. Correct answer: (b)

   Rationale: Ultrasound produces heat by means of conversion.

   Reference: Behrens, B., & Michlovitz, S. (1996). *Physical agents: Theory and practice for the physical therapist assistant* (p. 55). Philadelphia: FA Davis.

2. Correct answer: (c)

   Rationale: Phonophoresis is the application of medication through the skin using ultrasound.

   Reference: Prentice, W. (2002). *Therapeutic modalities for physical therapists* (2nd ed., p. 133). New York: McGraw-Hill.

3. Correct answer: (a)

   Rationale: Gel and water are required mediums for the application of therapeutic ultrasound. Without a medium, the acoustic waves may damage the ultrasound applicator.

   Reference: Prentice, W. (2002). *Therapeutic modalities for physical therapists* (2nd ed., p. 289). New York: McGraw-Hill.

4. Correct answer: (d)

   Rationale: Although there are thermal effects with pulsed ultrasound applications, vigorous heating does not occur in the pulsed mode.

   Reference: Behrens, B., & Michlovitz, S. (1996). *Physical agents: Theory and practice for the physical therapist assistant* (p. 96). Philadelphia: FA Davis.

5. Correct answer: (b)

   Rationale: These effects are both stimulated by soft tissue mobilization and therapeutic heating.

   Reference: Hayes, K. (2002). *Manual for physical agents* (5th ed., p. 3, 4). New York: Prentice.

6. Correct answer: (c)

   Rationale: The other choices are not contraindications as they are presented. Ultrasound should not be applied over the specific area of pregnancy or cancer.

   Reference: Michlovitz, S. (1990). *Thermal agents in rehabilitation* (2nd ed., pp. 162–164). Philadelphia: FA Davis.

7. Correct answer: (d)

   Rationale: The indirect application is indicated when treating an irregular portion of the extremity. All of the other statements are when using water as the coupling agent.

   Reference: Hayes, K. (2002). *Manual for physical agents* (5th ed., p. 46, 47). New York: Prentice Hall.

8. Correct answer: (c)

   Rationale: Although each of these needs to be addressed, corrected, and prevented when possible, only the BNR > 6.0 would pose the potential danger for some treatment areas of the skin receiving more than the input dosage.

   Reference: Prentice, W. (2002). *Therapeutic modalities for physical therapists* (2nd ed., p. 279). New York: McGraw-Hill.

9. Correct answer: (a)

   Rationale: With attenuation increased by the application of moist heat packs, there is less penetration of ultrasound following.

   Reference: Prentice, W. (2002). *Therapeutic modalities for physical therapists* (2nd ed., p. 301). New York: McGraw-Hill.

10. Correct answer: (a)

    Rationale: Application of ultrasound over the spinal cord is only a contraindication after removal of the lamina.

    Reference: Hayes, K. (2002). *Manual for physical agents* (5th ed., p. 45). New York: Prentice.

11. Correct answer: (b)

    Rationale: The irregular shape around the anatomical snuff-box would indicate use of indirect ultrasound application.

    Reference: Hayes, K. (2002). *Manual for physical agents* (5th ed., p. 46). New York: Prentice.

12. Correct answer: (c)

    Rationale: This is determined through calibration and is not apparent to visual inspection of the ultrasound applicator.

    Reference: Prentice, W. (2002). *Therapeutic modalities for physical therapists* (2nd ed., p. 275). New York: McGraw-Hill.

13. Correct answer: (d)

    Rationale: The higher, 3 megahertz setting produces a sound wave that is absorbed more superficially.
    Reference: Behrens, B., & Michlovitz, S. (1996). *Physical agents: Theory and practice for the physical therapist assistant* (p. 86). Philadelphia: FA Davis.

14. Correct answer: (a)

    Rationale: The intensity is expressed in watts per centimeter squared.
    Reference: Behrens, B., & Michlovitz, S. (1996). *Physical agents: Theory and practice for the physical therapist assistant* (p. 87). Philadelphia: FA Davis.

15. Correct answer: (a)

    Rationale: Ultrasound can be safely applied over metallic implants but not over methylmethacrylate cement.
    Reference: Cameron, M. (1999). *Physical agents in rehabilitation: From research to practice* (p. 291). Philadelphia: WB Saunders.

16. Correct answer: (c)

Rationale: At 4.0 centimeters of muscle, 70% of the energy has been attenuated.

Reference: Behrens, B., & Michlovitz, S. (1996). *Physical agents: Theory and practice for the physical therapist assistant* (p. 86). Philadelphia: FA Davis.

17. Correct answer: (d)

Rationale: This is a maximum intensity guideline for treating subacromial bursitis.

Reference: Prentice, W. (2002). *Therapeutic modalities for physical therapists* (2nd ed., p. 284, 285). New York: McGraw-Hill.

18. Correct answer: (b)

Rationale: Tendon tissue absorbs a greater amount of energy than skin, muscle, or fat.

Reference: Cameron, M. (1999). *Physical agents in rehabilitation: From research to practice* (p. 277). Philadelphia: WB Saunders.

19. Correct answer: (d)

Rationale: Traditionally the stationary technique has been used for small areas, however due to the undesired effects of fixed spatial-peak intensities, it is no longer recommended.

Reference: Prentice, W. (2002). *Therapeutic modalities for physical therapists* (2nd ed., p. 292). New York: McGraw-Hill.

20. Correct answer: (c)

Rationale: A 3 MHz setting is most appropriate for tissue that is 1–2 centimeters thick.

Reference: Cameron, M. (1999). *Physical agents in rehabilitation: From research to practice* (p. 292). Philadelphia: WB Saunders.

ELECTRICAL STIMULATION AND IONTOPHORESIS

Twenty-two Items

1. Correct answer: (a)

Rationale: The last choice is self-contradictory. The preferred current is interferential stimulation at 75–150 pulses per second during acute episodes of pain relief.

Reference: Behrens, B., & Michlovitz, S. (1996). *Physical agents: Theory and practice for the physical therapist assistant* (p. 339). Philadelphia: FA Davis.

2. Correct answer: (a)

Rationale: Sensory level, negative high-voltage, has been shown to inhibit wound infection.

Reference: Guccione, A. (2000). *Geriatric physical therapy* (2nd ed., p. 389). St. Louis: Mosby.

3. Correct answer: (c)

Rationale: Russian stimulation units provide carrier frequencies of 2400–2500 hertz.

Reference: Behrens, B., & Michlovitz, S. (1996). *Physical agents: Theory and practice for the physical therapist assistant* (p. 360). Philadelphia: FA Davis.

4. Correct answer: (d)

   Rationale: The tens unit is portable and user friendly, which allows the patient more control of the settings and application.

   Reference: Behrens, B., & Michlovitz, S. (1996). *Physical agents: Theory and practice for the physical therapist assistant* (pp. 348–350). Philadelphia: FA Davis.

5. Correct answer: (d)

   Rationale: Each of the statements regarding microcurrent is accurate.

   Reference: Prentice, W. (2002). *Therapeutic modalities for physical therapists* (2nd ed., p. 108). New York: McGraw-Hill.

6. Correct answer: (d)

   Rationale: Typically, high-voltage stimulators require the use of a dispersive pad.

   Reference: Hayes, K. (2002). *Manual for physical agents* (5th ed., p. 165). New York: Prentice.

7. Correct answer: (d)

   Rationale: Biphasic current at a medium range of bursts, and duration between 40 and 500 microseconds, has been shown to be effective in addressing motor weakness.

   Reference: Behrens, B., & Michlovitz, S. (1996). *Physical agents: Theory and practice for the physical therapist assistant* (p. 284, 285). Philadelphia: FA Davis.

8. Correct answer: (a)

   Rationale: A tens unit does not directly address vascular function, or volitional recruitment.

   Reference: Behrens, B., & Michlovitz, S. (1996). *Physical agents: Theory and practice for the physical therapist assistant* (p. 350). Philadelphia: FA Davis.

9. Correct answer: (a)

   Rationale: The cathode is negative and should be placed at the site of edema.

   Reference: Cameron, M. (1999). *Physical agents in rehabilitation: From research to practice* (p. 396). Philadelphia: WB Saunders.

10. Correct answer: (a)

    Rationale: A 200–300 microsecond pulse width, with a frequency of more than 30 hertz is effective in achieving muscle contraction.

    Reference: Hayes, K. (2002). *Manual for physical agents* (5th ed., p. 106). New York: Prentice.

11. Correct answer: (a)

    Rationale: Improving the moisture content of the skin will decrease the impedance and improve conductivity.

    Reference: Hayes, K. (2002). *Manual for physical agents* (5th ed., p. 106). New York: Prentice.

12. Correct answer: (d)

Rationale: Typically interferential stimulation is directed at a sensory level response, and requires four electrodes for the resultant interference. These currents at 0–5 beats per second may be capable of producing a minor motor response.

Reference: Hayes, K. (2002). *Manual for physical agents* (5th ed., p. 151). New York: Prentice.

13. Correct answer: (c)

Rationale: Low-voltage direct current is sufficient in producing the desired contraction.

Reference: Hayes, K. (2002). *Manual for physical agents* (5th ed., p. 110, 111). New York: Prentice.

14. Correct answer: (a)

Rationale: The cathode should be twice the size of the anode to reduce alkaline reactions in the skin. Some newer iontophoresis units prevent this with buffered medications.

Reference: Behrens, B., & Michlovitz, S. (1996). *Physical agents: Theory and practice for the physical therapist assistant* (p. 323). Philadelphia: FA Davis.

15. Correct answer: (b)

Rationale: Motor recruitment is better achieved at a 35–50 hertz frequency.

Reference: Behrens, B., & Michlovitz, S. (1996). *Physical agents: Theory and practice for the physical therapist assistant* (p. 360). Philadelphia: FA Davis.

16. Correct answer: (b)

Rationale: Direct current can produce twitch contractions; alternating current can produce tetanic contractions, and at least 5 milliamps is required for a motor response. The finger tips are capable of sensory stimulus at levels less than 1 milliamp.

Reference: Behrens, B., & Michlovitz, S. (1996). *Physical agents: Theory and practice for the physical therapist assistant* (p. 255). Philadelphia: FA Davis.

17. Correct answer: (d)

Rationale: Neuromuscular stimulation is effective in increasing peripheral circulation, endurance, and reducing spasticity.

Reference: Hayes, K. (2002). *Manual for physical agents* (5th ed., pp. 108–110). New York: Prentice.

18. Correct answer: (d)

Rationale: Targeting the painful tissue is difficult due to current density being greater under the location of the electrodes and the variation in tissue resistance.

Reference: Hayes, K. (2002). *Manual for physical agents* (5th ed., pp. 151, 153). New York: Prentice.

19. Correct answer: (c)

Rationale: A tens unit can be applied over a herniated disk. Each of the others is considered a contraindication for transcutaneous electrical nerve stimulation.

Reference: Hayes, K. (2002). *Manual for physical agents* (5th ed., p. 124). New York: Prentice.

20. Correct answer: (d)

Rationale: Neuromuscular stimulation can be effective in addressing spasticity.

Reference: Hayes, K. (2002). *Manual for physical agents* (5th ed., p. 109). New York: Prentice.

21. Correct answer: (b)

Rationale: The first and last choices are utilized to increase temperature and promote healing. The third choice is most appropriate in addressing pain.

Reference: Behrens, B., & Michlovitz, S. (1996). *Physical agents: Theory and practice for the physical therapist assistant* (p. 355). Philadelphia: FA Davis.

22. Correct answer: (c)

Rationale: Each of the other choices is a general contraindication for electrical stimulation. A person who is deconditioned is not specifically contraindicated for electrical stimulation.

Reference: Behrens, B., & Michlovitz, S. (1996). *Physical agents: Theory and practice for the physical therapist assistant* (p. 254). Philadelphia: FA Davis.

BIOFEEDBACK

Six Items

1. Correct answer: (c)

Rationale: Cleaning and abrading the skin increases detection of motor unit action potentials.

Reference: Hayes, K. (2002). *Manual for physical agents* (5th ed., p. 192). New York: Prentice.

2. Correct answer: (d)

Rationale: This is the only choice innervated by the median nerve.

Reference: Lippert, L. (2000). *Clinical kinesiology for physical therapist assistants* (3rd ed., p. 180). Philadelphia: FA Davis.

3. Correct answer: (a)

Rationale: Set the initial threshold just above the baseline and increase as necessary to encourage the person to increase recruitment.

Reference: Hayes, K. (2002). *Manual for physical agents* (5th ed., p. 192, 193). New York: Prentice.

4. Correct answer: (a)

Rationale: Any form of visual or auditory feedback can be described as biofeedback, including the traditional method of electrical myography. Open practice does not provide feedback.

Reference: Kisner, C., & Colby, L. (2002). *Therapeutic exercise: Foundations and techniques* (4th ed., p. 198). Philadelphia: FA Davis.

5. Correct answer: (a)

Rationale: The closer the detection electrodes, the lesser is the electrical noise detection.

Reference: Hayes, K. (2002). *Manual for physical agents* (5th ed., p. 192). New York: Prentice.

6. Correct answer: (a)

   Rationale: The inhibition application monitors the muscle that needs to relax (the agonist).

   Reference: Hayes, K. (2002). *Manual for physical agents* (5th ed., p. 193). New York: Prentice.

MECHANICAL MODALITIES—SPINAL TRACTION, TILT TABLE, STANDING FRAMES, AND CONTINUOUS PASSIVE MOTION DEVICES

Twenty-two Items

1. Correct answer: (a)

   Rationale: Injuries at or above T6 present risk of autonomic dysreflexia.

   Reference: Somers, M. (2001). *Spinal cord injury: Functional rehabilitation* (2nd ed., p. 35). New Jersey: Prentice Hall.

2. Correct answer: (d)

   Rationale: The application for traction to address discogenic pain should avoid prolonged pull times or duration, which may lead to an increase in intradiscal pressure.

   Reference: Hayes, K. (2002). *Manual for physical agents* (5th ed., p. 100). New York: Prentice.

3. Correct answer: (b)

   Rationale: A low velocity has been shown superior to higher velocities.

   Reference: Behrens, B., & Michlovitz, S. (1996). *Physical agents: Theory and practice for the physical therapist assistant* (p. 194). Philadelphia: FA Davis.

4. Correct answer: (c)

   Rationale: Of these choices, only osteoporosis is a precaution for mechanical pelvic traction.

   Reference: Prentice, W. (2002). *Therapeutic modalities for physical therapists* (2nd ed., p. 389). New York: McGraw-Hill.

5. Correct answer: (c)

   Rationale: 7 seconds has been shown to be the minimal time to achieve maximal vertebral separation.

   Reference: Behrens, B., & Michlovitz, S. (1996). *Physical agents: Theory and practice for the physical therapist assistant* (p. 168). Philadelphia: FA Davis.

6. Correct answer: (a)

   Rationale: Positioning can positively impact muscle tone, but standing does not result in extensor effects in the upper extremity.

   Reference: Campbell, S., et al. (2000). *Physical therapy for children* (2nd ed., p. 136). Philadelphia: WB Saunders.

7. Correct answer: (a)

   Rationale: A CPM does not increase tissue formation, rather facilitates mobility and alignment of the tissue.

   Reference: Cameron, M. (1999). *Physical agents in rehabilitation: From research to practice* (p. 81). Philadelphia: WB Saunders.

8. Correct answer: (c)

   Rationale: Each of these interventions is appropriate to address orthostatic hypotension, though the parallel bars are least tolerable early on.

   Reference: Pierson, F. (2002). *Principles and techniques of patient care* (3rd ed., p. 216). Philadelphia: WB Saunders.

9. Correct answer: (a)

   Rationale: Each of these statements is true about the standing frame, but monitoring their vital signs is most important.

   Reference: O'Sullivan. (2001). *Physical rehabilitation assessment and treatment* (4th ed., p. 909). Philadelphia: FA Davis.

10. Correct answer: (c)

    Rationale: Mechanical spinal traction can exacerbate medial disk protrusions and spinal hypermobility. Traction interventions are contraindicated for fused joints.

    Reference: Prentice, W. (2002). *Therapeutic modalities for physical therapists* (2nd ed., p. 389). New York: McGraw-Hill.

11. Correct answer: (d)

    Rationale: A 25° angle has been shown to best increase intervertebral space.

    Reference: Behrens, B., & Michlovitz, S. (1996). *Physical agents: Theory and practice for the physical therapist assistant* (p. 168). Philadelphia: FA Davis.

12. Correct answer: (b)

    Rationale: Recent spinal fractures are absolutely contraindicated; however, pregnancy and respiratory insufficiency are only relative contraindications. Spinal stenosis is an indication for spinal traction.

    Reference: Hayes, K. (2002). *Manual for physical agents* (5th ed., p. 92, 93). New York: Prentice.

13. Correct answer: (d)

    Rationale: A strap should not be placed over the cervical spine when using the tilt table. The head and neck can be stabilized with padded wedges, bolsters, or pillows.

    Reference: Minor, M., & Minor, S. (1999). *Patient care skills* (p. 311).

14. Correct answer: (b)

    Rationale: The physical therapist needs to reevaluate a patient who is pain free after one visit. The concern is that the traction may have increased the compression upon the nerve root.

Reference: Cameron, M. (1999). *Physical agents in rehabilitation: From research to practice* (p. 225). Philadelphia: WB Saunders.

15. Correct answer: (c)

Rationale: The vertebral arteries are protected within the cervical vertebrae. Certain pathologies involving these arteries may be considered precautions for many interventions.

Reference: Cameron, M. (1999). *Physical agents in rehabilitation: From research to practice* (p. 225). Philadelphia: WB Saunders.

16. Correct answer: (c)

Rationale: Function up to the eighth thoracic neurological level is typically required for adequate stabilization of the trunk and pelvis.

Reference: O'Sullivan. (2001). *Physical rehabilitation assessment and treatment* (4th ed., p. 909). Philadelphia: FA Davis.

17. Correct answer: (c)

Rationale: The tilt table affects the skin through a change of contact pressure; it also affects breathing and heart functions. The endocrine system is least affected.

Reference: Pierson, F. (2002). *Principles and techniques of patient care* (3rd ed., p. 216). Philadelphia: WB Saunders.

18. Correct answer: (a)

Rationale: The prone application of lumbar traction promotes the extension posture of the lumbar spine.

Reference: Cameron, M. (1999). *Physical agents in rehabilitation: From research to practice* (p. 231). Philadelphia: WB Saunders.

19. Correct answer: (c)

Rationale: Self-traction can be useful for low-load lumbar distraction. Self-traction is not used for the cervical region of the spine. Traction to address cervical disks is applied with a 60 second pull and a 20 second release.

Reference: Cameron, M. (1999). *Physical agents in rehabilitation: From research to practice* (p. 237, 238). Philadelphia: WB Saunders.

20. Correct answer: (c)

Rationale: A decrease in pedal pulse would more likely represent a lack of tolerance to the tilt table. An increase in pedal pulses may represent an increase in peripheral circulation.

Reference: Pierson, F. (2002). *Principles and techniques of patient care* (3rd ed., p. 216). Philadelphia: WB Saunders.

21. Correct answer: (c)

Rationale: Facing toward the door, with over-the-door home traction units, will promote cervical flexion.

Reference: Cameron, M. (1999). *Physical agents in rehabilitation: From research to practice* (p. 232). Philadelphia: WB Saunders.

22. Correct answer: (d)

    Rationale: Pressure on the spinal cord is considered a precaution for mechanical spinal traction.

    Reference: Behrens, B., & Michlovitz, S. (1996). *Physical agents: Theory and practice for the physical therapist assistant* (p. 178). Philadelphia: FA Davis.

WHIRLPOOLS AND HUBBARD TANKS

Seventeen Items

1. Correct answer: (c)

   Rationale: Circulatory insufficiency can be addressed by whirlpools, but active wound bleeding may be exacerbated with vasodilatation effects of the whirlpool.

   Reference: Cameron, M. (1999). *Physical agents in rehabilitation: From research to practice* (p. 191). Philadelphia: WB Saunders.

2. Correct answer: (b)

   Rationale: Hubbard tank treatments should not exceed 102°, especially since a larger portion of the person's body is typically submerged and they are less capable of dissipating heat from their body.

   Reference: Hayes, K. (2002). *Manual for physical agents* (5th ed., p. 28). New York: Prentice.

3. Correct answer: (b)

   Rationale: Open wounds are typically treated between 94° and 98°.

   Reference: Behrens, B., & Michlovitz, S. (1996). *Physical agents: Theory and practice for the physical therapist assistant* (p. 141). Philadelphia: FA Davis.

4. Correct answer: (c)

   Rationale: The correct concentration of chloramines-T is 50 grams per 60 gallons of water.

   Reference: Behrens, B., & Michlovitz, S. (1996). *Physical agents: Theory and practice for the physical therapist assistant* (p. 141). Philadelphia: FA Davis.

5. Correct answer: (d)

   Rationale: This is one example of an acceptable cleansing material.

   Reference: Hayes, K. (2002). *Manual for physical agents* (5th ed., p. 28). New York: Prentice.

6. Correct answer: (a)

   Rationale: Conduction of heat occurs with direct contact between two objects of differing temperature.

   Reference: Behrens, B., & Michlovitz, S. (1996). *Physical agents: Theory and practice for the physical therapist assistant* (p. 22). Philadelphia: FA Davis.

7. Correct answer: (b)

   Rationale: A person submerged in a whirlpool tank should not operate or assist with the operation of any of the electrical devices because they are not properly grounded.

   Reference: Hayes, K. (2002). *Manual for physical agents* (5th ed., p. 28). New York: Prentice.

8. Correct answer: (c)

   Rationale: A person being treated in a highboy tank must be able to flex their knee and hip to achieve a safe posture.

   Reference: Michlovitz, S. (1990). *Thermal agents in rehabilitation* (2nd ed., p. 118, 119). Philadelphia: FA Davis.

9. Correct answer: (d)

   Rationale: The correct suggested dilution ratio is one part sodium hypochlorite to one hundred parts water.

   Reference: Behrens, B., & Michlovitz, S. (1996). *Physical agents: Theory and practice for the physical therapist assistant* (p. 155). Philadelphia: FA Davis.

10. Correct answer: (a)

    Rationale: Wounds that are primarily closed, and have epithelialization and granulation, may suffer more damage than benefit from whirlpool intervention.

    Reference: Behrens, B., & Michlovitz, S. (1996). *Physical agents: Theory and practice for the physical therapist assistant* (p. 154). Philadelphia: FA Davis.

11. Correct answer: (c)

    Rationale: Each of the other choices are risks directly related to the use of an extremity tank, due to the person having to hang their extremity over the edge of the tank, in a dependent position.

    Reference: Behrens, B., & Michlovitz, S. (1996). *Physical agents: Theory and practice for the physical therapist assistant* (p. 155). Philadelphia: FA Davis.

12. Correct answer: (c)

    Rationale: Convection occurs when a medium such as air or water moves past an object of a different temperature. Convection produces a more rapid heat exchange than direct contact.

    Reference: Behrens, B., & Michlovitz, S. (1996). *Physical agents: Theory and practice for the physical therapist assistant* (p. 22). Philadelphia: FA Davis.

13. Correct answer: (b)

    Rationale: The choices provide 2.0, 1.2, 4.5, and 30 pounds per square inch, respectively.

    Reference: Cameron, M. (1999). *Physical agents in rehabilitation: From research to practice* (p. 185). Philadelphia: WB Saunders.

14. Correct answer: (c)

    Rationale: Whirlpool intervention provides nonselective mechanical debridement to open tissues.

    Reference: Behrens, B., & Michlovitz, S. (1996). *Physical agents: Theory and practice for the physical therapist assistant* (p. 151). Philadelphia: FA Davis.

15. Correct answer: (d)

    Rationale: Each of the other tissue conditions may benefit from whirlpool interventions. Cellulitis is contraindicated for whirlpool interventions.

    Reference: Behrens, B., & Michlovitz, S. (1996). *Physical agents: Theory and practice for the physical therapist assistant* (p. 151). Philadelphia: FA Davis.

16. Correct answer: (a)

    Rationale: Open wounds often have descriptive odors, color, shapes, and sizes present. Peripheral pressure is not necessary for documenting the status of the wound.

    Reference: Behrens, B., & Michlovitz, S. (1996). *Physical agents: Theory and practice for the physical therapist assistant* (p. 153). Philadelphia: FA Davis.

17. Correct answer: (b)

    Rationale: Malodorous or exudating wounds may benefit from hydrotherapy intervention for cleansing. Wounds with greater than 50% eschar, granulation, or cellulitis will not benefit from hydrotherapy interventions.

    Reference: Behrens, B., & Michlovitz, S. (1996). *Physical agents: Theory and practice for the physical therapist assistant* (p. 154). Philadelphia: FA Davis.

Procedural Interventions Group IV: Airway Clearance, Wound Care, Health and Wellness, Monitoring Patient Responses, and Modifying Interventions

OVERVIEW

This chapter includes questions covering procedural interventions included in the exam. There are 54 questions in this chapter that deal with airway clearance, wound care, skin integrity, monitoring patient responses, and modifying interventions.

KEY POINTS FOR REVIEW

Airway Clearance

- Breathing strategies
- Manual techniques
- Mechanical techniques
- Positioning

Wound Care and Skin Integrity

- Monitoring skin status
- Positioning to prevent pressure
- Protective equipment
- Dressing application and removal
- Topical agents
- Nonsharp debridement

Monitoring Patient Responses and Modifying Interventions Accordingly

- Modality adjustments
- Exercise progression/regression
- Medical precautions
- Body mechanics
- Muscle recruitment

Health and Wellness

- Health and prevention

AIRWAY CLEARANCE TECHNIQUES— BREATHING STRATEGIES

Six Items

1. Which intervention should be incorporated into patient education with someone at risk for cerebral vascular accidents or rupture of an aneurysm?

   _____ a. splinting

   _____ b. huffing

   _____ c. facilitated cough

   _____ d. paroxysmal cough

2. Which of the following should be included in the instructions for facilitating an effective cough?

   _____ a. sitting or leaning forward

   _____ b. contraction of the abdominals

   _____ c. have the person make a forceful "k" sound

   _____ d. all of these should be included

3. Which of the following is LEAST appropriate concerning airway clearance strategies?

   _____ a. incorporate anterior splinting for persons with recent unhealed abdominal incisions

   _____ b. utilize proper suctioning to clear the trachea and main stem bronchi

   _____ c. paroxysmal coughing will facilitate bronchial airway clearance

   _____ d. avoid suctioning which is contraindicated for persons with artificial airways

4. Which breathing strategy would be MOST beneficial for a person with chronic obstructive pulmonary disease (COPD)?

   _____ a. perform activities while pacing forced expirations

   _____ b. nonforceful, pursed-lip inspiration

____ c. nonforceful, pursed-lip expiration

____ d. forceful pursed-lip breathing

5. A person is performing therapeutic strengthening activities in the physical therapy area. Which strategy would BEST assist the person's performance during the exercise session?

____ a. involuntary breathing

____ b. accessory breathing

____ c. diaphragmatic breathing

____ d. segmental breathing

6. A person being treated with airway clearance interventions has chronic obstructive pulmonary disease. Which airway clearance technique produces the LEAST increase in intrathoracic pressure?

____ a. splinting

____ b. huffing

____ c. facilitated cough

____ d. paroxysmal cough

AIRWAY CLEARANCE TECHNIQUES—MANUAL AND MECHANICAL TECHNIQUES

Three Items

1. Which vibration technique is MOST appropriate for airway clearance interventions?

____ a. vibration is used in conjunction with postural drainage and percussive interventions

____ b. pressure is applied in the same direction that the chest wall is moving

____ c. vibration is used in conjunction with mechanical suctioning

____ d. pressure is applied with both hands directly upon the skin during the exhalation phase

2. Which manual airway clearance technique is MOST appropriate for percussive interventions?

____ a. providing percussive interventions only by mechanical equipment

____ b. percussive interventions should not be provided by a physical therapist assistant

____ c. applying percussive interventions continuously for several minutes, or until the patient needs to cough

____ d. utilizing percussive interventions to reduce pulmonary embolism

3. Which procedure must be done prior to suctioning a person on an artificial airway?

____ a. provide manual resuscitator bag to increase arterial oxygenation

____ b. monitor oxygen saturation and ensure it is greater than 90%

____ c. check to see if the person can exhale forcefully

____ d. donn sterile gloves

AIRWAY CLEARANCE TECHNIQUES—POSITIONING

Three Items

1. A person, 12 years of age, who has been diagnosed with cystic fibrosis, is delegated to you for postural drainage. Is this appropriate, and if so, how would you position the person to clear the lateral segments of the lower lobes?

   _____ a. no, this intervention is contraindicated

   _____ b. yes, this intervention is appropriate; position prone with the head slightly higher than the trunk

   _____ c. yes, this intervention is appropriate; position in sidelying with the head slightly lower than the trunk

   _____ d. this intervention is not contraindicated, but should only be performed by a physical therapist

2. A person was admitted to an inpatient physical therapy setting yesterday afternoon. After participating in an early morning therapy session, you return the person to their room. The person is tired and asks to return to bed and take a nap. Which condition is MOST likely to indicate that the person should avoid laying flat in bed?

   _____ a. dysphasia

   _____ b. dysphagia

   _____ c. recent lumbar laminectomy

   _____ d. cardiomyopathy

3. A person has a pulmonary condition that indicates postural drainage intervention. During treatment, where should the lung segment that you intend to aid by postural drainage be positioned?

   _____ a. horizontal

   _____ b. sagittal

   _____ c. frontal

   _____ d. vertical

WOUND CARE AND SKIN INTEGRITY— MONITOR SKIN STATUS

Three Items

1. A person recently suffered superficial partial thickness burns over their anterior left thigh, from a hot liquid. Which of the following descriptions is MOST correct about partial thickness burns?

   _____ a. healing typically occurs without evidence of scarring

   _____ b. the epidermis is involved but typically not the dermis

   _____ c. the area is typically discolored, blistered, with moderate to severe levels of pain

   _____ d. the dermis and epidermis are destroyed, with damage also to the subcutaneous fat layer

2. You are seeing a person bedside to address functional mobility. Upon rolling them onto their side to secure their pants, you observe an area of skin with erythema, which dissipates several minutes after the pressure has been removed. Which of these descriptions should be documented regarding this area of their skin?

    _____ a. stage one skin ulcer

    _____ b. stage two skin ulcer

    _____ c. stage three skin ulcer

    _____ d. macerated decubitus ulcer

3. A person presents with a plantar ulcer for whirlpool and sterile dressing interventions. After removing the wound dressing, you observe that the skin appears cold and pale with moderate drainage, but the person complains of no pain. Which condition MOST likely led to this type of wound?

    _____ a. acute arterial insufficiency

    _____ b. chronic venous insufficiency

    _____ c. chronic arterial insufficiency

    _____ d. acute venous insufficiency

WOUND CARE AND SKIN INTEGRITY—PATIENT POSITIONING AND USE OF ADAPTIVE AND PROTECTIVE DEVICES FOR PRESSURE RELIEF

Seven Items

1. A person, who experienced a flash-steam burn injury to the right axillary region, is being treated at your facility. What instructions should be given to the patient regarding positioning?

    _____ a. place in the position of comfort

    _____ b. place in the position of shoulder abduction, and flexion

    _____ c. place in the position of shoulder abduction, and extension

    _____ d. place in the position of shoulder adduction

2. A person with a burn at their left elbow should be placed in which positions to prevent undesired contractures?

    _____ a. humeroulnar extension and radioulnar supination

    _____ b. humeroulnar flexion and radioulnar pronation

    _____ c. humeroulnar extension and radioulnar pronation

    _____ d. humeroulnar flexion and radioulnar supination

3. A person who has been admitted to an extended care facility requires daily use of a wheelchair as their primary mode of mobility. Which approach is BEST for preventing the development of pressure lesions upon this person's skin during extended wheelchair use?

_____ a. have the person participate in a group exercise course to improve circulation and decrease body fat

_____ b. teach the person to perform weight-shifting every 2 hours

_____ c. order a high-back reclining wheelchair

_____ d. place two to three standard cushions in the seat of the wheelchair and include adjustable leg rests

4. When leaving a person in bed for a prolonged period of time, who is dependent in bed mobility and transfers, it is necessary to pad bony prominences. What is the primary purpose of padding bony prominences during prolonged static positioning?

_____ a. prevent contractures

_____ b. prevent skin breakdown

_____ c. promote patient comfort

_____ d. promote circulation

5. A person who spends a significant duration of time in a wheelchair is more susceptible to skin breakdown at the ischial tuberosities. Which intervention would be LEAST appropriate in addressing pressure relief goals for a person with an incomplete spinal cord injury at the tenth thoracic neurological level?

_____ a. wheelchair cushion

_____ b. wheelchair push-ups

_____ c. power wheelchair with tilt in space function

_____ d. regularly scheduled position changes

6. Which description is LEAST consistent with deep partial-thickness burns?

_____ a. there is damage to the epidermis

_____ b. the skin may have a mottled appearance

_____ c. there is only mild to no pain, due to nerve damage

_____ d. the skin may be red and moist

7. Burn injuries affecting the fingers are typically addressed with hand splints to prevent contractures. Which position is MOST likely to develop into contractures after burn injury to the fingers and hand?

_____ a. metacarpal phalangeal extension

_____ b. first digit abduction

_____ c. interphalangeal flexion

_____ d. radiocarpal extension

WOUND CARE AND SKIN INTEGRITY— DRESSING APPLICATION AND REMOVAL

Four Items

1. Which of the following methods of wound care should be utilized for effective dressing application?

_____ a. dressings applied to the lower extremity should conceal the toes and feet to catch any potential drainage

_____ b. dressing should extend at least 1″ beyond the border of the wound

_____ c. bandages that slip should be securely covered in place with an additional gauze wrap

_____ d. avoid overlapping of the gauze wrap with each turn to reduce wrinkles

2. You are preparing to apply a sterile wound dressing to a person after a pulsed-lavage treatment. What materials are needed first for preparing to apply a sterile wound dressing?

_____ a. sterile gauze and wrap

_____ b. sterile field

_____ c. sterile gloves

_____ d. sterile bandage scissors

3. Which technique is LEAST appropriate for removing a wound dressing from a person with an open wound adhering to the bandage?

_____ a. slowly removing the dressing while avoiding stimulating new bleeding

_____ b. allowing the dressing to soak in clean water

_____ c. lavaging the wound with sterile water

_____ d. placing the person in the whirlpool and turning the turbine on low

4. Which technique is MOST appropriate regarding wound dressings?

_____ a. observing for color changes in the distal segment of the extremity may indicate that the dressing is too tight

_____ b. using metal clips or additional taping to a person's skin if necessary to secure the dressing

_____ c. once a sterile dressing has covered the open wound, the clinician's gloves may be removed to improve dexterity

_____ d. sterile gauze wrap should be applied with the outside of the wrap facing toward the person's skin

WOUND CARE AND SKIN INTEGRITY— TOPICAL AGENTS APPLICATION

Three Items

1. Which of the following wound dressings have absorptive properties?

_____ a. wet to dry dressing

_____ b. impregnated gauze

_____ c. biosynthetics

_____ d. Unna's boot

2. Which characteristic is most accurate regarding wet to dry saline gauze applications?

_____ a. wet to dry applications have debridement and absorptive properties

_____ b. wet to dry applications have only absorptive properties

_____ c. wet to dry applications are contraindicated for stage four ulcerations

_____ d. wet to dry applications have only debridement properties

3. What is the appropriate thickness application for silvadene?

_____ a. 1–2 millimeters

_____ b. 6–8 millimeters

_____ c. 2–4 millimeters

_____ d. 8–10 millimeters

WOUND CARE AND SKIN INTEGRITY — DEBRIDEMENT TECHNIQUES EXCEPT SHARP

Two Items

1. A person who sustained a burn injury to the left forearm. Which of the following interventions is MOST appropriate for facilitation autolytic debridement?

_____ a. cathodal stimulation

_____ b. anodal stimulation

_____ c. biphasic stimulation

_____ d. quadripolar stimulation

2. A person has a diabetic ulcer at their left calcaneus. Which chemical debridement intervention is indicated for this person?

_____ a. hydrocolloids

_____ b. sterile saline

_____ c. pulsed lavage

_____ d. whirlpool

MONITORING PATIENT RESPONSES AND MODIFYING INTERVENTIONS

Seventeen Items

1. A person has received pulsed ultrasound intervention for 8 minutes at 1.5 watts per square centimeters to the lumbar erector spinae, followed by soft tissue mobilization, for 2 weeks. The patient

continues to tell you that the treatment has not made any significant changes in their symptoms at all. You will probably help the patient the MOST by doing which of the following?

_____ a. changing the ultrasound setting to continuous

_____ b. extending the ultrasound treatment time to 10 minutes

_____ c. increasing the ultrasound intensity to 1.8 watts per square centimeters

_____ d. discussing the lack of progress with the physical therapist

2. A person is performing therapeutic exercises to address lateral epicondylitis. Upon teaching the person how to actively perform wrist extension, you observe that their wrist deviates towards the radius during each repetition. After demonstrating the correct motion again, you see the same deviation during attempted wrist extension. Which muscle weakness would BEST explain this occurrence?

_____ a. flexor carpi ulnaris

_____ b. extensor carpi radialis

_____ c. flexor carpi radialis

_____ d. extensor carpi ulnaris

3. A person you instruct in therapeutic exercises for the shoulder demonstrates a lack of full overhead range into flexion during the first several repetitions. Which of the following is MOST often the cause of less than full active shoulder flexion?

_____ a. excess scapular upward rotation

_____ b. lack of scapular elevation

_____ c. excess scapular elevation

_____ d. lack of scapular downward rotation

4. You are treating a person with multiple sclerosis who appears agitated and tired during the middle of a treatment session. Which modification is MOST appropriate?

_____ a. no modifications are necessary; these observations are typical of a person with multiple sclerosis

_____ b. consult with the physical therapist about applying moist heat to relax the person and decrease agitation

_____ c. decrease the intensity of the activity and provide more rest periods

_____ d. encourage the person to complete the treatment session within a reasonable amount of time

5. A person is attempting to perform 35 repetitions of supine short arc quads with both of their lower extremities, and begins to experience and complain of anterior thigh soreness after repetition 25. Which of the following is MOST accurate about this occurrence?

_____ a. the symptom is due to ischemia; you should decrease the repetitions

_____ b. the symptom is due to delayed muscle soreness; you should decrease the repetitions

_____ c. the symptom is more likely to occur as a result of concentric muscle contraction; change to eccentric or isometric activity and decrease the repetitions

_____ d. the symptom is normal; continue through at least 35 repetitions

6. A person who recently had a coronary artery bypass graft complains of lightheadedness when rising from the supine position. They have been performing active range of motion with both of their lower extremities in supine, but have not yet tolerated active range of motion in sitting. Which modification is MOST appropriate to achieve this goal?

_____ a. increase repetitions in supine

_____ b. perform exercises in semirecumbent

_____ c. perform exercises in sidelying

_____ d. add arm exercises in supine

7. A person recently had a left total knee arthroplasty. In supine, you instruct the person to place their right knee in a flexed position, with their foot flat on the treatment table. Next, you have the person perform a left straight-leg raise. While observing the straight-leg raise, you notice the abdomen bulges up throughout the concentric and eccentric phases of each repetition. Which muscle is MOST likely weak or not being recruited to cause of this observation?

_____ a. rectus abdominus

_____ b. internal oblique

_____ c. erector spinae

_____ d. transverse abdominus

8. If a person is having difficulty performing a sit-up, you should make which modification?

_____ a. provide physical assistance by pulling on their arms

_____ b. place a pillow under the person's feet

_____ c. have them perform the sit-up in the horizontal plane

_____ d. move their arms down by their side

9. Heterotropic ossification can be a complication while recovering from a spinal cord injury. If a person with a spinal cord injury complained of increasing pain, in which of the following areas would you MOST likely suspect heterotropic ossification?

_____ a. dorsal foot

_____ b. biceps

_____ c. lateral hips

_____ d. spine

10. A physician orders the tilt table for a person with orthostatic hypotension. After an evaluation, the physical therapist delegates this intervention to you to begin this afternoon. After you have transferred the person onto the tilt table, secured the patient, and elevated to 60°, the patient has a loose bowel movement. Which of the following would be appropriate?

_____ a. recline after 5 minutes in that position

_____ b. continue the treatment until full upright is achieved and their vital signs are stable

_____ c. contact the physical therapist by phone

_____ d. remove the patient from the tilt table as soon as possible

11. Which of the following is NOT a potential outcome of therapeutic strength training?
_____ a. a reduced risk of coronary heart disease
_____ b. a decreased risk for some forms of cancer
_____ c. a decreased probability of fall in the elderly
_____ d. an increase in proprioception

12. You have been providing mechanical lumbar traction to a person with low back pain. On the patient's prior visit, they rated their symptoms on a zero to ten scale as a "six." Upon the patient's current visit, they rate their symptoms as an "eight." The neurological signs of their low back pain remain unchanged. What would be the MOST appropriate treatment modification?
_____ a. decrease duration of traction
_____ b. keep the duration of traction the same, and increase the traction force
_____ c. keep the duration of traction the same, and decrease the traction force
_____ d. keep the duration of traction the same, and keep the traction force the same

13. A physical therapist delegates a person to you for continuous ultrasound for 6 minutes at 1.5 watts per square centimeters. During the first ultrasound application, the person did not tolerate the intensity setting. Which parameter adjustments SHOULD be made in this situation?
_____ a. increase the ultrasound intensity
_____ b. decrease the attenuation
_____ c. increase the duration of exposure
_____ d. use a pulsed setting and increase intensity to 1.5 watts per squared centimeters

14. A person is recovering from a prolonged period of inactivity, which has resulted in severe weakness of the upper extremities and a general lack of endurance. Currently, the person is completing a strengthening program using the Daily Adjustable Progressive Resistance Exercise (DAPRE) method. During their fourth set, the person performs 15 repetitions using 10 pounds. Which adjustment should be made to their next exercise session?
_____ a. increase repetitions by five
_____ b. increase weight by 15 pounds
_____ c. increase weight by 5 pounds
_____ d. increase repetitions by 15

15. A person, who is recovering from a motor vehicle crash, is participating in therapeutic strengthening in a physical therapy setting. During their first set, using a 10 pound weight on a pulley system, they perform ten repetitions. Which progression would follow in the second set based upon the Oxford method of exercise progression?
_____ a. ten repetitions using a $7\frac{1}{2}$ pound weight
_____ b. 20 repetitions using a 6 pound weight
_____ c. ten repetitions using a 12 pound weight
_____ d. ten repetitions using a 1 pound weight

16. A person is performing therapeutic strengthening based upon the Daily Adjustable Progressive Resistance Exercise model. During their third set, using 9 pounds, they achieved five repetitions. Based upon this information, which adjustments should be made to the fourth set?

_____ a. increase to ten repetitions using the same weight

_____ b. perform five repetitions using a 7 pound weight

_____ c. perform as many repetitions as possible using a 9 pound weight

_____ d. increase to ten repetitions using a 5 pound weight

17. You are applying an ice massage to a person to address lateral epicondylitis. During the intervention, you observe that the skin is beginning to consistently blanche and the person reports numbness. Which action is MOST appropriate?

_____ a. cease the application of the ice massage

_____ b. continue until full complete blanching of the epidermis is achieved

_____ c. continue until 8 minutes of intervention are completed

_____ d. check with the physical therapist

HEALTH AND WELLNESS—PREVENTION, INSTRUCTION, AND INTERVENTIONS

Six Items

1. A person has just recovered from their fifth ankle sprain in 12 years. Which therapeutic exercise intervention can BEST prevent recurrent lateral ankle sprains?

_____ a. soleus stretching

_____ b. peroneal stretching

_____ c. soleus strengthening

_____ d. peroneal strengthening

2. Which activity is MOST appropriate to reduce the physical strain that occurs with a forward head posture?

_____ a. scapular adduction

_____ b. chin tucks

_____ c. scapular downward rotation

_____ d. cervical flexion

3. Which intervention promotes relaxation, reduces muscle tension, increases tolerance to activities, and improves ventilation?

_____ a. active inhibition

_____ b. segmental breathing

_____ c. productive huffing

_____ d. diaphragmatic breathing

4. You are teaching a person the habits of a good standing posture. The person is under the care of the physical therapist to address lumbar spinal stenosis. Which statement is appropriate for effective standing posture for this person?

    _____ a. posterior pelvic tilting to reduce intervertebral foraminal narrowing

    _____ b. scapular retraction to reduce discogenic symptoms

    _____ c. cervical retraction to reduce facet symptoms

    _____ d. lateral flexion of the spine to reduce fascial symptoms

5. A person is required to perform repeated bilateral reaching across a surface directly in front of them at their workstation. At their workstation, they are unable to step any closer to this work surface to decrease their reaching distance. What instructions would prevent excessive strain to their body?

    _____ a. instruct the person to stand and avoid stabilizing their pelvis against the work surface

    _____ b. instruct the person to climb on top of their work surface

    _____ c. instruct the person to stand and stabilize their pelvis against the work surface

    _____ d. instruct the person to stabilize against the work surface with one upper extremity

6. A woman is participating in a supervised home wellness program in order to improve cardiovascular and endocrine function. Based upon this information, which goal is MOST appropriate for this woman?

    _____ a. decrease capillary refill response

    _____ b. reduce body-fat percentage to 18%

    _____ c. reduce body-fat percentage to 15%

    _____ d. reduce body-fat percentage to 22%

ANSWERS AND RATIONALE

AIRWAY CLEARANCE TECHNIQUES— BREATHING STRATEGIES

Six Items

1. Correct answer: (b)

    Rationale: Huffing is used to clear airway with less chance of producing the Valsalva effect.

    Reference: Kisner, C., & Colby, L. (2002). *Therapeutic exercise: Foundations and techniques* (4th ed., p. 758). Philadelphia: FA Davis.

2. Correct answer: (d)

    Rationale: Each of these is necessary to facilitate effective cough.

    Reference: Kisner, C., & Colby, L. (2002). *Therapeutic exercise: Foundations and techniques* (4th ed., p. 677). Philadelphia: FA Davis.

3. Correct answer: (d)

   Rationale: Suctioning is indicated for all persons with artificial airways.

   Reference: Kisner, C., & Colby, L. (2002). *Therapeutic exercise: Foundations and techniques* (4th ed., p. 679). Philadelphia: FA Davis.

4. Correct answer: (c)

   Rationale: Forceful expiration should be avoided with COPD.

   Reference: Kisner, C., & Colby, L. (2002). *Therapeutic exercise: Foundations and techniques* (4th ed., p. 672). Philadelphia: FA Davis.

5. Correct answer: (c)

   Rationale: Diaphragmatic breathing will reduce energy expenditure.

   Reference: Kisner, C., & Colby, L. (2002). *Therapeutic exercise: Foundations and techniques* (4th ed., p. 750). Philadelphia: FA Davis.

6. Correct answer: (b)

   Rationale: Huffing is performed differently than a cough, in that the abdominals pull up and in, with less resistance to the expiration of air.

   Reference: Kisner, C., & Colby, L. (2002). *Therapeutic exercise: Foundations and techniques* (4th ed., p. 702). Philadelphia: FA Davis.

AIRWAY CLEARANCE TECHNIQUES—MANUAL AND MECHANICAL TECHNIQUES

Three Items

1. Correct answer: (d)

   Rationale: Pressure is applied directly upon the skin during the exhalation phase.

   Reference: Kisner, C., & Colby, L. (2002). *Therapeutic exercise: Foundations and techniques* (4th ed., p. 762). Philadelphia: FA Davis.

2. Correct answer: (c)

   Rationale: Percussive interventions can be applied manually or mechanically by a physical therapist or physical therapist assistant. Pulmonary embolism is a contraindication for percussive interventions. Percussive interventions are applied continuously for several minutes or until the patient needs to cough.

   Reference: Kisner, C., & Colby, L. (2002). *Therapeutic exercise: Foundations and techniques* (4th ed., p. 762). Philadelphia: FA Davis.

3. Correct answer: (c)

   Rationale: Each of these is a fundamental step to follow prior to suctioning a person on an artificial airway. The first step is checking to see if the person can exhale forcefully; if so, do not apply suction.

Reference: Hillegass, E., & Sadowsky, H. (2001). *Essentials of cardiopulmonary physical therapy* (2nd ed., p. 653, 654). Philadelphia: WB Saunders.

AIRWAY CLEARANCE TECHNIQUES—POSITIONING

Three Items

1. Correct answer: (c)

   Rationale: The lateral segments of the lower lobes are placed in the gravity-oriented plane when the head is 30°–45° lower than the trunk.

   Reference: Kisner, C., & Colby, L. (2002). *Therapeutic exercise: Foundations and techniques* (4th ed., p. 764). Philadelphia: FA Davis.

2. Correct answer: (b)

   Rationale: Dysphagia is difficulty in swallowing. A person who lies flat and has dysphagia is at risk for choking or aspiration.

   Reference: O'Sullivan. (2001). *Physical rehabilitation assessment and treatment* (4th ed., p. 534). Philadelphia: FA Davis.

3. Correct answer: (d)

   Rationale: Align the lung segment vertical to enable the force of gravity to drain fluids.

   Reference: Kisner, C., & Colby, L. (2002). *Therapeutic exercise: Foundations and techniques* (4th ed., p. 764). Philadelphia: FA Davis.

WOUND CARE AND SKIN INTEGRITY— MONITOR SKIN STATUS

Three Items

1. Correct answer: (c)

   Rationale: Partial thickness burns have moderate levels of pain due to the partially intact nerve endings. Discoloration and blistering are consistent with partial thickness burns.

   Reference: Rothstein J., et al. (1998). *The rehabilitation specialist's handbook* (2nd ed., p. 1115). Philadelphia: FA Davis.

2. Correct answer: (a)

   Rationale: Stage one skin ulcers still have the epidermis intact.

   Reference: Anemaet, W., et al. (2000). *Home rehabilitation: Guide to clinical practice* (p. 474). St. Louis: Mosby.

3. Correct answer: (b)

Rationale: These signs are typical of chronic venous insufficiency. The wounds are typically shallow with good granulation.

Reference: Goodman, C., & Snyder, T. (2000). *Differential diagnosis in physical therapy* (3rd ed., p. 463). Philadelphia: WB Saunders.

WOUND CARE AND SKIN INTEGRITY— PATIENT POSITIONING AND USE OF ADAPTIVE AND PROTECTIVE DEVICES FOR PRESSURE RELIEF

Seven Items

1. Correct answer: (b)

Rationale: Person with axillary burns injuries are susceptible to shoulder adduction contractures.

Reference: Anemaet, W., et al. (2000). *Home rehabilitation: Guide to clinical practice* (p. 480). St. Louis: Mosby.

2. Correct answer: (a)

Rationale: The elbow is most susceptible to flexion and pronation contractures.

Reference: Anemaet, W., et al. (2000). *Home rehabilitation: Guide to clinical practice* (p. 480). St. Louis: Mosby.

3. Correct answer: (b)

Rationale: Weight-shifting is the primary method of preventing skin breakdown.

Reference: O'Sullivan. (2001). *Physical rehabilitation assessment and treatment* (4th ed., p. 883). Philadelphia: FA Davis.

4. Correct answer: (b)

Rationale: Padding bony prominences disperses pressure upon those areas of skin susceptible to breakdown as a result of compression ischemia.

Reference: Pierson, F. (2002). *Principles and techniques of patient care* (3rd ed., p. 90). Philadelphia: WB Saunders.

5. Correct answer: (c)

Rationale: A person with function above T10 should be independent in positioning themselves, and not require tilt in space wheelchair function.

Reference: Nixon, V., & Schneider, F. (1985). *Spinal cord injury: A guide to functional outcomes in physical therapy management* (p. 75). Maryland: Aspen.

6. Correct answer: (c)

Rationale: Extreme pain is more common as free nerve endings are exposed with deep partial-thickness burns.

Reference: Anemaet, W., et al. (2000). *Home rehabilitation: Guide to clinical practice* (p. 168). St. Louis: Mosby.

7. Correct answer: (a)

Rationale: Burn injuries to the fingers are at risk to develop contractures into MCP extension, first digit adduction, and IP extension.

Reference: Anemaet, W., et al. (2000). *Home rehabilitation: Guide to clinical practice* (p. 480). St. Louis: Mosby.

WOUND CARE AND SKIN INTEGRITY— DRESSING APPLICATION AND REMOVAL

Four Items

1. Correct answer: (b)

Rationale: The bandage should extend beyond the wound bed for absorbing drainage and securing to health skin. All of the other choices are invalid.

Reference: Pierson, F. (2002). *Principles and techniques of patient care* (3rd ed., p. 310). Philadelphia: WB Saunders.

2. Correct answer: (b)

Rationale: Each of the sterile materials is needed, beginning with the sterile field to establish a clean working surface.

Reference: Pierson, F. (2002). *Principles and techniques of patient care* (3rd ed., p. 308). Philadelphia: WB Saunders.

3. Correct answer: (d)

Rationale: The dressing should be removed prior to powering the turbine to prevent the material becoming stuck in the turbine.

Reference: Pierson, F. (2002). *Principles and techniques of patient care* (3rd ed., p. 308). Philadelphia: WB Saunders.

4. Correct answer: (a)

Rationale: All of the other statements are accurate. Color changes distal to the wound dressing indicate that the dressing is too tight.

Reference: Pierson, F. (2002). *Principles and techniques of patient care* (3rd ed., p. 308). Philadelphia: WB Saunders.

WOUND CARE AND SKIN INTEGRITY— TOPICAL AGENTS APPLICATION

Three Items

1. Correct answer: (a)

   Rationale: Wet to dry dressings have absorptive properties, and the other choices do not.

   Reference: Anemaet, W., et al. (2000). *Home rehabilitation: Guide to clinical practice* (pp. 481–483). St. Louis: Mosby.

2. Correct answer: (d)

   Rationale: Wet to dry saline applications have debridement and absorptive properties, and are indicated for stage one to four ulcerations.

   Reference: Anemaet, W., et al. (2000). *Home rehabilitation: Guide to clinical practice* (p. 483). St. Louis: Mosby.

3. Correct answer: (c)

   Rationale: Silvadene is applied in a film 2–4 millimeters thick.

   Reference: Rothstein J., et al. (1998). *The rehabilitation specialist's handbook* (2nd ed., p. 1125). Philadelphia: FA Davis.

WOUND CARE AND SKIN INTEGRITY— DEBRIDEMENT TECHNIQUES EXCEPT SHARP

Two Items

1. Correct answer: (a)

   Rationale: Autolytic debridement can be facilitated with cathodal (negative) stimulation.

   Reference: Myers, B. (2004). *Wound management, principles and practice* (p. 163, 164). Upper Saddle River, NJ: Prentice Hall.

2. Correct answer: (a)

   Rationale: Saline, lavage, and whirlpools are not chemical debridement interventions. Saline does not perform debridement, the other two are mechanical sources, unless a chemical is added to the water. Hydrocolloids have enzymes that facilitate wound debridement.

   Reference: O'Sullivan. (2001). *Physical rehabilitation assessment and treatment* (4th ed., p. 603, 604). Philadelphia: FA Davis.

MONITORING PATIENT RESPONSES AND MODIFYING INTERVENTIONS

Seventeen Items

1. Correct answer: (d)

   Rationale: Major modifications to the treatment plan require a physical therapist.

   Reference: Pagliarulo, M. (2001). *Introduction to physical therapy* (2nd ed., p. 55). St. Louis: Mosby.

2. Correct answer: (d)

   Rationale: The extensor carpi ulnaris and radialis should contract together to produce a balanced extension of the wrist. With weakness of the ulnaris muscle the pull of the radialis will cause movement into extension and towards the radius.

   Reference: Kendall, F., et al. (1993). *Muscles: Testing and function* (4th ed., p. 261). Baltimore: Williams & Wilkins.

3. Correct answer: (b)

   Rationale: The scapula must fully elevate, upwardly rotate, and protract to achieve full active shoulder flexion.

   Reference: Sahrmann, S. (2002). *Diagnosis and treatment of movement impairment syndromes* (p. 203). St. Louis: Mosby.

4. Correct answer: (c)

   Rationale: Persons with multiple sclerosis should be educated and encouraged in utilizing energy conservation approaches.

   Reference: O'Sullivan. (2001). *Physical rehabilitation assessment and treatment* (4th ed., p. 729). Philadelphia: FA Davis.

5. Correct answer: (a)

   Rationale: Acute muscle soreness is typically due to ischemia. Delayed onset of muscle soreness does not occur until after the treatment session. Eccentric muscle activity produces more delayed muscle soreness than concentric activity.

   Reference: Kisner, C., & Colby, L. (2002). *Therapeutic exercise: Foundations and techniques* (4th ed., pp. 63–65). Philadelphia: FA Davis.

6. Correct answer: (b)

   Rationale: Orienting the person to greater elevation of the head and body will address their tolerance to sitting.

   Reference: O'Sullivan. (2001). *Physical rehabilitation assessment and treatment* (4th ed., p. 92). Philadelphia: FA Davis.

7. Correct answer: (d)

   Rationale: The transverse abdominus functions to compress the abdomen.

   Reference: Sahrmann, S. (2002). *Diagnosis and treatment of movement impairment syndromes* (p. 135). St. Louis: Mosby.

8. Correct answer: (d)

   Rationale: Placing the person's arms at their side decreases the resistance arm of the upper body.

   Reference: Kendall, F., et al. (1993). *Muscles: Testing and function* (4th ed., p. 163). Baltimore: Williams & Wilkins.

9. Correct answer: (c)

   Rationale: Heterotropic ossification most commonly occurs in the hips and knees.

   Reference: Martin, S., & Kessler, M. (2000). *Neurologic intervention for physical therapist assistants* (p. 190). Philadelphia: WB Saunders.

10. Correct answer: (d)

    Rationale: The patient's dignity and infection control should remain priorities throughout all interactions.

    Reference: Somers, M. (2001). *Spinal cord injury: Functional rehabilitation* (2nd ed., p. 31). New Jersey: Prentice Hall.

11. Correct answer: (d)

    Rationale: Each of the other choices are potential outcomes of therapeutic strengthening.

    Reference: Guccione, A. (2000). *Geriatric physical therapy* (2nd ed., p. 52). St. Louis: Mosby.

12. Correct answer: (d)

    Rationale: An increase in symptoms may be an indication of less impingement of the nerve root. Keep the parameters the same and allow the patient time to improve or for clinical signs to change.

    Reference: Hayes, K. (2000). *Manual for physical agents* (5th ed., p. 100). New Jersey: Prentice Hall.

13. Correct answer: (c)

    Rationale: Continuous ultrasound is used primarily for its thermal effects. Any decreases in intensity must be compensated for in treatment duration.

    Reference: Prentice, W. (2002). *Therapeutic modalities for physical therapists* (2nd ed., p. 283). New York: McGraw-Hill.

14. Correct answer: (b)

    Rationale: The resistance in the fourth set was insufficient based upon the DAPRE method.

    Reference: Kisner, C., & Colby, L. (2002). *Therapeutic exercise: Foundations and techniques* (4th ed., p. 126). Philadelphia: FA Davis.

15. Correct answer: (a)

    Rationale: The Oxford method of exercise progression uses a set of 10 at the ten repetition maximum resistance, followed by a set of 10 at 75% of the ten repetition maximum.

Reference: Kisner, C., & Colby, L. (2002). *Therapeutic exercise: Foundations and techniques* (4th ed., p. 125). Philadelphia: FA Davis.

16. Correct answer: (c)

    Rationale: The weight is kept the same in this fourth set when five or six repetitions are achieved in the third set.

    Reference: Kisner, C., & Colby, L. (2002). *Therapeutic exercise: Foundations and techniques* (4th ed., p. 126). Philadelphia: FA Davis.

17. Correct answer: (a)

    Rationale: Cryotherapy should never exceed the point of anesthesia.

    Reference: Hayes, K. (2000). *Manual for physical agents* (5th ed., p. 62). New Jersey: Prentice Hall.

HEALTH AND WELLNESS—PREVENTION, INSTRUCTION, AND INTERVENTIONS

Six Items

1. Correct answer: (d)

    Rationale: The peroneal tendons resist the varus forces, which in excess produces injury to the anterior talofibular ligament.

    Reference: Evans, R. (2001). *Illustrated orthopedic physical assessment* (2nd ed., p. 843). St. Louis: Mosby.

2. Correct answer: (b)

    Rationale: Cervical retraction decreases the forward head posture.

    Reference: Kisner, C., & Colby, L. (2002). *Therapeutic exercise: Foundations and techniques* (4th ed., p. 643). Philadelphia: FA Davis.

3. Correct answer: (d)

    Rationale: Diaphragmatic breathing can facilitate tolerance, ventilation, and relaxation.

    Reference: Kisner, C., & Colby, L. (2002). *Therapeutic exercise: Foundations and techniques* (4th ed., p. 750). Philadelphia: FA Davis.

4. Correct answer: (a)

    Rationale: Posterior pelvic tilting will promote better lumbar alignment and pressure upon the spinal cord.

    Reference: Norkin, C., & Levangie, P. (1992). *Joint structure and function: A comprehensive analysis* (2nd ed., p. 436). Philadelphia: FA Davis.

5. Correct answer: (c)

   Rationale: Stabilizing their pelvis against the work surface allows a decrease in resistance level arm length. Although not ideal workstation arrangement, this technique will reduce the stresses upon their body.

   Reference: Nordin, M., & Frankel, V. (2001). *Basic biomechanics of the musculoskeletal system* (3rd ed., p. 425). Philadelphia: Lippincott Williams & Wilkins.

6. Correct answer: (d)

   Rationale: The ideal body-fat composition percentage for adult women is 20–22%.

   Reference: Thibodeau, G., & Patton, K. (2002). *The human body in health and disease* (3rd ed., p. 52). St. Louis: Mosby.

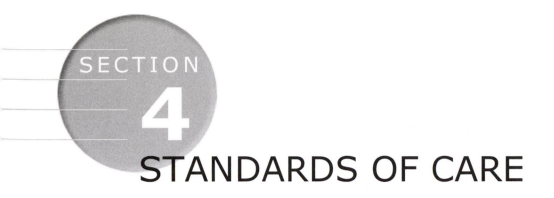

SECTION 4

STANDARDS OF CARE

Standards of Care: Patient Confidentiality, Professional Issues, Legal/Ethical Issues, Body Mechanics, Positioning, Safety, First Aid, Cardiopulmonary Resuscitation, Sterile Technique, Universal Precautions, and Equipment Preparation

OVERVIEW

This chapter includes questions covering professional standards of care included in the exam. There are 168 questions in this chapter, which is the most diverse content area dealt with by the exam. Content includes patient confidentiality, safety, autonomy, and consent, working within state laws, under supervision of a physical therapist, and within the skill level of a physical therapist assistant. Also, this section covers body mechanics, positioning, draping, clinical decision making, aseptic techniques, universal precautions, first aid, and emergency procedures.

KEY POINTS FOR REVIEW

Patient Care Standards

- Autonomy
- Patients' Bill of Rights
- Informed refusal
- Restraints
- Age of consent
- Medical directives
- Confidentiality
- Personal health information
- Informed consent
- Documentation

Physical Therapist Assistance Practice Standards

- Supervision by the physical therapist
- Guide to Physical Therapist Practice
- Standards of Conduct for the Affiliate Member
- Responsibilities that cannot be delegated
- Americans with Disabilities Act
- Occupational Health and Safety Administration
- American Physical Therapy Association
- Normative Model for Physical Therapist Assistant Education
- Clinical decision making

Safety Standards

- Body mechanics
- Positioning and draping
- Preventing contractures
- Ensuring patient safety
- Medical precautions
- Patient observations
- First aid procedures
- Emergency procedures
- Cardiopulmonary resuscitation

Universal Precaution Standards

- Aseptic technique
- Personal protective equipment
- Hand washing
- Discarding soiled and nonsoiled items
- Assembling materials for aseptic technique

MAINTAINING PATIENT CONFIDENTIALITY

Thirteen Items

1. You greet a person whom the physical therapist has delegated to you to apply ultrasound therapy. What must be shared with the patient prior to applying this intervention, in order to gain informed consent?

    _____ a. explanation of physician's referral, insurance coverage for this intervention, alternative payment plans, indications and contraindications, and answer any questions

    _____ b. allow patient to view written documentation of evaluation, answer any questions, explain intervention in laymen terms, and check contraindications

    _____ c. findings of evaluation, explanation of intervention, answer any questions, reasonable alternatives to treatment, and expected benefits/risks of intervention

    _____ d. nothing must be discussed, as patients treated in physical therapy may give implied consent

2. If an adult patient expresses that they are falling in love with their health care provider, can the provider reciprocate their emotion?

    _____ a. no, the health care provider is not allowed to fall in love with patients; it violates most practice acts

    _____ b. no, the health care provider is considered singularly responsible for the relationship, since patients can be emotionally vulnerable during treatment

    _____ c. yes, since the patient initiated the emotional exchange and the provider is only acknowledging their true feelings

    _____ d. yes, the relationship is legally consensual

3. Which of the following is not considered necessary to be included when gaining informed consent for treatment?

    _____ a. explanation of expected outcome of receiving no treatment intervention

    _____ b. checking for contraindications

    _____ c. answering questions

    _____ d. explaining difficult procedures in lay terms

4. Incident reports are completed as directed by your employer when injuries, potential injuries, or variations in procedures occur. Which statement is most accurate concerning incident reports?

    _____ a. when the incident involves a patient, document in either SOAP or narrative format in the patient's record that an incident report has been properly completed and filed with the facility

    _____ b. you should include a personal perspective about the reason why you think the deviation or injury occurred, to facilitate the follow up on the report

    _____ c. when completing an incident report, give one copy to your supervisor and one to the patient, or person involved

    _____ d. you should clearly label the report for use as a quality care, or patient safety improvement document

5. A person files a claim for injury sustained in a physical therapy session with you. In conjunction, they include the hospital as liable, and it is determined they have vicarious liability. Which of the following is MOST accurate regarding vicarious liability?

_____ a. you may be financially responsible for damages to the plaintiff

_____ b. the hospital may be financially responsible for damages to the plaintiff

_____ c. the hospital has the right to seek compensation from you for their costs

_____ d. you and the hospital may be financially responsible for damages to the plaintiff, which the hospital has the right to seek compensation for from you

6. Which of the conditions is not guaranteed in the Patients' Bill of Rights by the American Hospital Association?

_____ a. you have the right to know if this hospital has relationships with outside parties that may influence your treatment and care

_____ b. you have the right to privacy

_____ c. you have the right to expect that treatment records are confidential unless you have given permission to release the information

_____ d. you have the right to a private room

7. A person refuses an intervention after receiving a clear explanation of the procedure and offers informed consent. Which of the following should occur?

_____ a. document in the patient's record as given informed consent, and noncompliant

_____ b. document in the patient's record as noncompliant

_____ c. document in the patient's record as giving an informed refusal

_____ d. document in the patient's record as noncompliant and recommend discharge to physical therapist

8. Health care professionals, who approach ethical dilemmas by primarily considering the duty of practitioners in those situations, are using which approach to ethics?

_____ a. casuistry approach

_____ b. teleological approach

_____ c. inductive approach

_____ d. deontological approach

9. A patient's daughter wants to look at her father's medical record. He has recently been admitted for insidious onset of low back pain. What should you do as a physical therapist assistant?

_____ a. allow her to read the physical therapy portion of her father's record and answer any questions

_____ b. tell her to request permission from the physician

_____ c. tell her that she must have permission from her father before she can view his record

_____ d. tell her that she cannot see the chart because she may not understand the terminology and may misinterpret the documentation

10. A group of three co-workers are at lunch in the hospital employees' cafeteria. They are quietly discussing a current patient's diagnosis and plan of care. Which of the following is occurring?

     _____ a. informed consent standards are being breached

     _____ b. confidentiality standards are being breached

     _____ c. legal release standards are being breached

     _____ d. they are not breaching any standards

11. A physical therapist assistant is discussing a patient's progress and treatment with the supervisory physical therapist. Which of the following is a violation of a patient's confidentiality?

     _____ a. describing the patient by height or weight

     _____ b. describing the patient by their occupation

     _____ c. discussing a personal story the patient shared with you

     _____ d. discussing a lack of attendance to scheduled appointments

12. After writing a progress note on a person, a physical therapist assistant files the note in the person's record. Which statement MOST accurately describes the rule of confidentiality?

     _____ a. no other person is allowed to read the progress note

     _____ b. any ethical person employed at the facility may review the progress note

     _____ c. only the persons providing direct patient care may review the progress note

     _____ d. some persons do not have the qualifications to read the progress note

13. A person is waiting in the reception area for their appointment time. The physical therapist assistant is prepared to begin the treatment session a few minutes prior to the scheduled appointment. Which action is MOST appropriate?

     _____ a. go and greet the person in the reception area

     _____ b. go introduce yourself and confirm the patient's name

     _____ c. go introduce yourself, and confirm the patient's name and diagnosis

     _____ d. go introduce yourself, and confirm the patient's name, diagnosis, and plan of care

MAINTAINING PATIENT AUTONOMY AND OBTAINING CONSENT

Thirteen Items

1. Prior to treating a person, you review their medical record and discover that they have been placed in physical restraints. Which of the following is LEAST accurate regarding physical restraints?

     _____ a. physical restraints may be used as a form of discipline

     _____ b. physical restraints may be used for person who exhibit safety concerns to themselves or others

     _____ c. physical restraints require documentation and regular patient safety assessments

     _____ d. physical restraints must be used only when other less restraining strategies have failed

2. Prior to treating a person bedside, you review their medical record and discover that they have been placed in physical restraints. Which of the following materials is considered a physical restraint?

_____ a. seat belts on a wheelchair

_____ b. wrist cuffs

_____ c. any material that restricts a person's mobility

_____ d. bedding materials

3. Which of the following is MOST appropriate in legally identifying a person to make health care decisions on behalf of the patient, only in the event that the patient is unable to personally and competently render consent?

_____ a. advanced directive for health care

_____ b. living will

_____ c. informed consent document

_____ d. durable power of attorney for health care

4. Through professional quality improvement programs, some medical delivery systems have changed their approaches to health services. Instead of having the patient transported to various specialties within a hospital, the patient can be located in an area where MOST of the services are available. Which quality improvement model does this describe?

_____ a. patient-focused care

_____ b. critical pathways

_____ c. direct access

_____ d. evidence-based practice

5. A person in an inpatient medical treatment facility is participating in physical therapy. Today the physical therapist assistant reviews their medical record and discovers that they have been placed in physical restraints. Which of the following is not considered a physical restraint?

_____ a. lap belts on a wheelchair

_____ b. medications

_____ c. sheets and linens

_____ d. arm trough attachment for a wheelchair

6. Patients can maintain autonomy by providing an informed consent prior to any intervention. Which of the following is the preferred method for obtaining informed consent?

_____ a. asking the person if they have any questions, seeking permission after providing rationales, and documenting patient consent prior to intervention

_____ b. a thorough health questionnaire and waiver completed prior to or during the evaluation by the physical therapist

_____ c. asking a patient if it is okay to precede with an intervention

_____ d. checking for contraindications, explaining the rationale, and describing the intervention

7. A person speaks with a physical therapist assistant at the beginning of a treatment session. The person states that they are afraid of the electrical stimulation equipment used during the previous treatment session. After speaking with the physical therapist, they continue to state that they do not wish to have that intervention any more. Which action is MOST appropriate in this case?

   _____ a. inform the person better about the intervention, eventually obtaining compliance

   _____ b. discontinue the treatment session and allow the person to decide if physical therapy is right for them

   _____ c. allow the person to continue with physical therapy if they will comply with the plan of care

   _____ d. allow the person to choose whether or not to have the intervention

8. A person 30 years of age, who recently suffered a brain injury, is classified as a Stage IV on the Rancho Los Amigos Scale. The person has no known family members. How is consent for interventions or medical actions granted for this person?

   _____ a. medical personnel are allowed to implement standard interventions based upon medical review board decisions

   _____ b. no care may be rendered until a legal relative provides consent

   _____ c. a surrogate decision maker should be legally named to make decisions for the person

   _____ d. since the person is legally brain dead, no consent is required

9. Physical therapist assistants often deal with a variety of age groups. According to Erikson's Theory of Psychosocial Development, at what age do people FIRST begin to engage in autonomous behavior?

   _____ a. 2–4 years of age

   _____ b. 12–18 years of age

   _____ c. 21–32 years of age

   _____ d. 32–40 years of age

10. A person has been participating in physical therapy at an inpatient facility for 1 week. Today, the person is refusing to participate in one of the interventions because they do not think it is necessary or worthwhile. Which of the following is MOST appropriate in this situation?

   _____ a. proceed with the other interventions

   _____ b. inform the person that they are financially responsible for the physical therapy care, based upon noncompliance

   _____ c. proceed with the intervention

   _____ d. proceed with the interventions free of charge

11. Prior to touching a person during a treatment session, the physical therapist assistant ensures that the person is aware and consenting to the contact. After contacting the person's body, the person appears to be very uncomfortable. The person feels that the touch had a sexual connotation. Which of the following may be MOST legally applicable?

_____ a. the person may have been physically assaulted

_____ b. the person may have been physically battered

_____ c. the person may have been sexually assaulted

_____ d. the person may have been sexually battered

12. When a person is admitted to the hospital, they sign a document regarding Advanced Care Medical Directive. Which of the following is LEAST appropriate regarding this document?

_____ a. the document allows the person to refuse interventions, even if refusal leads to death of the person

_____ b. the document is legal only if completed by a person who is mentally competent

_____ c. patients must be informed of their rights to make this decision

_____ d. the medical facility may change the content of the form based upon corporate policy

13. A person, who is hospitalized in an acute care setting, is visited by a team of physicians and the physical therapist. Which of the following documents establishes the requirement for health professionals to identify themselves by name and title?

_____ a. Emergency Medical Treatment and Labor Act

_____ b. Omnibus Budget Reconciliation Act

_____ c. Patients' Bill of Rights

_____ d. Health Insurance Privacy and Accountability Act

WORK UNDER THE SUPERVISION AND DIRECTION OF A PHYSICAL THERAPIST IN AN ETHICAL, LEGAL, AND SAFE MANNER

Nine Items

1. A new physician in your town contacts a physical therapist assistant's acquaintance with the intention of increasing their patient referral base. The physician promises to give the physical therapist assistant unlimited access to a luxury box at the local sports stadium if they send referrals from the physical therapy clinic where they are employed. Which of the following responses is MOST appropriate for the assistant?

_____ a. agree to accept the offer, but only if the assistant can reimburse the physician for the cost of the luxury box seats

_____ b. speak with the director or financial officer of the clinic prior to accepting the offer

_____ c. thank the physician for the offer, politely decline and inform local authorities

_____ d. thank the physician for the offer and accept

2. A patient in a convalescent center who had a cerebral vascular accident 7 years ago affecting the left extremities underwent a right total hip arthroplasty 5 days ago. The physical therapist evaluated the patient and rated their bed mobility as poor. The patient has been unable to transfer from bed to chair without maximal assistance of two persons. You are to treat the person for the first time by yourself on the weekend. Which of the following is your BEST action in this case?

   _____ a. refuse to perform the treatment since you are alone

   _____ b. ask for assistance from other patient care staff

   _____ c. inform the physician that you are unable to perform the treatment today, but that intervention will continue during full staffing periods

   _____ d. document that the patient refused

3. While operating a therapeutic modality, the machine falls off the wheeled cart and lands on your left foot. You immediately experience extreme pain and have difficulty in walking. Based on this information, what are you required to do?

   _____ a. pursue litigation

   _____ b. complete an incident report and report the event to your supervisor

   _____ c. sit down until asymptomatic

   _____ d. document the event in the patient's medical record as an interruption to treatment

4. One day at a physical therapy setting, you notice that a clinical student is spending a lot of time with a patient during and after the treatment session discussing things not related to the patient's care. What is your MOST appropriate action?

   _____ a. confront the student immediately, one on one

   _____ b. reschedule the patient with another caregiver on subsequent sessions

   _____ c. discuss the event with the student's clinical instructor

   _____ d. disregard the observation

5. A physical therapist assistant and a physical therapist are having a conference in review of their current patient load. During the discussion, one of the clinicians makes a sexually oriented remark related to a physical attraction they have towards one of the patients. The other clinician becomes uncomfortable and asks to end the conference early. Which situation has potentially occurred during the conference?

   _____ a. quid pro quo

   _____ b. sexual harassment

   _____ c. sexual abuse

   _____ d. hostile work environment

6. A physical therapist assistant is transfer training a person who recently experienced a cerebral vascular accident, resulting in global aphasia and minimal right hemiparesis. During the transfer from the bed to the wheelchair, the wheelchair locks failed, the patient fell to the floor and was injured. Which of the following statements is LEAST relevant in this situation regarding why the patient or their family may have grounds for a negligence suit?

_____ a. the physical therapist assistant failed to use a safe wheelchair and may be found liable by acts of omission

_____ b. maintenance of the wheelchair may have been insufficient and the hospital may be found liable by respondeat superior

_____ c. the patient did not check the wheelchair brakes and may be determined to have contributory negligence

_____ d. the supervising physical therapist may have failed to properly train the physical therapist assistant and may be found liable

7. Which of the following is established for a health care provider to be LEAST likely to be found legally liable for an incident?

_____ a. the provider had a duty to act

_____ b. the action of the provider caused harm

_____ c. the actions of the provider were reasonably prudent

_____ d. the provider omitted a pertinent step

8. A person has been delegated to a physical therapist assistant for therapeutic exercise interventions. Which of the following events LEAST often require that the physical therapist personally see the patient?

_____ a. upon discharge from care

_____ b. upon initial evaluation

_____ c. upon minor modifications to a person's treatment

_____ d. upon acute changes in a person's medical status

9. A profession is defined as having at least five characteristics. Which characteristic of a profession does the American Physical Therapy Association function as?

_____ a. lifetime commitment

_____ b. representative organization

_____ c. specialized education

_____ d. service to clients

KNOWING AND WORKING WITHIN APPLICABLE STATE LAWS AND RULES GOVERNING PHYSICAL THERAPY

Twelve Items

1. Which of the following documents legally govern the utilization of physical therapist assistants?

_____ a. the document on responsibilities that cannot be delegated

_____ b. State Practice Acts

_____ c. Guide for Ethical Conduct

_____ d. Vision 2020 statement

2. The Americans with Disabilities Act applies to private sector businesses that employ what number of employees?

_____ a. 15 or more

_____ b. 50 or more

_____ c. 150 or more

_____ d. 1500 or more

3. The Occupational Safety and Health Administration requires healthcare employers to provide which of the following?

_____ a. personal protective equipment to all persons involved in patient care

_____ b. personal protective equipment to all persons exposed to patients in emergency medical care

_____ c. personal protective equipment to all persons exposed to patients with incontinence

_____ d. personal protective equipment to all persons exposed to bodily fluids

4. After graduation, a physical therapist assistant attends a job interview. During the interview, the employer should not ask which of the following questions?

_____ a. How long have you been a physical therapist assistant?

_____ b. What hours are you available to work?

_____ c. What pay range are you looking for?

_____ d. Do you have any children?

5. The American Physical Therapy Association is recognized as the primary representative organization for physical therapy, at the national level. Which is the highest policy making body within the American Physical Therapy Association?

_____ a. Combined Sections

_____ b. Affiliate Assembly

_____ c. Board of Directors

_____ d. House of Delegates

6. Some states have Good Samaritan laws affecting the response to persons in emergency situations. What is the purpose of Good Samaritan laws?

_____ a. prevent people with good intentions from injuring victims

_____ b. limit liability of caregivers who act reasonably

_____ c. initiate lawsuits against plaintiffs

_____ d. eliminate lawsuits against health care providers

7. In reference to laws, a _____ is set forth by a legislative body, whereas a _____ is established by one or a series of court decisions.

_____ a. statute, common law

_____ b. statute, regulation

_____ c. regulation, policy

_____ d. common law, policy

8. A person is participating in an outpatient physical therapy rehabilitation program. They have informed their current employer of their need for accessibility and modification to their workstation, based upon recommendations by the physical therapist. Which of the following is an appropriate reason for the employer to deny the person's request?

   _____ a. the accommodation is not needed by other current employees

   _____ b. the accommodation directly impairs the operation of the company

   _____ c. the accommodation is expensive

   _____ d. the employee will be terminated after completion of worker's compensation funding

9. The following four individuals are being treated in physical therapy setting. Which of them would not be covered under the Americans with Disabilities Act?

   _____ a. a person, 13 years of age, who is blind

   _____ b. a person, 40 years of age, who has severe mental retardation

   _____ c. a person, 26 years of age, who is a naturalized citizen from China

   _____ d. a person, 72 years of age, with severe learning impairment

10. When reviewing a treatment session with the supervisory physical therapist, they suggest that an incident report be completed based upon an event with the patient. What is the primary reason for completing an incident report?

    _____ a. the report provides a memorandum about the alleged incident

    _____ b. the report protects the person causing the alleged incident

    _____ c. the report serves as a legal defense for the alleged defendant

    _____ d. the report allows the person to document the cause of the alleged incident

11. In cases of determining legal negligence involving health care providers, a preponderance of evidence must be established for which of the following parameters?

    _____ a. duty to act and causation of harm

    _____ b. breach of duty and causation of harm

    _____ c. causation of harm and incurred damages

    _____ d. duty to act, causation of harm, or breach of duty

12. Incident reports should establish a record and description of the event. Which of the following SHOULD be omitted from an incident report?

    _____ a. speculation on the potential cause of the incident with recommendations for the prevention of future incidents

    _____ b. objective, first-hand accounts observed by the writer of the incident report

    _____ c. concise and thorough description of the incident

    _____ d. time and date of occurrence and the names of any witnesses

PERFORMING ONLY THOSE TASKS WITHIN A PHYSICAL THERAPIST ASSISTANT'S KNOWLEDGE AND SKILL LEVEL

Nine Items

1. Regularly scheduled equipment checks are performed to ensure all equipment is calibrated, lubricated, and adjusted according to the manufacturer's guidelines. Which the following procedures is LEAST appropriate for physical therapist assistants?

   _____ a. training physical therapist assistants to do simple repairs on all nonelectrical magnetic spectrum emitting equipment if a breakdown should occur

   _____ b. supervising new physical therapist assistants and students is the use of all newly purchased equipment

   _____ c. physical therapist assistants documenting all preventative and repair services performed upon the equipment

   _____ d. conducting in-house educational sessions for physical therapist assistants regarding the indications and contraindications for all equipment

2. When one health care provider performs the skills and techniques of another profession, it is referred to as which of the following terms?

   _____ a. professional encroachment

   _____ b. professional negligence

   _____ c. professional impingement

   _____ d. professional misconduct

3. Who is responsible for determining which tasks may be directed to other physical therapy personnel?

   _____ a. the supervising physical therapist assistant

   _____ b. the supervising physical therapist

   _____ c. the director of physical therapy

   _____ d. each individual caregiver

4. Who is responsible for completing the initial evaluation of a patient?

   _____ a. the supervising physical therapist assistant

   _____ b. the supervising physical therapist

   _____ c. the director of physical therapy

   _____ d. each individual caregiver

5. Who is responsible for ensuring that all individuals are treated with dignity and with the high professional standards of the physical therapy profession?

   _____ a. the supervising physical therapist assistant

   _____ b. the supervising physical therapist

   _____ c. the director of physical therapy

   _____ d. each individual caregiver

6. A person is treated in a physical therapy setting. The person has been referred to physical therapy by a physician, evaluated by the physical therapist, and directed to the physical therapist assistant for treatment. Which individual has the primary responsibility for gaining informed consent prior to applying physical therapy interventions?

   _____ a. each caregiver

   _____ b. the physical therapist assistant

   _____ c. the physical therapist

   _____ d. the physician

7. Which physical therapy employment setting is LEAST appropriate for a physical therapist assistant?

   _____ a. a home health setting, with the physical therapist assistant providing the majority of interventions, and monthly reexamination of the patient by the physical therapist

   _____ b. an inpatient hospital setting, with the physical therapist assistant providing physical therapy interventions, and the physical therapist available in the same building

   _____ c. an elementary school setting, with the physical therapist assistants providing the majority of interventions, and initiating contact with the physical therapist, as the assistant deems necessary

   _____ d. a residential rehabilitative setting, with the physical therapist assistant and the physical therapist each seeing the same patients daily

8. Which physical therapy interventions is considered LEAST appropriate for a physical therapist assistant?

   _____ a. modification of a group of therapeutic exercises

   _____ b. nonselective sharp wound debridement

   _____ c. selective sharp wound debridement

   _____ d. peripheral joint mobilization

9. Which activities are LEAST appropriate for a physical therapist assistant?

   _____ a. modify an intervention based upon a patient's personality

   _____ b. perform interventions in a safe and effective manner

   _____ c. perform wound dressing interventions

   _____ d. modify the patient's plan of care

UTILIZING CLINICAL DECISION MAKING IN DATA COLLECTION AND INTERVENTION

Eleven Items

1. Which data collection technique BEST reflects the available length of a person's muscle?

   _____ a. active goniometric measurement of the agonist motion

   _____ b. passive goniometric measurement of the antagonist motion

   _____ c. manual muscle testing of the antagonist motion

   _____ d. anatomical palpation during active versus passive range agonist motion

2. A person, 47 years of age, is participating in cardiac rehabilitation. What target heart rate range, not to exceed 70% of maximal heart rate, is MOST indicated to promote cardiopulmonary endurance?

   _____ a. 33–47 beats per minute

   _____ b. 153–173 beats per minute

   _____ c. 91–121 beats per minute

   _____ d. 70–90 beats per minute

3. A person, who had a surgical release of the transverse carpal ligament to address carpal tunnel syndrome 4 weeks ago, now complains of severe night pain and sensitivity to temperature. What is a probable explanation for this information?

   _____ a. they could possibly have reflex sympathetic dystrophy

   _____ b. they could have a localized infection

   _____ c. this is typical up to 6 weeks after a surgical release

   _____ d. they are possibly inflicting self-harm to their affected upper extremity

4. Upon checking a person's progress since their last therapy session, you find they have right elbow range of motion of 44°–148°. Which active inhibition technique is most appropriate for a person with a right elbow flexion contracture?

   _____ a. passively extend the elbow, resist a triceps contraction, relax, and repeat

   _____ b. passively extend the elbow, resist a triceps contraction, relax, take further into extension range, and repeat

   _____ c. passively extend the elbow, resist a biceps contraction, relax, take further into flexion range, and repeat

   _____ d. passively flex the elbow, resist the biceps contraction, relax, take further into range, and repeat

5. A physical therapist assistant applies a stretch to a person's gastrocnemius. Immediately after the stretch, the assistant finds no change in available dorsiflexion range of motion. The intervention is repeated several times a day, in therapy and at home by the patient. After several weeks, the person has gained 7° of dorsiflexion. Which of the following properties of muscles and tendons has been demonstrated?

   _____ a. contractility

   _____ b. extensibility

   _____ c. plasticity

   _____ d. elasticity

6. A person, who is recovering from an arthroscopic debridement of their knee, demonstrates left knee active range of motion at 6°–120° and passive range of motion at 4°–138°. Which intervention is MOST appropriate?

   _____ a. strengthen the quadriceps and stretch the hamstrings

   _____ b. strengthen the hamstrings only

   _____ c. stretch the quadriceps and strengthen the hamstrings

   _____ d. strengthen the quadriceps only

7. A person is manual muscle tested and found to have 4−/5 strength in their right quadriceps femoris. Which intervention is MOST indicated to improve their strength?

_____ a. 20–30 minutes of Russian stimulation, patient resting in supine

_____ b. 3 sets of 15 repetitions, submaximal eccentric quadriceps contraction

_____ c. 3 sets of 10 repetitions, maximal isometric quadriceps contraction

_____ d. 3 sets of 20 repetitions, concentric quadriceps contraction

8. Which intervention is MOST appropriate for a person's right knee with 3+/5 strength of the vastus medialis, 15°–138° actively and 4°–140° passively?

_____ a. strengthen the quadriceps and stretch the hamstrings

_____ b. strengthen the hamstrings only

_____ c. stretch the quadriceps and strengthen the hamstrings

_____ d. strengthen the quadriceps only

9. A person is having difficulty with a muscular endurance activity. Which of the following sets of exercise parameters is MOST effective in addressing endurance?

_____ a. 3 sets of 15 repetitions, with minimal rest periods

_____ b. 3 sets of 10 repetitions, with 2 minute periods

_____ c. 10 sets of 3 repetitions, with 10 second rest periods

_____ d. 4 sets of 30 repetitions, with 30 second rest periods

10. A person has a stiff or short left hamstring. Which intervention is MOST indicated?

_____ a. apply a stretch into hip flexion with the knee extended

_____ b. apply a stretch into hip flexion with the knee flexed

_____ c. apply a stretch into knee flexion with the person in sitting

_____ d. apply a stretch into hip flexion with the person in supine

11. If a person is flexing their left knee to strengthen their hamstrings, they may have a tendency to dorsiflex their left ankle in order to achieve which of the following?

_____ a. achieve full knee extension

_____ b. activate their soleus muscle

_____ c. activate their gastrocnemius muscle

_____ d. place their hamstrings in midrange

UTILIZING, TEACHING, REINFORCING, AND OBSERVING BODY MECHANICS

Fourteen Items

1. A physical therapist assistant is observing a person lifting a moderate-sized object from the floor and carrying it across a room. Which strategy for effective body mechanics BEST applies to this task?

_____ a. carrying the object to one side

_____ b. keeping the object close and up towards the chest

_____ c. carrying the object close to the body with both arms

_____ d. keeping the object as close to the shoulders as possible

2. A physical therapist assistant is positioning a person with bilateral upper extremity paresis in sitting at the edge of an adjustable mat table. Which body mechanics strategy will achieve the greatest amount of stability to facilitate the sitting posture?

_____ a. distribute their weight between their feet, avoiding weight bearing through their upper extremities

_____ b. lean the person back onto a wedge, and use pillows that establish a 70° angle

_____ c. maximally extend the elbows with the person bearing weight through their arms

_____ d. lower the mat table to the lowest possible position to facilitate lower trunk contribution

3. You are gait training a person in the use of a wheeled walker with partial weight bearing on their left lower extremity. Where would you position yourself for safety when assisting a person to stand from the mat table?

_____ a. in front of the person

_____ b. to the person's left

_____ c. to the person's right

_____ d. behind the person

4. As you observe a person using a standard walker, you note that the assistive device is too short. This will MOST likely produce which of the following alterations?

_____ a. increase base of support

_____ b. flat low back posture

_____ c. decrease base of support

_____ d. kyphotic posture

5. A person has been primarily bedridden for 3 years prior to residing at your skilled nursing facility. When performing a dependent transfer technique, it is important to use the components of effective body mechanics. Which of the following strategies is LEAST effective for safely performing a dependent transfer technique?

_____ a. keep a controlled speed over the weight that you are lifting

_____ b. elevate the patient higher than your center of gravity

_____ c. large and stronger muscles should perform the majority of the work effort

_____ d. maintain center of gravity over your base of support

6. You are performing a stand-pivot transfer from a wheelchair to a bed with a person who has myelopathy primarily affecting the lower extremities. Which of the following is an effective strategy for proper body mechanics?

_____ a. keep your feet aligned parallel when blocking the person's knees

_____ b. keep your feet together for a stable base of support

_____ c. ensure that the person does not let go of the chair during the transfer

_____ d. use an offset stance

7. A person states that they are experiencing an exacerbation of low back pain at their place of employment. What should the patient be instructed regarding effective body mechanics to MOST effectively reduce the risk of lumbar strain?

_____ a. bend at the knees

_____ b. keep your back straight

_____ c. avoid end range of the lumbar spine

_____ d. avoid holding your breath

8. A person is participating in body mechanics skills training in a work-hardening setting of physical therapy. During lifting movements, it is important to increase intraabdominal pressure to improve stability of the lumbar spine. Contraction of which muscle is MOST effective at increasing intraabdominal pressure?

_____ a. transverse abdominus

_____ b. rectus abdominus

_____ c. bilateral external obliques

_____ d. latissimus dorsi

9. When instructing a person in the use of an assistive device to facilitate ambulation, cues regarding proper body mechanics and safety are also addressed. Which of the following statements is LEAST accurate regarding the utilization of assistive devices?

_____ a. use of an assistive device that is too short will increase flexion forces upon the spine

_____ b. use of a unilateral assistive device limits the amount of total body weight that can be supported

_____ c. use of a four-footed cane provides greater stability during gait than a standard cane

_____ d. use of a standard walker requires higher energy expenditure than not using an assistive device

10. A person is performing therapeutic exercise interventions to improve body mechanics and reduce thoracolumbar strain. Which activity is MOST effective in improving lumbar function and preventing thoracolumbar injury?

_____ a. double knee to chest

_____ b. prone extension using the arms

_____ c. standing lateral bends

_____ d. hip and knee stretching

11. A person is having difficulty with sitting stability when attempting sitting balance on the edge of a mat table. The physical therapist assistant is providing the person with strategies to facilitate sitting stability through upper extremity body mechanics. Which joint position provides the greatest stability at the radiocarpal joint?

_____ a. position in full wrist extension with full ulnar deviation

_____ b. position in full wrist extension with full supination

_____ c. position in neutral position of the wrist with the fingers in a fisted position

_____ d. position in a fisted position of the fingers with supination

12. A physical therapist has instructed a physical therapist assistant to perform therapeutic exercises with a patient to improve body mechanics. Which exercise intervention is MOST appropriate for a person with spinal lordosis and an anterior tilted pelvis?

_____ a. single knee to chest

_____ b. posterior pelvic tilt

_____ c. double knee to chest

_____ d. stabilization of the spine in neutral

13. A person is working with a physical therapist assistant to improve their techniques of lifting and carrying objects. Which instruction for patient education regarding prevention of lumbar strain and injury is MOST appropriate?

_____ a. keep the load slightly anterior to the surface of the body

_____ b. keep the load close to the upper thoracic region of the spine

_____ c. keep the load close to the lower thoracic region of the spine

_____ d. keep the load close to the lumbar region of the spine

14. A person is performing exercise interventions to address a glenohumeral joint condition. Specifically, the physical therapist has prescribed therapeutic exercises in the scapular plane. What should the clinician observe to assure the desired quality of full overhead motion using the shoulder in the scapular plane?

_____ a. the first 30° of humeral motion occurs without movement of the scapula

_____ b. scapulohumeral motion occurs at a 2:1 ratio

_____ c. there is greater than 160° of total overhead motion

_____ d. there is 180° of scaption

POSITIONING, DRAPING, AND STABILIZING PATIENTS

Twelve Items

1. A person in a prolonged supine position is LEAST likely to develop contractures in which of the following muscles?

_____ a. hamstrings

_____ b. iliopsoas

_____ c. deep hip external rotators

_____ d. rectus femoris

2. A person who has recently had a cerebral vascular accident is positioned in sidelying to address tone. Which of the following joint contractures is LEAST likely to occur in repeated prolonged sidelying positioning?

_____ a. iliofemoral flexion, and knee flexion

_____ b. iliofemoral adduction and internal rotation

_____ c. glenohumeral adduction and external rotation

_____ d. glenohumeral adduction

3. Which positioning technique will allow a person with neurological impairment of strength to generate the greatest amount of muscle force?

_____ a. place the muscle in a lengthened position

_____ b. place the muscle in a shortened position

_____ c. place the muscle in its mid overall length

_____ d. place the muscle in a position just slightly more lengthened than midrange

4. In normal short-sitting, the greatest amount of body weight pressure is located over which anatomical landmark(s)?

_____ a. ischial tuberosities

_____ b. sacrum

_____ c. lumbar spinous processes

_____ d. linea aspera of femurs

5. Which positioning technique is MOST appropriate for preparing a person for an intervention to be applied to the skin over the distal quadriceps?

_____ a. sidelying with the knees flexed and a pillow between the knees

_____ b. prone with the knees, pelvis, and head on a pillow

_____ c. supine, with a pillow under the head and knees

_____ d. sitting with a pillow at the popliteal crease

6. A person is being positioned in bed for an extended period due to the medical order for bed rest. Which of the following guidelines is not appropriate?

_____ a. reposition the person every 2 hours

_____ b. place the head of the bed in an elevation position

_____ c. maintain at least 1" of support between the mattress and the bed

_____ d. use pillows or wedges to prevent direct contact between bony prominences

7. Which parameter is LEAST appropriate when positioning a person in prone?

_____ a. knees flexed to 90°

_____ b. ankles at 90°

_____ c. hips abducted to 15°

_____ d. trunk in neutral

8. A person enters a treatment area to receive interferential stimulation to the lumbar paraspinal muscles with a moist heat pack for 20 minutes. Which positioning technique is MOST appropriate to prepare the person for this intervention?

_____ a. sitting with their back supported on a chair

_____ b. supine with a pillow under their knees and head

_____ c. prone with a pillow under their feet, pelvis, and head

_____ d. semirecumbent, supported by pillows, and slight flexion of the knees and feet

9. Which position will cause the greatest limitation for achieving neutral head alignment with a person who is neurologically impaired?

_____ a. prone

_____ b. supine

_____ c. sitting

_____ d. sidelying

10. Which of the following positions requires the LEAST amount of energy expenditure?

_____ a. supine

_____ b. prone

_____ c. sitting supported

_____ d. modified plantar grade

11. A person is receiving a combination of ultrasound and high-voltage direct current to the right thoracic paraspinal muscles. Which patient positioning technique is MOST appropriate for this intervention?

_____ a. sitting, leaning towards the left onto pillows placed on the treatment plinth

_____ b. sidelying, with pillows under the feet and upper trunk

_____ c. prone, with pillows under the feet and upper trunk

_____ d. sidelying, with pillows under the feet, head, and upper trunk

12. A person arrives at a physical therapy setting for therapeutic electrical stimulation interventions with moist heat to the middle and upper trapezius. What is the MOST appropriate positioning and draping technique for applying these interventions?

_____ a. sidelying, with a pillow under their humerus and between their knees, with draping below the tenth thoracic vertebrae

_____ b. supine, with a pillow under their head and knees, with draping below the inferior angles of the scapulae

_____ c. prone, with a pillow under their trunk and feet, with draping below the twelfth thoracic vertebrae

_____ d. sitting, leaning against the table onto several pillows, with draping below the inferior angles of the scapulae

ENSURING PATIENT SAFETY AND SAFE APPLICATION OF PATIENT CARE

Eight Items

1. Which of the following is not included in postsurgical precautions after rotator cuff repair?
   _____ a. avoid glenohumeral flexion greater than 140°
   _____ b. avoid glenohumeral external rotation greater than 30°
   _____ c. avoid glenohumeral internal rotation greater than 15°
   _____ d. avoid glenohumeral abduction greater than 90°

2. A person who had an elective left total hip arthroplasty SHOULD be directed to avoid which position?
   _____ a. iliofemoral abduction less than 40°
   _____ b. iliofemoral neutral rotation
   _____ c. iliofemoral flexion greater than 90°
   _____ d. iliofemoral adduction greater than 0°

3. A person who recently had a spinal cord injury at the sixth thoracic level is being trained for sliding board transfers. During the treatment session, the person becomes hypertensive, bradycardic, and complains of difficulty with their vision. What would be your BEST response?
   _____ a. place the patient in upright sitting and consult the supervising physical therapist about using a mechanical lift during the next treatment session
   _____ b. place the patient in upright sitting monitor the patient's vitals signs, and contact the patient's nurse or physician immediately
   _____ c. lay the patient supine, contact the physical therapist, and monitor the patient's vital signs
   _____ d. lay the patient supine, monitor and record the patient's vital signs, and inform the patient's nurse after therapy is completed

4. A person has been referred to physical therapy, evaluated by the physical therapists, and prescribed treatments for low back pain. The therapist has ordered ultrasound with electrical stimulation. Prior to today's session, the patient informs you that she may be pregnant. Which of the following is MOST appropriate?
   _____ a. after today's treatment, consult the patient's physical therapist
   _____ b. apply the ultrasound only without the electrical stimulation and consult the patient's physical therapist
   _____ c. consult the patient's physical therapist prior to applying today's treatment
   _____ d. refer the patient back to her physician

5. Upon reading a patient's evaluation form completed by the physical therapist, you find that the patient has been diagnosed as having insulin-dependent diabetes. Which of the following is true about the effects of insulin?
   _____ a. insulin decreases cellular uptake of amino acids
   _____ b. insulin decreases cellular uptake of glucose

_____ c. insulin increases cellular uptake of amino acids

_____ d. insulin increases cellular uptake of glucose

6. You are seeing a person bedside after a left anterior cruciate ligament reconstruction. Prior to beginning the exercise and ambulation interventions, you ask them how their knee is feeling. The person complains of severe pain in their left calf muscle that kept them awake all the night. Upon palpation they have a moderate increase in symptoms. Which of the following would be MOST appropriate?

_____ a. notify their nurse immediately of a potential thrombus formation

_____ b. instruct them to increase repetitions with their active ankle range of motion, which will decrease their gastrosoleus spasms at night

_____ c. perform the active knee range of motion prior to the ambulation, to relax the patient

_____ d. let them know that this is common after an anterior cruciate ligament repair, and typically subsides within 2–3 days

7. A person with a confirmed medical history of angina and diabetes is currently participating in cardiac rehabilitation. Their current short-term goal is to ambulate 250′ without a rest period. The person is ambulating without an assistive device or physical assistance, and so far has surpassed 220′. If the person complains of slight chest pain at this point, which of the following would be MOST immediately appropriate?

_____ a. decrease cadence and continue 30′ more

_____ b. sit the person down

_____ c. have the person use a wheeled walker to complete the last 30′

_____ d. administer a nitroglycerin tablet if available and walk further if the person's symptoms subside

8. A person had a total joint replacement earlier in the week. Today you observe the status of the limb prior to beginning the treatment session at the person's bedside. Which of the following is LEAST concerning regarding the potential presence of postsurgical infection?

_____ a. pain around the joint

_____ b. erythema around the surgical site

_____ c. warmth of the extremity

_____ d. drainage from the surgical site

PERFORMING FIRST AID

Ten Items

1. A person is practicing transfers from the mat table to the wheelchair. During the third attempt, the person receives a laceration injury upon their left thigh, which is bleeding significantly. Which is the MOST immediate action you should take for the person's safety?

_____ a. leave the person to get a pair of gloves

_____ b. apply direct pressure using the pillow case

_____ c. wrap the gait belt around the person's femur

_____ d. apply pressure to the popliteal artery

2. Which anatomical location is an effective place for applying direct pressure to decrease arterial bleeding?

_____ a. jugular

_____ b. brachial

_____ c. popliteal

_____ d. tracheal

3. A person receives a partial thickness cut injury to the dorsal surface of the right forearm. A staff member applies direct compression using a sterile gauze while wearing a pair of disposable gloves. What is the MOST appropriate time frame for this body part to stop bleeding?

_____ a. 15–30 seconds

_____ b. 1–3 minutes

_____ c. 4–5 minutes

_____ d. 6–10 minutes

4. A person has fallen in the bathroom of an outpatient physical therapy facility, and is found unconscious. Which actions are LEAST appropriate when responding to this event?

_____ a. move the person to the hallway to accurately assess them

_____ b. contact emergency medical services

_____ c. assess the person's airway, breathing, and circulation

_____ d. attempt to arouse the person verbally and with noxious stimulation

5. Which type of wound is LEAST likely to require stitches?

_____ a. laceration

_____ b. avulsion

_____ c. puncture

_____ d. incision

6. Direct pressure applied over the femoral artery can be effective in reducing moderate bleeding in the leg. Which anatomical location is correct for applying pressure at the femoral artery pressure point?

_____ a. posterior aspect of the knee

_____ b. just superior to the pes anserine of the medial leg

_____ c. at the inguinal crease

_____ d. approximately one to inches superior to the base of the patella

7. A person is bleeding from their left lower leg. After applying direct pressure, the bleeding does not stop. Pressure should then be applied to which anatomical location?

_____ a. posterior to the lateral malleolus

_____ b. posterior to the medial malleolus

_____ c. just medial to the distal biceps femoris

_____ d. just inferior to the inguinal crease of the same leg

8. Which first aid technique is MOST appropriate for a person who sustained a minor burn to their hand?

_____ a. apply a margarine product with no butter content

_____ b. cover the area with a dry sterile dressing and bandage

_____ c. immerse the injured area in cool water

_____ d. rub ice onto the injured area

9. A person is eating lunch during a physical therapy inservice. Suddenly, they reach for their throat and complain that they are choking. Which of the following is MOST appropriate?

_____ a. observe the person and monitor their ability to breathe

_____ b. apply five upward thrusts below the xiphoid process while standing behind the person

_____ c. lean the person over a chair or table and assist in applying abdominal thrusts until the object is dislodged

_____ d. apply upward thrusts between the umbilicus and xipoid process until the object becomes dislodged

10. Which of the following statements is LEAST true regarding a first aid response for a person who has just splashed a chemical into their eyes and is complaining that it is burning?

_____ a. if the chemical is acidic, flush with water for at least 10 minutes

_____ b. flush the eye from the inner corner towards the outer corner

_____ c. if the chemical is alkaline, flush with water for at least 20 minutes

_____ d. the head should be tilted away from the injured side if only one eye is affected

PERFORMING EMERGENCY PROCEDURES

Ten Items

1. Your patient, who is 31 years of age, suddenly collapses to the floor during gait training, is unresponsive, is not breathing, and has no pulse. What is the first thing you should do?

_____ a. use ammonia inhalants to arouse consciousness

_____ b. start chest compressions

_____ c. establish an airway

_____ d. contact emergency medical services

2. A person performing gait training with a standard walker suddenly collapses to the floor and has a convulsive seizure. What is the first thing you should do?

_____ a. manually restrain the person safely and begin cardiopulmonary resuscitation

_____ b. strap the person to a wooden board and begin cardiopulmonary resuscitation

_____ c. position in sidelying, check for open airway, and protect them until seizure is completed

_____ d. position in supine, check for open airway, and protect them until seizure is completed

3. A person is performing therapeutic exercises in sidelying on the mat table. Suddenly, the person is unresponsive, their eyes are open, and they are relatively still. With which type of seizure are these signs consistent?

_____ a. simple partial seizure

_____ b. tonic-clonic seizure

_____ c. absence seizure

_____ d. atonic seizure

4. A person performing lower extremity exercises on a mat table in a crowded inpatient physical therapy treatment area suddenly loses consciousness. What should you do FIRST?

_____ a. ask someone to call 9-1-1

_____ b. check to see if the person is oriented to person, place, or time

_____ c. ask someone to alert the in-house emergency response staff

_____ d. begin chest compression, and establish an airway

5. Rescue respiration must be provided to victims in order to reduce damage to vital organs. Potential irreversible brain damage occurs with the absence of oxygen within how many minutes?

_____ a. 1–3 minutes

_____ b. 3–5 minutes

_____ c. longer than 10 minutes

_____ d. 4–6 minutes

6. A person has been participating in physical therapy for 10 days. Some time after their arrival today, the person is found unconscious in the restroom. The person has a patent airway and is breathing. Since it is documented that the person is diabetic, which of the following responses is MOST appropriate?

_____ a. lay person on their side and cushion their head

_____ b. initiate cardiopulmonary resuscitation

_____ c. administer a sugar source

_____ d. administer insulin dose

7. A person is performing rescue breathing technique for an unconscious, unresponsive person with an open airway. Which of the following is MOST accurate regarding the correct execution of rescue breathing?

_____ a. ventilation should be 1–$1\frac{1}{2}$ seconds in duration when assisting adults

_____ b. ventilation should be $1\frac{1}{2}$–2 seconds in duration when assisting adults

_____ c. ventilation should be 3–5 seconds in duration when assisting adults

_____ d. ventilation should be $\frac{1}{2}$–3 seconds in duration when assisting adults

8. A person is found unconscious, is not breathing, and has a patent airway. What is the correct rate for performing rescue respirations to an adult person who is not breathing?

_____ a. 12 ventilations per minute

_____ b. 16 ventilations per minute

_____ c. 20 ventilations per minute

_____ d. 24 ventilations per minute

9. A person in a staff break area appears to be choking. They are unable to produce an audible sign and are holding their throat. What is the correct method for performing abdominal thrusts to someone who is choking?

_____ a. close to the xiphoid process, well above the umbilicus

_____ b. midway between the xiphoid process and the umbilicus

_____ c. above the umbilicus, well below the xiphoid process

_____ d. below the umbilicus and below the xiphoid process

10. A person is seen choking. What is the correct method of assisting a person who is choking?

_____ a. once the person becomes unconscious, initiate cardiopulmonary resuscitation

_____ b. once the person becomes unconscious, lower them to the floor, and continue abdominal thrusts

_____ c. once the person becomes unconscious, lay them onto their side to keep the airway clear from emesis

_____ d. once the person becomes unconscious, lean the person over the back of a chair or table, and apply the thrusts over the lumbar region

PERFORMING CPR

Twelve Items

1. A person is unresponsive, not breathing, but has a patent airway. Since they have no heart rate, emergency medical services are notified and chest compressions are initiated. When performing cardiopulmonary resuscitation to an adult, which of the following parameters is MOST accurate?

_____ a. the rescuer should keep their arms flexed, with their back aligned straight

_____ b. applying the chest compressions at a rate higher than one hundred compressions per minute

_____ c. the rescuer should position themselves straddling the person, avoiding contact with the xiphoid process

_____ d. applying chest compressions at a depth of $1^1/_2''$–$2''$

2. A person is performing cardiopulmonary resuscitation to an unconscious victim. What is the correct rate for providing rescue respirations?

_____ a. two initial breaths, then fifteen per minute for an infant

_____ b. two initial breaths, then twenty per minute for a child

_____ c. two initial breaths, then twenty per minute for an adult

_____ d. two initial breaths, then thirty per minute for a child

3. An adult is supine on a plinth performing straight leg raises. You realize that they are gagging on their chewing gum. What should be your FIRST response in this situation?

    _____ a. ask someone to contact emergency medical services

    _____ b. inform the person not to chew gum when performing supine therapeutic exercises

    _____ c. ask the person if they can speak or cough

    _____ d. approach the person from behind and apply abdominal thrusts

4. A person is performing cardiopulmonary resuscitation. What is the correct ratio of chest compressions to respirations for an adult?

    _____ a. 12:2

    _____ b. 10:1

    _____ c. 15:2

    _____ d. 5:1

5. What is the correct ratio of chest compressions to respirations when performing cardiopulmonary resuscitation to an infant?

    _____ a. 12:2

    _____ b. 10:1

    _____ c. 15:2

    _____ d. 5:1

6. Which of the following is MOST accurate about responding to a person who is choking?

    _____ a. abdominal thrusts can be administered from behind a person only

    _____ b. an emergency response should begin with patting a person who is choking on the back

    _____ c. adults who choke often lose consciousness and heart rate

    _____ d. children who choke often lose consciousness and heart rate

7. A person is performing cardiopulmonary resuscitation. After several minutes the rescuer notices that the abdomen is bulging. Which of the following explanations is MOST likely?

    _____ a. no oxygen is reaching the brain

    _____ b. ventilation is being applied with excessive pressure

    _____ c. the ribs are fractured due to excessive compression

    _____ d. the person is in ventricular fibrillation

8. A person is performing wall slides in a physical therapy exercise area, when suddenly they suffer cardiac arrest, become unconscious, and are not breathing. What is the BEST positioning to assist this person?

    _____ a. supine on a padded surface

    _____ b. sidelying on the closest treatment table

    _____ c. sitting in the nearest chair

    _____ d. supine on the floor

9. What is the correct ratio of chest compressions to respirations when performing cardiopulmonary resuscitation to a child?

    _____ a. 12:2

_____ b. 10:1

_____ c. 15:2

_____ d. 5:1

10. What is the correct rate of chest compressions for a child during cardiopulmonary resuscitation?

_____ a. 100 per minute

_____ b. 60–80 per minute

_____ c. 90 per minute

_____ d. 120 per minute

11. When performing cardiopulmonary resuscitation to a child, respirations are provided at which of the following rates?

_____ a. one breath every second

_____ b. one breath every 3 seconds

_____ c. one breath every 5 seconds

_____ d. fifteen breaths every minute

12. During a physical therapy visit to a person's home, an infant, 10 months of age, appears to have choked on a small object. Which of the following superficial sites is MOST reliable and accessible for assessing their heart rate?

_____ a. pericardial

_____ b. carotid

_____ c. femoral

_____ d. brachial

STERILE PROCEDURES

Seven Items

1. In a physical therapy clinical setting, which of the following is considered the MOST reasonable practice for preventing the spread of infection?

_____ a. surgical asepsis

_____ b. medical asepsis

_____ c. sterile environment

_____ d. contamination

2. When preparing a sterile field for an open wound care, which of the following guidelines is MOST accurate?

_____ a. a 1" border at the edges of the field is considered to be unsterile

_____ b. a 2" border at the edges of the field is considered to be unsterile

_____ c. a 3" border at the edges of the field is considered to be unsterile

_____ d. a 4" border at the edges of the field is considered to be unsterile

3. Which of the following should be avoided in techniques to maintain a sterile field during an aseptic technique?

_____ a. wear a mask and avoid sneezing or coughing across the field

_____ b. avoid reaching over or across the field

_____ c. ensure that the surface the field is placed upon is aseptic prior to placement

_____ d. open each of the packages prior to beginning the aseptic technique

4. Which of the following is MOST accurate regarding sterile gloving techniques?

_____ a. closed-glove techniques are more practical than open-glove techniques

_____ b. open-glove techniques provide a better chance of preventing contamination of the gloves

_____ c. it is easier to doff gloves after the open-glove technique

_____ d. it is easier to contaminate the gloves with the open technique

5. Which statement is MOST accurate regarding the establishment and maintenance of a sterile field for aseptic procedures?

_____ a. sterile items maintain their cleanliness for up to 2 hours after use

_____ b. all items placed upon the sterile field are considered sterile

_____ c. contamination occurs with momentary contact between sterile and nonsterile items

_____ d. each package placed upon the sterile field is considered cleaner on its exterior

6. Which technique is MOST effective for wearing personal protective equipment during aseptic procedures?

_____ a. the gloves should be placed over the sleeves of the gown

_____ b. the gown should be placed over the sleeves of the gloves

_____ c. the gown and gloves should not overlap

_____ d. the gown and gloves may or may not overlap

7. Which technique is acceptable for maintaining an aseptic condition during wound care interventions?

_____ a. don sterile gloves and gown, remove old wound dressing, discard off the materials, place the extremity in a whirlpool tank, and remove the gloves; afterwards, remove the patient, dry, apply sterile dressing, and discard the gloves, gown, and mask

_____ b. don gloves, gown, and mask, remove old wound dressing, place materials in approved bodily wastes container, place the extremity in a whirlpool tank; afterwards, remove the patient, dry, apply sterile dressing, discard the gloves, gown, and mask, and wash hands

_____ c. don gloves, gown, and mask, remove old wound dressing, discard in approved bodily waste container, and wash hands; afterwards, remove the patient, dry, apply sterile dressing, discard the gloves, gown, and mask, and wash hands

_____ d. don gloves, remove old wound dressing, discard the used materials, and place the extremity into whirlpool tank; afterwards, remove patient, dry, apply sterile dressing, and discard the gloves in approved soiled wastes container

DEMONSTRATING APPROPRIATE SEQUENCING OF EVENTS RELATED TO UNIVERSAL PRECAUTIONS

Seven Items

1. A person's medical record states that they have acquired a nosocomial infection. Based upon this information, which of the following is most accurate?

   _____ a. the infection was acquired in a hospital setting

   _____ b. the infection is the result of their body's rejection of a recent blood transfusion

   _____ c. they are most likely on reverse precautions

   _____ d. they are most likely on respiratory precautions

2. A physical therapist assistant has a small area of dermatitis on the dorsum of their hand with moderate exudate. They are scheduled to treat a patient with human immunodeficiency virus for management of an open wound. Which action is MOST appropriate?

   _____ a. continue with treatment as scheduled, and wash hands thoroughly before and after the treatment session

   _____ b. double glove and treat as scheduled, and wash hands thoroughly before and after the treatment session

   _____ c. use sterile precautions including mask and gloves, and wash hands thoroughly before and after the treatment session

   _____ d. assist with scheduling someone else to treat the patient

3. Wet-to-dry wound dressings can be indicated for devitalized wound beds. When applying a wet-to-dry wound dressing, which of the following is the correct sequence of application?

   _____ a. apply a single layer of sterile saline-soaked gauze and wrap in sterile dressing

   _____ b. apply a single layer of sterile saline-soaked gauze, cover with a single layer of dry gauze, and wrap in sterile dressing

   _____ c. apply a wet sterile saline-soaked wrap, cover with dry sterile gauze, and carefully secure with paper tape

   _____ d. apply sterile saline irrigation to the wound bed, cover with sterile gauze, and wrap in sterile dressing

4. What is the correct sequence for preparing to enter a person's room that is on protective isolation?

   _____ a. don the mask, then the cap, then the sterile gloves, and then the gown

   _____ b. don the gloves, then the gown, and then the cap

   _____ c. wash the hands, don sterile gloves, then the mask, then the gown, and then the cap

   _____ d. don the cap, then the mask, wash the hands, then don the sterile gloves, and then the gown

5. What is the correct sequence for preparing to exit a person's room on respiratory isolation?

_____ a. remove the mask and then wash hands

_____ b. wash hands and then remove the mask

_____ c. used gloved hands to remove the mask and then wash hands

_____ d. remove the gloves and then the mask

6. What is the correct sequence for preparing to exit a person's hospital room who is on contact isolation?

_____ a. doff the gloves, wash the hands, remove the gown, and then wash the hands

_____ b. doff the gloves and then the gown

_____ c. doff the gown, remove the gloves, and then wash the hands

_____ d. wash the hands, remove the gloves and gown, and then wash the hands

7. What is the correct sequence for preparing to exit a person's room who is in protective isolation?

_____ a. remove the gown first

_____ b. remove the mask last

_____ c. remove the gloves first

_____ d. remove the mask first

DEMONSTRATING ASEPTIC TECHNIQUE

Seven Items

1. Which of the following would BEST minimize the transmission of hepatitis B pathogens?

_____ a. don patient in gloves, gown, and mask to protect staff and visitors from infection

_____ b. wear gloves when treating the person

_____ c. wear a mask when treating the person

_____ d. wear gloves, gown, and mask when treating the person

2. Which personal protective equipment is essential for safely treating a person with a diagnosed contagious respiratory infection?

_____ a. mask

_____ b. gown

_____ c. gloves

_____ d. hair cover

3. Which technique is LEAST appropriate for effective hand washing for medical asepsis?

_____ a. wet your hands with your hands held lower than your elbows

_____ b. scrub the hands with a detergent for 30 seconds

_____ c. scrub the palms with a circular pattern of friction

_____ d. rinse the wrists and hands for at LEAST 10 seconds each

4. Which statement is LEAST accurate regarding effective hand washing techniques?

_____ a. an antimicrobial soap is recommended after working with a person who has methicillin-resistant staphylococcus aureus

_____ b. an antimicrobial soap is recommended after working with a person who has streptococcus

_____ c. an antimicrobial soap is recommended after working with a person who has vancomycin-resistant enterococca

_____ d. handwashing is the singlemost effective means of preventing the spread of infection

5. Which personal protective garment is necessary for applying nonimmersion wound irrigation?

_____ a. mask, cap, and gloves

_____ b. gloves, goggles, and gown

_____ c. gown, gloves, cap, and mask

_____ d. gown, gloves, goggles, and mask

6. When preparing sterile materials for an aseptic procedure, which of the following should be considered FIRST?

_____ a. the cost of replacing the sterile material

_____ b. if the packaging has maintained its integrity

_____ c. the color of the packaging

_____ d. if the package contains a sharp instrument

7. When opening a sterile package, which location is considered the LEAST aseptic?

_____ a. edges of packaging

_____ b. the inner lining of the packaging

_____ c. the middlemost portion of the packaging

_____ d. the potion most distal from the clinician

PROPERLY DISCARDING SOILED ITEMS

Seven Items

1. You are preparing a person for pulsed lavage. After removing a wound dressing, which of the following is MOST appropriate?

_____ a. double bag the material

_____ b. place the material in a single plastic bag, double bag if the outer portion of the bag may have been contaminated

_____ c. place the material in a common waste can and transport to the incinerator at the end of the day

_____ d. place the material in a single plastic bag

2. A physical therapist assistant has just completed a sterile dressing. After removing their personal protective equipment, which activity should follow?

_____ a. wash hands, with at least 10 seconds of rubbing lathered hands

_____ b. use nearly hot water, lather for at least 30 seconds, and scrub dry on a cotton towel

_____ c. wash hands with at least 5 seconds of rubbing lathered hands

_____ d. use cool to cold water, lather for at least 15 seconds, and pat dry with a sterile towel

3. A physical therapist assistant is cleaning a treatment area after a person has their wound cleaned and redressed. Which of the following items should be single bagged prior to disposal?

_____ a. used scalpel blades

_____ b. used tweezers

_____ c. used needles

_____ d. used syringes

4. Which sequence is MOST appropriate when preparing to perform a sterile technique?

_____ a. don gloves first and then the gown

_____ b. don one glove first, then the gown, and then the other glove

_____ c. don gown first and then the gloves

_____ d. don gloves up to thenar eminences, then the gown, and fold over the gloves

5. Upon entering a person's hospital room, you discover an uncapped needle and full syringe on the bedside table. Which action is MOST appropriate?

_____ a. remove the needle from the syringe, dispose in a puncture-resistant box, and then contact the nurse

_____ b. contact the nurse

_____ c. place the syringe and needle in a puncture-resistant box and then contact the nurse

_____ d. place the cap upon the needle and then contact the nurse

6. After removing a wound dressing in preparation for placing the person's body part in a whirlpool, which of the following is MOST appropriate?

_____ a. have the person sit in the whirlpool and then dispose of the dressing

_____ b. place the dressing in a plastic disposal bag

_____ c. hold the dressing until the person is stabilized in the whirlpool

_____ d. place the dressing upon a the sterile field until the person is safely stabilized in the whirlpool

7. A person on contact isolation has a bowel movement in bed while you are assisting them with lower extremity range of motion. Which of the following is LEAST appropriate?

_____ a. the physical therapist assistant assists the staff with turning the person in order for them to be properly cleaned

_____ b. all potentially soiled linens are removed from the person and the bed

_____ c. the linens are prerinsed in the sink and placed in a plastic disposal bag

_____ d. the physical therapist assistant dons a clean glove and gown prior to providing any assistance

DETERMINING EQUIPMENT TO BE USED AND ASSEMBLING ALL MATERIALS

Seven Items

1. Which statement is the primary element of universal precautions?
   _____ a. avoid contact with bloody substances
   _____ b. treat all persons as potentially infectious
   _____ c. avoid wiping your nose
   _____ d. wash your hands thoroughly before and after treatment session

2. A clinician is preparing to perform wound care interventions, including mechanical debridement, for a person with an open wound. Which item does not need to be assembled prior to applying this intervention?
   _____ a. sterile forceps
   _____ b. sterile saline
   _____ c. sterile brush
   _____ d. pulsed lavage machine

3. A person is receiving wound care interventions in a physical therapy setting. Which material is LEAST appropriate for addressing a person with a minor, noninfected burn wound?
   _____ a. hydrocolloids
   _____ b. calcium alginates
   _____ c. hydrogels
   _____ d. wet to dry dressing

4. A person who has an open wound is being treated in physical therapy. Currently, the person is wearing a moisture barrier/skin sealant. Which of the following is LEAST accurate regarding the use of moisture barriers or skin sealants?
   _____ a. the barriers are used to increase maceration
   _____ b. the barriers are used to protect the surrounding skin from adhesions
   _____ c. the sealants increase the oily content of the skin
   _____ d. the sealants can be left in place for 5 days

5. A person, who has a burn wound, is currently experiencing heavy drainage from the wound bed. Which wound care materials are MOST appropriate for this person?
   _____ a. wet to dry dressing
   _____ b. alginate dressing
   _____ c. topical antimicrobial
   _____ d. hydrocolloids

6. When treating persons who are on isolation precautions it is important to understand which type of protective equipment is indicated. Which clinical condition does not indicate the use of gloves?

_____ a. methicillin-resistant staphylococcus aureus

_____ b. vancomycin-resistant entercoccus

_____ c. clostridium difficile

_____ d. rubella

7. When preparing to enter a person's hospital room, you don the appropriate personal protective equipment. Which type of personal protective equipment is MOST indicated when working with persons on airborne precautions with tuberculosis?

_____ a. over the ear surgical mask

_____ b. negative air flow mask

_____ c. T-280 disposable mask

_____ d. N-95 dust mist mask

ANSWERS AND RATIONALE

MAINTAINING PATIENT CONFIDENTIALITY

Thirteen Items

1. Correct answer: (c)

   Rationale: The findings of the evaluation, explanation of proposed interventions, benefits and risks, and reasonable alternatives to interventions must be addressed to the patient.

   Reference: Scott, R. (1997). *Promoting legal awareness in physical and occupational therapy* (p. 124). St. Louis: Mosby.

2. Correct answer: (b)

   Rationale: Based upon case law, the health care provider is considered primarily responsible, and held to a higher expectation than the patient.

   Reference: Scott, R. (1997). *Promoting legal awareness in physical and occupational therapy* (p. 103). St. Louis: Mosby.

3. Correct answer: (b)

   Rationale: Although necessary prior to applying any intervention, contraindications are not a part of informed consent.

   Reference: Scott, R. (1999). *Health care malpractice, a primer on legal issues for professionals* (2nd ed., p. 40). New York: McGraw-Hill.

4. Correct answer: (d)

   Rationale: Case law has established that documents designated for improving the quality of care and patient safety within a systematic review program are often exempted from involuntary release to litigants. Failure to clearly label such documents may allow their release without the facility's permission.

   Reference: Scott, R. (1997). *Promoting legal awareness in physical and occupational therapy* (p. 71). St. Louis: Mosby.

5. Correct answer: (d)

   Rationale: Each of these events is possible with the establishment of vicarious liability.

   Reference: Scott, R. (1997). *Promoting legal awareness in physical and occupational therapy* (p. 54). St. Louis: Mosby.

6. Correct answer: (d)

   Rationale: The other three conditions are included in the Patients' Bill of Rights.

   Reference: Scott, R. (1997). *Promoting legal awareness in physical and occupational therapy* (p. 118, 119). St. Louis: Mosby.

7. Correct answer: (c)

   Rationale: By documenting that the patient has given an informed choice, it shows that the provider has made the person aware of expected benefits and risks, with and without this intervention. This covers the caregiver better legally than simply stating the person was noncompliant. It also appears less slanderous of the patient.

   Reference: Scott, R. (1997). *Promoting legal awareness in physical and occupational therapy* (p. 124). St. Louis: Mosby.

8. Correct answer: (d)

   Rationale: Deonto means duty. An approach to ethical situations focusing on the duty of professionals to act.

   Reference: Purtillo, R., & Haddad, A. (2002). *Health professional and patient interaction* (6th ed., p. 29). Philadelphia: WB Saunders.

9. Correct answer: (c)

   Rationale: The right to privacy is guaranteed by the Patients' Bill of Rights. Recently, the protection of personal health information is further protected by the Health Insurance Portability and Accountability Act.

   Reference: Scott, R. (1997). *Promoting legal awareness in physical and occupational therapy* (p. 118, 119). St. Louis: Mosby.

10. Correct answer: (b)

    Rationale: Patient's confidentiality is breached when potential identifiers, or information not necessary, are discussed. Generally, you should not discuss patients with a person not involved in their treatment. You should also avoid discussion patients in nonprivate areas.

Reference: Purtillo, R., & Haddad, A. (2002). *Health professional and patient interaction* (6th ed., p. 152). Philadelphia: WB Saunders.

11. Correct answer: (c)

    Rationale: Describing a person by height or weight may be useful toward a person's function, or to identify the person to their physical therapist. The physical therapist does not have a need to know about a personal story the patient shared with you.

    Reference: Purtillo, R., & Haddad, A. (2002). *Health professional and patient interaction* (6th ed., p. 152). Philadelphia: WB Saunders.

12. Correct answer: (c)

    Rationale: Only the persons involved in direct patient care of that person should review the progress note.
    Reference: Lukan, M. (2001). *Documentation for physical therapist assistants* (2nd ed., p. 119). Philadelphia: FA Davis.

13. Correct answer: (b)

    Rationale: Avoid discussing the person's condition and status in the reception area. Introduction of their names is appropriate in a public area.
    Reference: Purtillo, R., & Haddad, A. (2002). *Health professional and patient interaction* (6th ed., p. 117). Philadelphia: WB Saunders.

MAINTAINING PATIENT AUTONOMY AND OBTAINING CONSENT

Thirteen Items

1. Correct answer: (a)

   Rationale: Physical restraints are used to protect the patient, or others, and may not be used for disciplinary purposes.
   Reference: Scott, R. (1997). *Promoting legal awareness in physical and occupational therapy* (p. 252). St. Louis: Mosby.

2. Correct answer: (c)

   Rationale: Any material used to prevent the mobility and freedom of a person is considered a physical restraint.
   Reference: Scott, R. (1997). *Promoting legal awareness in physical and occupational therapy* (p. 252). St. Louis: Mosby.

3. Correct answer: (d)

   Rationale: The durable power of attorney for health care designates a surrogate decision maker to take effect when the person is no longer legally competent to make decisions for them.

Reference: Scott, R. (1997). *Promoting legal awareness in physical and occupational therapy* (p. 252). St. Louis: Mosby.

4. Correct answer: (a)

   Rationale: Patient-focused care is an approach that arranges the health care delivery around the patient, instead of vice versa.

   Reference: Pagliarulo, M. (2001). *Introduction to physical therapy* (2nd ed., p. 126). St. Louis: Mosby.

5. Correct answer: (b)

   Rationale: Medications are considered a chemical form of restraint.

   Reference: Scott, R. (1997). *Promoting legal awareness in physical and occupational therapy* (p. 252). St. Louis: Mosby.

6. Correct answer: (a)

   Rationale: The elements of obtaining informed consent include clear explanations, addressing any questions, and documenting the occurrence.

   Reference: Ramsden, E. (1999). *The Person as patient, psychosocial perspectives for the health care professional* (p. 208, 209). Philadelphia: WB Saunders.

7. Correct answer: (d)

   Rationale: Under the ethical principles of patient autonomy, patients are credited with being the best judge of what is good or acceptable for them.

   Reference: Ramsden, E. (1999). *The person as patient, psychosocial perspectives for the health care professional* (p. 214). Philadelphia: WB Saunders.

8. Correct answer: (c)

   Rationale: Surrogate consent is required when a person has compromised cognitive function.

   Reference: Scott, R. (1999). *Health care malpractice, a Primer on legal issues for professionals* (2nd ed., p. 47). New York: McGraw-Hill.

9. Correct answer: (a)

   Rationale: Age 2–4 years is described as the autonomy versus shame and doubt stage. Although too young to provide legal consent for their care, it is important to involve patients even at very young ages.

   Reference: Ramsden, E. (1999). *The person as patient, psychosocial perspectives for the health care professional* (p. 14). Philadelphia: WB Saunders.

10. Correct answer: (a)

    Rationale: A patient is considered to have an inherent right to control and self-determination.

    Reference: Scott, R. (1997). *Promoting legal awareness in physical and occupational therapy* (p. 253). St. Louis: Mosby.

11. Correct answer: (c)

    Rationale: Any intentional contact for arousal or gratification of the person or caregiver may qualify as sexual battery.

Reference: Scott, R. (1999). *Professional ethics: A guide for rehabilitation professionals* (p. 134). St. Louis: Mosby.

12. Correct answer: (d)

Rationale: The hospital must address applicable state laws, and provide written policies used in the facility and state the person's informed choices regarding these issues.

Reference: Scott, R. (1997). *Promoting legal awareness in physical and occupational therapy* (p. 252, 253). St. Louis: Mosby.

13. Correct answer: (c)

Rationale: The Patients' Bill of Rights states that you have the right to know which providers are responsible for your health care.

Reference: Scott, R. (1999). *Health care malpractice, a primer on legal issues for professionals* (2nd ed., p. 19, 20). New York: McGraw-Hill.

WORK UNDER THE SUPERVISION AND DIRECTION OF A PHYSICAL THERAPIST IN AN ETHICAL, LEGAL, AND SAFE MANNER

Nine Items

1. Correct answer: (c)

Rationale: Health care professionals should avoid the perception of inappropriate conduct.

Reference: Bottomley, J. (2000). *Quick reference dictionary for physical therapy* (p. 255). Thorofare, NJ: Slack Incorporated.

2. Correct answer: (b)

Rationale: Protection of the patient's safety, their interests, and health is the first priority and the correct choice.

Reference: Edge, R., & Groves, J. (1999). *Ethics of health care: A guide for clinical practice* (2nd ed., p. 65). Albany: Delmar.

3. Correct answer: (b)

Rationale: Incident reports are required for all deviations in patient care, or work-related procedures. This document establishes a memorandum of an event.

Reference: Scott, R. (1994). *Legal aspects of documenting patient care* (2nd ed., p. 161). Maryland: Aspen.

4. Correct answer: (c)

Rationale: The clinical instructor has a responsibility regarding the student. They can further determine what type of response the event requires.

Reference: Scott, R. (1997). *Promoting legal awareness in physical and occupational therapy* (p. 182, 183). St. Louis: Mosby.

5. Correct answer: (d)

   Rationale: Quid pro quo is typically a request or offered exchange for sexual conduct. Sexual harassment is a general term used to apply to quid pro quo or hostile work environment. Sexual abuse is an unwanted physical act, without consent.

   Reference: Nosse, L., et al. (1999). *Managerial and supervisory principles for physical therapists* (p. 263). Baltimore: Williams & Wilkins.

6. Correct answer: (c)

   Rationale: A person with global aphasia would not be found contributing to negligence.

   Reference: Scott, R. (1997). *Promoting legal awareness in physical and occupational therapy* (p. 33). St. Louis: Mosby.

7. Correct answer: (d)

   Rationale: Any of the other choices are grounds for establishing negligence. With cases filed to investigate negligence, a peer review will establish what is considered reasonably prudent.

   Reference: Scott, R. (1997). *Promoting legal awareness in physical and occupational therapy* (p. 34). St. Louis: Mosby.

8. Correct answer: (c)

   Rationale: Minor modifications to treatment do not require personal contact with the patient.

   Reference: Pagliarulo, M. (2001). *Introduction to physical therapy* (2nd ed., p. 58). St. Louis: Mosby.

9. Correct answer: (b)

   Rationale: The American Physical Therapy Association (APTA) is the primary representative organization for physical therapy.

   Reference: Pagliarulo, M. (2001). *Introduction to physical therapy* (2nd ed., p. 8). St. Louis: Mosby.

KNOWING AND WORKING WITHIN APPLICABLE STATE LAWS AND RULES GOVERNING PHYSICAL THERAPY

Twelve Items

1. Correct answer: (b)

   Rationale: State practice acts are laws; the other documents are policies, and are not directly legally binding.

   Reference: Pagliarulo, M. (2001). *Introduction to physical therapy* (2nd ed., p. 55). St. Louis: Mosby.

2. Correct answer: (a)

   Rationale: The American with Disabilities Act applies to private sector employers with more than 15 employees.

   Reference: Bottomley, J. (2000). *Quick reference dictionary for physical therapy* (p. 452). Thorofare, NJ: Slack Incorporated.

3. Correct answer: (d)

   Rationale: Individuals are treated based upon universal precautions. Employees should be provided personal protective equipment (PPE) when potentially exposed to bodily fluids.

   Reference: Pierson, F. (2002). *Principles and techniques of patient care* (3rd ed., p. 44). Philadelphia: WB Saunders.

4. Correct answer: (d)

   Rationale: Personal information should not be solicited during an employment interview.

   Reference: Scott, R. (1997). *Promoting legal awareness in physical and occupational therapy* (p. 211). St. Louis: Mosby.

5. Correct answer: (d)

   Rationale: The House of Delegates is the highest policy-making body of the American Physical Therapy Association.

   Reference: Pagliarulo, M. (2001). *Introduction to physical therapy* (2nd ed., p. 82). St. Louis: Mosby.

6. Correct answer: (b)

   Rationale: The laws do not eliminate lawsuits or affect the actions of rescuers; they are directed to protecting persons who act reasonable for the aid of another person.

   Reference: Scott, R. (1997). *Promoting legal awareness in physical and occupational therapy* (p. 246, 247). St. Louis: Mosby.

7. Correct answer: (a)

   Rationale: Statutes are a legislative function, where common law is derived from judicial proceedings.

   Reference: Pagliarulo, M. (2001). *Introduction to physical therapy* (2nd ed., p. 93). St. Louis: Mosby.

8. Correct answer: (b)

   Rationale: Employers are required to make reasonable accommodation, except those that fundamentally alter the operation of business. There are varying financial limitations to the employer's responsibility, but choice (c) is vague.

   Reference: Scott, R. (1997). *Promoting legal awareness in physical and occupational therapy* (p. 195, 196). St. Louis: Mosby.

9. Correct answer: (c)

   Rationale: Race, gender, or sexual orientation is not applicable under the American with Disabilities Act.

   Reference: Scott, R. (1997). *Promoting legal awareness in physical and occupational therapy* (p. 197). St. Louis: Mosby.

10. Correct answer: (a)

    Rationale: This is the primary reason for completing an incident report. An incident report is intended to serve as a quality improvement document, and may not necessarily protect individuals from legal grievance.

    Reference: Scott, R. (1997). *Promoting legal awareness in physical and occupational therapy* (p. 161, 162). St. Louis: Mosby.

11. Correct answer: (d)

    Rationale: Negligence can be established from any of these given parameters.

    Reference: Scott, R. (1999). *Health care malpractice, a primer on legal issues for professionals* (2nd ed., p. 22). New York: McGraw-Hill.

12. Correct answer: (a)

    Rationale: Incident reports should be written without speculation, or attempts to describe potential cause.

    Reference: Scott, R. (1997). *Promoting legal awareness in physical and occupational therapy* (p. 162). St. Louis: Mosby.

PERFORMING ONLY THOSE TASKS WITHIN A PHYSICAL THERAPIST ASSISTANT'S KNOWLEDGE AND SKILL LEVEL

Nine Items

1. Correct answer: (a)

   Rationale: Biomedical equipment maintenance and repair is not within the scope of physical therapy personnel, and qualifies as a material risk.

   Reference: Scott, R. (1997). *Promoting legal awareness in physical and occupational therapy* (p. 122). St. Louis: Mosby.

2. Correct answer: (a)

   Rationale: Professional encroachment occurs when a person performs the skills of another profession, and may be in violation of some laws.

   Reference: Pagliarulo, M. (2001). *Introduction to physical therapy* (2nd ed., p. 124). St. Louis: Mosby.

3. Correct answer: (b)

   Rationale: This is one of the responsibilities that cannot be delegated by the supervisory physical therapist.

   Reference: Pagliarulo, M. (2001). *Introduction to physical therapy* (2nd ed., p. 55). St. Louis: Mosby.

4. Correct answer: (b)

   Rationale: This is one of the responsibilities that cannot be delegated by the physical therapist.

   Reference: Pagliarulo, M. (2001). *Introduction to physical therapy* (2nd ed., p. 55). St. Louis: Mosby.

5. Correct answer: (d)

Rationale: Each physical therapy provider is responsible for ensuring the professional standards are maintained with each person.

Reference: Scott, R. (1997). *Promoting legal awareness in physical and occupational therapy* (pp. 291–295). St. Louis: Mosby.

6. Correct answer: (c)

Rationale: The physical therapist has sole responsibility for obtaining informed consent.

Reference: Scott, R. (1999). *Health care malpractice, a primer on legal issues for professionals* (2nd ed., p. 41). New York: McGraw-Hill.

7. Correct answer: (c)

Rationale: The physical therapist should make regular supervisory visits, at least monthly, but at the determination of the therapist. The assistant is only indicated to request additional supervisory visits as needed.

Reference: Pagliarulo, M. (2001). *Introduction to physical therapy* (2nd ed., p. 58). St. Louis: Mosby.

8. Correct answer: (c)

Rationale: The American Physical Therapy Association provides policy guidance regarding these interventions. Though it is not specified in most state laws, the policy likely has influence in legal proceedings. The use of selective sharp debridement includes the choice of leaving or taking potentially healthy tissue. Within physical therapy, this is considered the exclusive domain of the physical therapist.

Reference: Myers, B. (2004). *Wound management, principles and practice* (p. 72). Upper Saddle River, NJ: Prentice Hall.

9. Correct answer: (d)

Rationale: The plan of care should not be modified without the direction of the supervising physical therapist.

Reference: (1999). *A normative model of physical therapist assistant education: Version 99* (p. 177). Alexandria, VA: American Physical Therapy Association.

UTILIZING CLINICAL DECISION MAKING IN DATA COLLECTION AND INTERVENTION

Eleven Items

1. Correct answer: (b)

Rationale: A muscle reaches passive insufficiency in length when passively taking it through the motion of its antagonist.

Reference: Smith, L., et al. (1996). *Brunnstrom's clinical kinesiology* (5th ed., p. 135). Philadelphia: FA Davis.

2. Correct answer: (c)

   Rationale: This person's maximal heart rate is 173 beats per minute; 70% is 121 beats per minute.

   Reference: Hillegass, E., & Sadowsky, H. (2001). *Essentials of cardiopulmonary physical therapy* (2nd ed., p. 695). Philadelphia: WB Saunders.

3. Correct answer: (a)

   Rationale: These symptoms are the telltale signs of the potential presence of reflex sympathetic dystrophy.

   Reference: Magee, D. J. (2002). *Orthopedic physical assessment* (4th ed., p. 360). Philadelphia: WB Saunders.

4. Correct answer: (b)

   Rationale: This is an accurate description of an active inhibition technique, specifically agonist contraction.

   Reference: Kisner, C., & Colby, L. (2002). *Therapeutic exercise: Foundations and techniques* (4th ed., p. 195). Philadelphia: FA Davis.

5. Correct answer: (c)

   Rationale: Plastic changes in muscles in tendons allow for lengthening to increase available range of motion.

   Reference: Lieber, R. (2002). *Skeletal muscle structure, function & plasticity* (2nd ed., p. 173). Philadelphia: Lippincott Williams & Wilkins.

6. Correct answer: (b)

   Rationale: The person has full available range of motion into flexion and extension. They are unable to complete available left knee flexion, which indicates a need to strengthen the hamstrings.

   Reference: Lesh, S. (2000). *Clinical orthopedics for the physical therapist assistant* (p. 362). Philadelphia: FA Davis.

7. Correct answer: (d)

   Rationale: Russian stimulation is more indicated for 2−/5 to 3+/5 strength. Submaximal eccentric and isometric contractions are indicated for less than 3/5 strength.

   Reference: Kisner, C., & Colby, L. (2002). *Therapeutic exercise: Foundations and techniques* (4th ed., p. 84, 85). Philadelphia: FA Davis.

8. Correct answer: (d)

   Rationale: The person has full available right knee range of motion. Both 3+/5 vastus medialis oblique strength and their inability to actively extend their right knee beyond 15° are indications for quadriceps strengthening.

   Reference: Kisner, C., & Colby, L. (2002). *Therapeutic exercise: Foundations and techniques* (4th ed., p. 59). Philadelphia: FA Davis.

9. Correct answer: (d)

   Rationale: This choice offers the highest repetitions, and sets, with the least between set rest duration.

   Reference: Kisner, C., & Colby, L. (2002). *Therapeutic exercise: Foundations and techniques* (4th ed., p. 75). Philadelphia: FA Davis.

10. Correct answer: (a)

   Rationale: The hamstrings actively produce hip extension and knee flexion. Stretching is applied in the opposite direction of its actions.

   Reference: Kisner, C., & Colby, L. (2002). *Therapeutic exercise: Foundations and techniques* (4th ed., p. 493). Philadelphia: FA Davis.

11. Correct answer: (c)

   Rationale: With dorsiflexion the gastrocnemius is lengthened at the ankle and enabled to contribute in a knee flexion force.

   Reference: Bottomley, J. (2000). *Quick reference dictionary for physical therapy* (p. 509). Thorofare, NJ: Slack Incorporated.

UTILIZING, TEACHING, REINFORCING, AND OBSERVING BODY MECHANICS

Fourteen Items

1. Correct answer: (c)

   Rationale: Carrying an object too high or on one side will create greater musculoskeletal strain.

   Reference: Nordin, M., & Frankel, V. (2001). *Basic biomechanics of the musculoskeletal system* (3rd ed., p. 272). Philadelphia: Lippincott Williams & Wilkins.

2. Correct answer: (c)

   Rationale: This is the closed-packed position of the ulnar-humeral joint, which is the most stable position for the elbow. Lowering the mat will often reduce the lower trunk contribution.

   Reference: Rothstein, J., et al. (1998). *The rehabilitation specialist's handbook* (2nd ed., p. 108). Philadelphia: FA Davis.

3. Correct answer: (b)

   Rationale: The PTA should stand on the person's involved side during sitting to and from standing, and gait training with an assistive device.

   Reference: Pierson, F. (2002). *Principles and techniques of patient care* (3rd ed., p. 225). Philadelphia: WB Saunders.

4. Correct answer: (d)

   Rationale: Bending forward to reach the device will increase postural flexion, resulting in a more kyphotic posture.

   Reference: Pierson, F. (2002). *Principles and techniques of patient care* (3rd ed., p. 222). Philadelphia: WB Saunders.

5. Correct answer: (b)

   Rationale: More effective is to keep the person closer to your center of gravity. Each of the other choices is a component of effective body mechanics.

   Reference: Pierson, F. (2002). *Principles and techniques of patient care* (3rd ed., p. 69). Philadelphia: WB Saunders.

6. Correct answer: (d)

   Rationale: This posture prepares the clinician for safety support of the person in each plane where the person may lose their balance.

   Reference: Pierson, F. (2002). *Principles and techniques of patient care* (3rd ed., p. 73). Philadelphia: WB Saunders.

7. Correct answer: (c)

   Rationale: End range of lumbar motion creates the greatest amount of spinal stress. Bending the hips and knees is common but less effective methods of improving body mechanics.

   Reference: Dvir, Z. (2000). *Clinical biomechanics* (p. 129). New York: Churchill Livingstone.

8. Correct answer: (a)

   Rationale: The transverse abdominus generally lies in the horizontal plane, attaches to the dorsal lumbar fascia, and is most effective of the lumbar muscle in increasing intraabdominal pressure.

   Reference: Nordin, M., & Frankel, V. (2001). *Basic biomechanics of the musculoskeletal system* (3rd ed., p. 278). Philadelphia: Lippincott Williams & Wilkins.

9. Correct answer: (c)

   Rationale: Evidence has shown that a four-footed cane may provide greater stability in stance, but not ambulation, than a standard cane.

   Reference: Dvir, Z. (2000). *Clinical biomechanics* (p. 178). New York: Churchill Livingstone.

10. Correct answer: (d)

    Rationale: Hip and knee mobility has been shown to be the most effective exercise of the choices in reducing risk of recurrent injury.

    Reference: Dvir, Z. (2000). *Clinical biomechanics* (p. 131). New York: Churchill Livingstone.

11. Correct answer: (a)

    Rationale: Full extension with full ulnar deviation places the wrist in the closed-packed position, which is the position with greatest stability for the wrist.

    Reference: Rothstein J., et al. (1998). *The rehabilitation specialist's handbook* (2nd ed., p. 108). Philadelphia: FA Davis.

12. Correct answer: (d)

    Rationale: Posterior pelvic tilts are often considered the standard response. However, posterior tilting also increases spinal loads. Spinal stabilization in a neutral position is most appropriate with the least amount of spinal stress.

    Reference: Dvir, Z. (2000). *Clinical biomechanics* (p. 130). New York: Churchill Livingstone.

13. Correct answer: (d)

    Rationale: Loads should be kept as close as possible to the lumbar segment of the spinal column.

    Reference: Dvir, Z. (2000). *Clinical biomechanics* (p. 129). New York: Churchill Livingstone.

14. Correct answer: (a)

    Rationale: The humerus should move first and most with flexion, scaption, and abduction of the shoulder.

    Reference: Dvir, Z. (2000). *Clinical biomechanics* (p. 178). New York: Churchill Livingstone.

POSITIONING, DRAPING, AND STABILIZING PATIENTS

Twelve Items

1. Correct answer: (d)

   Rationale: In supine, people are susceptible to flexion postures of the hip and knee, while the feet tends to turn out into external rotation.

   Reference: Pierson, F. (2002). *Principles and techniques of patient care* (3rd ed., p. 37). Philadelphia: WB Saunders.

2. Correct answer: (c)

   Rationale: Glenohumeral adduction and external rotation would occur with contracture of the posterior cuff or posterior deltoid muscles. These muscles rarely develop contractures.

   Reference: Pierson, F. (2002). *Principles and techniques of patient care* (3rd ed., p. 37). Philadelphia: WB Saunders.

3. Correct answer: (a)

   Rationale: Placing a muscle in an elongated position allows a person with neurogenic paresis to generate greater muscle force.

   Reference: Dvir, Z. (2000). *Clinical biomechanics* (p. 171). New York: Churchill Livingstone.

4. Correct answer: (a)

   Rationale: Answers (b) and (c) occur with excessive posterior pelvic tilt, (d) is an invalid choice, and (a) is the correct location in normal sitting.

   Reference: Pierson, F. (2002). *Principles and techniques of patient care* (3rd ed., p. 37). Philadelphia: WB Saunders.

5. Correct answer: (c)

   Rationale: The quadriceps are on the anterior surface of the body, and require the supine position for adequate access.

Reference: Minor, M., & Minor, S. (1999). *Patient care skills* (4th ed., p. 118). Norwalk, CT: Appleton & Lange.

6. Correct answer: (b)

Rationale: Elevation of the bed will increase pressure contact for the lower body. Elevation should only be integrated for persons with respiratory impairment.

Reference: Anemaet, W., et al. (2000). *Home rehabilitation: Guide to clinical practice* (p. 479). St. Louis: Mosby.

7. Correct answer: (a)

Rationale: In the prone position, excessive knee flexion is avoided to prevent anterior pressure of lower limbs.

Reference: Anemaet, W., et al. (2000). *Home rehabilitation: Guide to clinical practice* (p. 479). St. Louis: Mosby.

8. Correct answer: (c)

Rationale: The pillow under the feet may be optional. The paraspinal are located on the posterior surface of the trunk, which requires the prone position.

Reference: Minor, M., & Minor, S. (1999). *Patient care skills* (4th ed., p. 122). Norwalk, CT: Appleton & Lange.

9. Correct answer: (a)

Rationale: In the prone position, it is difficult to place the head in a neutral position, since the head is face down.

Reference: Anemaet, W., et al. (2000). *Home rehabilitation: Guide to clinical practice* (p. 94). St. Louis: Mosby.

10. Correct answer: (b)

Rationale: The prone position requires the least amount of energy expenditure.

Reference: Anemaet, W., et al. (2000). *Home rehabilitation: Guide to clinical practice* (p. 92, 93). St. Louis: Mosby.

11. Correct answer: (c)

Rationale: Either sitting or prone is appropriate for the application of ultrasound-electrical stimulation combination to the thoracic paraspinals. Sidelying upon pillows is more likely to stress the thoracic paraspinal muscles.

Reference: Minor, M., & Minor, S. (1999). *Patient care skills* (4th ed., p. 122). Norwalk, CT: Appleton & Lange.

12. Correct answer: (d)

Rationale: In this position, the body can be accessed, and the person sufficiently supported, without trapping the heat of the hot pack.

Reference: Andrade, C., & Clifford, P. (2001). *Outcome-based massage* (p. 104). Philadelphia: Lippincott Williams & Wilkins.

ENSURING PATIENT SAFETY AND SAFE APPLICATION OF PATIENT CARE

Eight Items

1. Correct answer: (c)

   Rationale: Answers (a), (b), and (d) cause stress to the glenohumeral joint capsule.

   Reference: Shankman, G. (1997). *Fundamental orthopedic management for the physical therapist assistant* (p. 248). St. Louis: Mosby.

2. Correct answer: (c)

   Rationale: This posture exceeds common postsurgical precautions after a total hip arthroplasty.

   Reference: Kisner, C., & Colby, L. (2002). *Therapeutic exercise: Foundations and techniques* (4th ed., p. 480). Philadelphia: FA Davis.

3. Correct answer: (b)

   Rationale: The patient is likely suffering an episode of autonomic dysreflexia. This is common for spinal injuries at or above the level of T6, and are a potential medical emergency.

   Reference: Martin, S., & Kessler, M. (2000). *Neurologic intervention for physical therapist assistants* (p. 189). Philadelphia: WB Saunders.

4. Correct answer: (c)

   Rationale: Each of these modalities is considered contraindicated, or at least precautionary with pregnancy.

   Reference: Cameron, M. (1999). *Physical agents in rehabilitation: From research to practice* (p. 9). Philadelphia: WB Saunders.

5. Correct answer: (d)

   Rationale: Insulin increases the metabolism of sugars, proteins, and fats.

   Reference: (1997). *Taber's cyclopedic medical dictionary* (19th ed., p. 1107). Philadelphia: FA Davis.

6. Correct answer: (a)

   Rationale: Pain in the calf, which increases with Homan's sign is a potential blood clot, in which case active exercise is contraindicated.

   Reference: Cipriano, J. (2003). *Photographic manual of regional orthopedic and neurologic Tests* (4th ed., p. 425). Philadelphia: Lippincott Williams & Wilkins.

7. Correct answer: (b)

   Rationale: Physical activity should cease if a person with angina begins to complain of chest pain. Physical therapist assistants should not administer medications.

   Reference: Kisner, C., & Colby, L. (2002). *Therapeutic exercise: Foundations and techniques* (4th ed., p. 152). Philadelphia: FA Davis.

8. Correct answer: (a)

Rationale: Pain is normal within a week of a total joint replacement. The other observations should be more concerning in regard to the potential presence of postsurgical infection.

Reference: Anemaet, W., et al. (2000). *Home rehabilitation: Guide to clinical practice* (p. 547). St. Louis: Mosby.

PERFORMING FIRST AID

Ten Items

1. Correct answer: (b)

Rationale: This question is about the person's safety. In general, direct pressure applied while wearing gloves or providing pressure over the femoral artery is most appropriate, but is not what this item is asking or offering.

Reference: (1987). *Emergency care and transportation of the sick and injured* (4th ed., p. 125). Park Ridge, IL: American Association of Orthopedic Surgeons.

2. Correct answer: (b)

Rationale: The brachial location is a major arterial pressure point, the others are superficial venous points, and the tracheal area is not for vascular compression.

Reference: (1987). *Emergency care and transportation of the sick and injured* (4th ed., p. 33). Park Ridge, IL: American Association of Orthopedic Surgeons.

3. Correct answer: (d)

Rationale: Bleeding should normally cease as a result of intrinsic processes within 6–10 minutes.

Reference: (1987). *Emergency care and transportation of the sick and injured* (4th ed., p. 125). Park Ridge, IL: American Association of Orthopedic Surgeons.

4. Correct answer: (a)

Rationale: Avoid moving unconscious persons before assessing if they have an injury, or are in cardiac or respiratory arrest.

Reference: (1987). *Emergency care and transportation of the sick and injured* (4th ed., p. 75). Park Ridge, IL: American Association of Orthopedic Surgeons.

5. Correct answer: (c)

Rationale: Puncture injuries typically produce a small entrance wound. The size and penetration of the wound is the primary determinant for the requirement of stitches.

Reference: (1987). *Emergency care and transportation of the sick and injured* (4th ed., p. 154). Park Ridge, IL: American Association of Orthopedic Surgeons.

6. Correct answer: (c)

Rationale: The femoral artery pressure point is located at the inguinal crease.

Reference: (1987). *Emergency care and transportation of the sick and injured* (4th ed., p. 33). Park Ridge, IL: American Association of Orthopedic Surgeons.

7. Correct answer: (c)

Rationale: This is the correct location for popliteal pressure point.

Reference: Anemaet, W., et al. (2000). *Home rehabilitation: Guide to clinical practice* (p. 569). St. Louis: Mosby.

8. Correct answer: (c)

Rationale: The burn should be cooled in water or with ice, however the ice should not be rubbed upon the wound.

Reference: Anemaet, W., et al. (2000). *Home rehabilitation: Guide to clinical practice* (p. 572). St. Louis: Mosby.

9. Correct answer: (a)

Rationale: A person who can speak should not receive abdominal thrusts until their airway is more obstructed. The application of abdominal thrusts may cause the object to obstruct the airway further. If they are unable to breathe or speak, then abdominal thrusts are applied.

Reference: Anemaet, W., et al. (2000). *Home rehabilitation: Guide to clinical practice* (p. 564). St. Louis: Mosby.

10. Correct answer: (d)

Rationale: Each of the other statements is true. If only one eye is affected, the head should be tilted toward the injured eye to prevent spread to the unaffected eye.

Reference: Anemaet, W., et al. (2000). *Home rehabilitation: Guide to clinical practice* (p. 273). St. Louis: Mosby.

PERFORMING EMERGENCY PROCEDURES

Ten Items

1. Correct answer: (c)

Rationale: The adult is likely to need medical services, and probably cardiopulmonary resuscitation in this case. The first thing that must be established is an airway, followed by attempts to ventilate the body to prevent irreversible damage.

Reference: (1987). *Emergency care and transportation of the sick and injured* (4th ed., p. 76, 77). Park Ridge, IL: American Association of Orthopedic Surgeons.

2. Correct answer: (c)

Rationale: Protect the person from harm, but avoid forcing or restraining their body as it may cause a more significant harm. The sidelying position can be used to prevent aspiration in the case of emesis during the seizure.

Reference: (1987). *Emergency care and transportation of the sick and injured* (4th ed., p. 382). Park Ridge, IL: American Association of Orthopedic Surgeons.

3. Correct answer: (c)

Rationale: An absence seizure is also known as a petit mal seizure, and is characterized as nonconvulsive, with the person staring or blinking unresponsively.

Reference: Martin, S., & Kessler, M. (2000). *Neurologic intervention for physical therapist assistants* (p. 369). Philadelphia: WB Saunders.

4. Correct answer: (c)

Rationale: In an inpatient setting, have someone notify the emergency medical staff, then establish an airway and implement CPR if necessary.

Reference: Anemaet, W., et al. (2000). *Home rehabilitation: Guide to clinical practice* (p. 527). St. Louis: Mosby.

5. Correct answer: (d)

Rationale: Loss of oxygen, for this period of time, and longer, may result in irreversible brain and vital tissue damage.

Reference: (1987). *Emergency care and transportation of the sick and injured* (4th ed., p. 74). Park Ridge, IL: American Association of Orthopedic Surgeons.

6. Correct answer: (c)

Rationale: If it is not known whether the person is suffering from insulin shock or diabetic coma, it is recommended to administer a sugar source.

Reference: (1987). *Emergency care and transportation of the sick and injured* (4th ed., p. 338). Park Ridge, IL: American Association of Orthopedic Surgeons.

7. Correct answer: (a)

Rationale: 1 to 1.5 seconds is the proper duration for adults.

Reference: (1987). *Emergency care and transportation of the sick and injured* (4th ed., p. 81). Park Ridge, IL: American Association of Orthopedic Surgeons.

8. Correct answer: (a)

Rationale: One ventilation every 5 seconds, or twelve per minute, is the correct rate of rescue breathing.

Reference: (1987). *Emergency care and transportation of the sick and injured* (4th ed., p. 81). Park Ridge, IL: American Association of Orthopedic Surgeons.

9. Correct answer: (c)

Rationale: The appropriate location for applying abdominal thrusts is above the umbilicus, well below the xiphoid, secondary to the risk of fracture, and resultant injury.

Reference: (1987). *Emergency care and transportation of the sick and injured* (4th ed., p. 84). Park Ridge, IL: American Association of Orthopedic Surgeons.

10. Correct answer: (b)

    Rationale: Abdominal thrusts are delivered in a series of six to ten thrusts, then check to see if their airway has been cleared. Repeat as needed. If the person becomes unconscious, lower them to the floor, straddle the person, and continue to apply the abdominal thrusts.

    Reference: (1987). *Emergency care and transportation of the sick and injured* (4th ed., p. 84). Park Ridge, IL: American Association of Orthopedic Surgeons.

PERFORMING CPR

Twelve Items

1. Correct answer: (d)

   Rationale: For an adult, the chest is manually compressed 1.5"–2" through extended arms.

   Reference: (1987). *Emergency care and transportation of the sick and injured* (4th ed., p. 103). Park Ridge, IL: American Association of Orthopedic Surgeons.

2. Correct answer: (b)

   Rationale: The correct rate of respirations for an infant and a child is 20; for an adult it is 12 per minute.

   Reference: Anemaet, W., et al. (2000). *Home rehabilitation: Guide to clinical practice* (p. 566). St. Louis: Mosby.

3. Correct answer: (c)

   Rationale: Abdominal thrusts should not be applied to a person who can speak or cough.

   Reference: (1987). *Emergency care and transportation of the sick and injured* (4th ed., p. 84). Park Ridge, IL: American Association of Orthopedic Surgeons.

4. Correct answer: (c)

   Rationale: Fifteen chest compressions are applied for every two respirations with an adult.

   Reference: (1987). *Emergency care and transportation of the sick and injured* (4th ed., p. 103). Park Ridge, IL: American Association of Orthopedic Surgeons.

5. Correct answer: (d)

   Rationale: Infants, up to 1 year of age, are given five chest compressions for every one breath during CPR.

   Reference: Anemaet, W., et al. (2000). *Home rehabilitation: Guide to clinical practice* (p. 566). St. Louis: Mosby.

6. Correct answer: (d)

   Rationale: This is common with choking infants and small children.

   Reference: (1987). *Emergency care and transportation of the sick and injured* (4th ed., p. 90). Park Ridge, IL: American Association of Orthopedic Surgeons.

7. Correct answer: (b)

   Rationale: This is a common occurrence with the application of rescue breathing.

   Reference: (1987). *Emergency care and transportation of the sick and injured* (4th ed., p. 83). Park Ridge, IL: American Association of Orthopedic Surgeons.

8. Correct answer: (d)

   Rationale: For CPR to be effective, it must be performed with the person supine on a flat firm surface.

   Reference: (1987). *Emergency care and transportation of the sick and injured* (4th ed., p. 77). Park Ridge, IL: American Association of Orthopedic Surgeons.

9. Correct answer: (d)

   Rationale: A child, 1–8 years of age, should receive five chest compressions for every one respiration.

   Reference: (1987). *Emergency care and transportation of the sick and injured* (4th ed., p. 107). Park Ridge, IL: American Association of Orthopedic Surgeons.

10. Correct answer: (a)

    Rationale: Chest compressions for a child, 1–8 years of age, is applied at a rate of 100 per minute.

    Reference: (1987). *Emergency care and transportation of the sick and injured* (4th ed., p. 103). Park Ridge, IL: American Association of Orthopedic Surgeons.

11. Correct answer: (b)

    Rationale: Rescue respirations are provided at a rate of 20 per minute.

    Reference: Anemaet, W., et al. (2000). *Home rehabilitation: Guide to clinical practice* (p. 566). St. Louis: Mosby.

12. Correct answer: (d)

    Rationale: The brachial pulse is the correct location for assessing the presence of a pulse in an infant.

    Reference: (1987). *Emergency care and transportation of the sick and injured* (4th ed., p. 106). Park Ridge, IL: American Association of Orthopedic Surgeons.

STERILE PROCEDURES

Seven Items

1. Correct answer: (b)

   Rationale: Medical asepsis is the practice of reducing the number and spread of infection.

   Reference: Pierson, F. (2002). *Principles and techniques of patient care* (3rd ed., p. 25). Philadelphia: WB Saunders.

2. Correct answer: (a)

   Rationale: Typically, a 1″ border at the edges of the field is considered to be nonsterile.

   Reference: Pierson, F. (2002). *Principles and techniques of patient care* (3rd ed., p. 297). Philadelphia: WB Saunders.

3. Correct answer: (d)

   Rationale: All of the other statements are true. Packages should only be opened when needed to maintain the best aseptic conditions.

   Reference: Pierson, F. (2002). *Principles and techniques of patient care* (3rd ed., p. 297). Philadelphia: WB Saunders.

4. Correct answer: (d)

   Rationale: The open-glove technique is more practical, but creates a greater risk for contamination.

   Reference: Pierson, F. (2002). *Principles and techniques of patient care* (3rd ed., p. 41, 42). Philadelphia: WB Saunders.

5. Correct answer: (c)

   Rationale: Any contact with nonsterile items compromises the sterility of another item.

   Reference: Pierson, F. (2002). *Principles and techniques of patient care* (3rd ed., p. 296). Philadelphia: WB Saunders.

6. Correct answer: (a)

   Rationale: The gloves should cover the sleeves of the gown.

   Reference: Minor, M., & Minor, S. (1999). *Patient care skills* (4th ed., p. 69). Norwalk, CT: Appleton & Lange.

7. Correct answer: (c)

   Rationale: The clinician should change gloves between procedures, even when it is the same person.

   Reference: Myers, B. (2004). *Wound management, principles and practice* (p. 109). Upper Saddle River, NJ: Prentice Hall.

DEMONSTRATING APPROPRIATE SEQUENCING OF EVENTS RELATED TO UNIVERSAL PRECAUTIONS

Seven Items

1. Correct answer: (a)

   Rationale: A nosocomial infection is acquired in a hospital setting.

   Reference: (1997). *Taber's cyclopedic medical dictionary* (19th ed.). Philadelphia: FA Davis.

2. Correct answer: (d)

   Rationale: The patient is immunocompromised and at a higher risk of contamination by the moderate exudate coming from their open wound. The person must be protected from harm with any reasonable accommodation.

   Reference: Pierson, F. (2002). *Principles and techniques of patient care* (3rd ed., p. 31). Philadelphia: WB Saunders.

3. Correct answer: (a)

   Rationale: This is the correct sequence of applying a wet-to-dry wound dressing.

   Reference: Myers, B. (2004). *Wound management, principles and practice* (p. 80, 81). Upper Saddle River, NJ: Prentice Hall.

4. Correct answer: (d)

   Rationale: The face and hair are covered to reduce contamination of the gown and gloves. The hands are then washed, sterile gloves are donned, and then the gown is worn.

   Reference: Pierson, F. (2002). *Principles and techniques of patient care* (3rd ed.). Philadelphia: WB Saunders.

5. Correct answer: (c)

   Rationale: This is the most preventative method. An acceptable second choice is the removal of the mask without gloves and then washing the hands.

   Reference: Goodman, C., et al. (2003). *Pathology implications for the physical therapist* (2nd ed., p. 202). Philadelphia: WB Saunders.

6. Correct answer: (c)

   Rationale: The gloves are used to remove the gown, to prevent contamination of the clothes or body.

   Reference: Goodman, C., et al. (2003). *Pathology implications for the physical therapist* (2nd ed., p. 202). Philadelphia: WB Saunders.

7. Correct answer: (a)

   Rationale: Upon exiting a person's room, who is on isolation, the gown is carefully removed first.

   Reference: Pierson, F. (2002). *Principles and techniques of patient care* (3rd ed., p. 39). Philadelphia: WB Saunders.

DEMONSTRATING ASEPTIC TECHNIQUE

Seven Items

1. Correct answer: (b)

   Rationale: Hepatitis B is typically spread through contact with feces or saliva.

   Reference: Goodman, C., et al. (2003). *Pathology implications for the physical therapist* (2nd ed.). Philadelphia: WB Saunders.

2. Correct answer: (a)

   Rationale: The primary mode of transmission is through the respiratory tracts.

   Reference: Goodman, C., et al. (2003). *Pathology implications for the physical therapist* (2nd ed., p. 202). Philadelphia: WB Saunders.

3. Correct answer: (b)

   Rationale: The palms typically take up to 30 seconds, with another 20 seconds for the backs of the hands, and for the fingers.

   Reference: Weiss, R. (1999). *Physical therapy aide: A worktext* (2nd ed., p. 152). Albany: Delmar.

4. Correct answer: (b)

   Rationale: All of the other statements are true. An antibacterial soap is sufficient for washing hands after working with someone with streptococcus.

   Reference: Goodman, C., et al. (2003). *Pathology implications for the physical therapist* (2nd ed., p. 200). Philadelphia: WB Saunders.

5. Correct answer: (d)

   Rationale: There is a significant risk for splash contamination when performing pulsed lavage.

   Reference: Cameron, M. (1999). *Physical agents in rehabilitation: From research to practice* (p. 204). Philadelphia: WB Saunders.

6. Correct answer: (b)

   Rationale: The integrity of the package is considered the first priority.

   Reference: Minor, M., & Minor, S. (1999). *Patient care skills* (4th ed., p. 53). Norwalk, CT: Appleton & Lange.

7. Correct answer: (a)

   Rationale: The edges are the parts that has had contact with gloves, etc.

   Reference: Minor, M., & Minor, S. (1999). *Patient care skills* (4th ed., p. 53). Norwalk, CT: Appleton & Lange.

PROPERLY DISCARDING SOILED ITEMS

Seven Items

1. Correct answer: (b)

   Rationale: Solid wastes are sufficiently contained in a single layer bag, unless contaminated on the outer surface.

   Reference: Minor, M., & Minor, S. (1999). *Patient care skills* (4th ed., p. 89). Norwalk, CT: Appleton & Lange.

2. Correct answer: (a)

   Rationale: Ten seconds is the minimum suggested time for lathering hands. Avoid using excessive hot water or abrasive materials which may compromise the resistant properties of hands. There are differences in the recommended duration for handwashing.

   Reference: Minor, M., & Minor, S. (1999). *Patient care skills* (4th ed., p. 58). Norwalk, CT: Appleton & Lange.

3. Correct answer: (d)

   Rationale: Syringes are the tubes that needles are connected to. All other items belong in a sharps box, except tweezers which should be sterilized, not discarded.

   Reference: Minor, M., & Minor, S. (1999). *Patient care skills* (4th ed., p. 89). Norwalk, CT: Appleton & Lange.

4. Correct answer: (c)

   Rationale: The gown is donned first and then the gloves.

   Reference: Minor, M., & Minor, S. (1999). *Patient care skills* (4th ed., p. 65, 66). Norwalk, CT: Appleton & Lange.

5. Correct answer: (b)

   Rationale: Syringes with content should be reported immediately to the nurse. Do not attempt to remove or recap needles.

   Reference: Minor, M., & Minor, S. (1999). *Patient care skills* (4th ed., p. 89). Norwalk, CT: Appleton & Lange.

6. Correct answer: (b)

   Rationale: Wound dressings should be placed in a plastic disposal bag immediately after removal.

   Reference: Minor, M., & Minor, S. (1999). *Patient care skills* (4th ed., p. 89). Norwalk, CT: Appleton & Lange.

7. Correct answer: (c)

   Rationale: The Center for Disease Control recommends that linens should not be prerinsed in patient care areas.

   Reference: Minor, M., & Minor, S. (1999). *Patient care skills* (4th ed., p. 91). Norwalk, CT: Appleton & Lange.

DETERMINING EQUIPMENT TO BE USED AND ASSEMBLING ALL MATERIALS

Seven Items

1. Correct answer: (b)

   Rationale: Universal precaution treats all persons as having potentially infectious bodily fluids.

   Reference: Pierson, F. (2002). *Principles and techniques of patient care* (3rd ed., p. 31). Philadelphia: WB Saunders.

2. Correct answer: (a)

   Rationale: The use of forceps is considered sharp debridement.

   Reference: Myers, B. (2004). *Wound management, principles and practice* (p. 81, 82). Upper Saddle River, NJ: Prentice Hall.

3. Correct answer: (d)

   Rationale: Hydrocolloids or hydrogels are indicated for small, noninfected burn wounds.

   Reference: Myers, B. (2004). *Wound management, principles and practice* (p. 341). Upper Saddle River, NJ: Prentice Hall.

4. Correct answer: (a)

   Rationale: The barriers are used to prevent maceration of the surrounding skin.

   Reference: Myers, B. (2004). *Wound management, principles and practice* (p. 135). Upper Saddle River, NJ: Prentice Hall.

5. Correct answer: (b)

   Rationale: The use of alginate type dressings is appropriate for heavily draining wounds.

   Reference: Myers, B. (2004). *Wound management, principles and practice* (p. 341). Upper Saddle River, NJ: Prentice Hall.

6. Correct answer: (d)

   Rationale: Rubella is a pathogen spread through droplet transmission, the primary indication is to wear a mask within 3′ of the person. Other personal protective equipment can be optionally requested.

   Reference: Pierson, F. (2002). *Principles and techniques of patient care* (3rd ed., p. 33). Philadelphia: WB Saunders.

7. Correct answer: (d)

   Rationale: The N-95 dust mist respirator is required for properly filtering quality against tuberculosis. The person should be in a private room, with the door closed, and with negative airflow.

   Reference: Pierson, F. (2002). *Principles and techniques of patient care* (3rd ed., p. 32, 33). Philadelphia: WB Saunders.

Appendix

Table A1 | Muscles of Facial Expression

Muscle	Function
Occipitalis	Draws scalp backward
Frontalis	Elevates eyebrows, wrinkles skin of forehead
Zygomaticus minor	Draws upper lip upward and outward
Levator labii superioris	Elevates upper lip
Levator labii superioris alaeque nasi	Raises upper lip and dilates nostril
Buccinator	Compresses cheek and retracts angle
Zygomaticus major	Pulls angle of mouth upward and backward when laughing
Mentalis	Raises and protrudes lower lip as when in doubt
Orbicularis oris	Closes lips

Table A2 | Muscles of Mastication and the Muscles That Move the Eyes

Muscle	Function
Muscles of mastication	
Masseter	Closes jaw
Temporalis	Raises mandible and closes mouth; draws mandible backward
Medial pterygoid	Raises mandible; closes mouth
Lateral pterygoid (two-headed)	Brings jaw forward
Muscles of the eye	
Superior rectus	Rolls eyeball upward
Inferior rectus	Rolls eyeball downward
Medial rectus	Rolls eyeball medially
Lateral rectus	Rolls eyeball laterally
Superior oblique	Rotates eyeball on axis

Table A3	The Cranial Nerves

Number	Name	Function
I	Olfactory	Sensory: smell
II	Optic	Sensory: vision
III	Oculomotor	Motor: movement of the eyeball, regulation of the size of the pupil
IV	Trochlear	Motor: eye movements
V	Trigeminal	Sensory: sensations of head and face, muscle sense
		Motor: mastication
		Note: divided into three branches: the ophthalmic branch, the maxillary branch, and the mandibular branch
VI	Abducens	Motor: movement of the eyeball, particularly abduction
VII	Facial	Sensory: taste
		Motor: facial expressions, secretions of saliva
VIII	Vestibulocochlear	Sensory: balance, hearing
		Note: divided into two branches: the vestibular branch responsible for balance and the cochlear branch responsible for hearing
IX	Glossopharyngeal	Sensory: taste
		Motor: swallowing, secretion of saliva
X	Vagus	Sensory: sensation of organs supplied
		Motor: movement of organs supplied
		Note: supplies the head, pharynx, bronchus, esophagus, liver, and stomach
XI	Accessory	Motor: shoulder movement, turning of head, voice production
XII	Hypoglossal	Motor: tongue movements

Table A4	Disorders of Joints

Common Disease, Disorder or Condition

Bursitis

Bursitis (burr-SIGH-tis) is an inflammation of the synovial bursa that can be caused from excessive stress or tension placed on the bursa. Playing tennis for long periods of time causes tennis elbow. It is an example of bursitis in the elbow joint caused by excessive stress. You may experience "canoist" elbow if you go canoeing and paddle for long hours. This is, of course, temporary. The elbow and the shoulder are common sites of bursitis. It can also be caused by a local or systemic inflammatory process. If bursitis persists, as in chronic bursitis, the muscles in the joint can eventually degenerate or atrophy and the joint can become stiff even though the joint itself is not diseased.

Arthritis

Arthritis (ahr-THRY-tis) is an inflammation of the whole joint. It usually involves all the tissues of the joint: cartilage, bone, muscles, tendons, ligaments, nerves, blood supply, and so on. There are well over 100 varieties of arthritis and 10% of the population experiences this disorder, which has no cure. Pain relief is common through analgesics but these only relieve a symptom of arthritis, the pain.

Rheumatic fever

Rheumatic fever is a disease involving a mild bacterial infection. If undetected in childhood, the bacterium can be carried by the bloodstream to the joints, resulting in a development of rheumatoid arthritis.

Rheumatoid arthritis

Rheumatoid arthritis is a connective tissue disorder resulting in severe inflammation of small joints. It is severely

debilitating and can destroy the joints of the hands and feet. The cause is unknown. A genetic factor may be involved or an autoimmune reaction in which an immune reaction develops against a person's own tissues. The synovial membranes of the joints and connective tissues grow abnormally to form a layer in the joint capsule. This layer grows into the articulating surfaces of the bones, destroying cartilage and fusing the bones of the joint.

Primary fibrositis

Primary fibrositis is an inflammation of the fibrous connective tissue in a joint. It is commonly called rheumatism by the layman. If it is in the lower back, it is commonly called lumbago.

Osteoarthritis

Osteoarthritis, sometimes referred to as degenerative joint disease, occurs with advancing age especially in people in their seventies. It is more common in overweight individuals and affects the weight-bearing joints. Mild exercising can prevent joint deterioration and increases the ability to maintain movement at joints.

Gout

Gout (GOWT) is an accumulation of uric acid crystals in the joint at the base of the large toe and other joints of the feet and legs. It is more common in men than in women. These waste product crystals can also accumulate in the kidneys causing kidney damage.

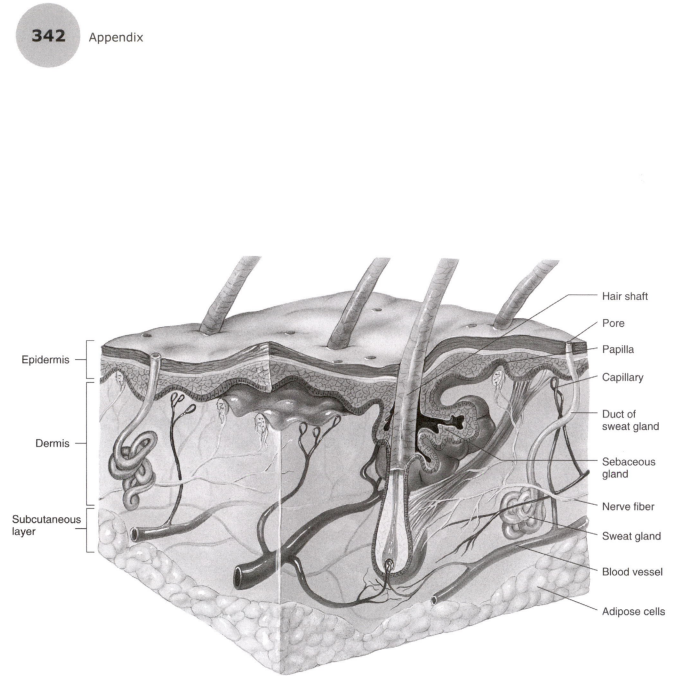

Figure A1. The layers of the skin and some of its appendages.

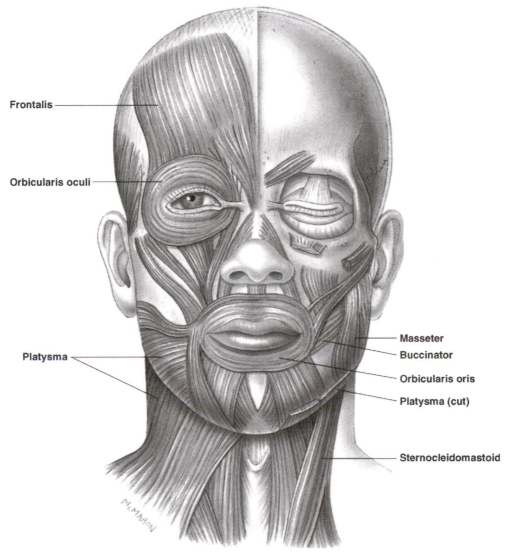

Figure A2. Some muscles of the head and neck (anterior view).

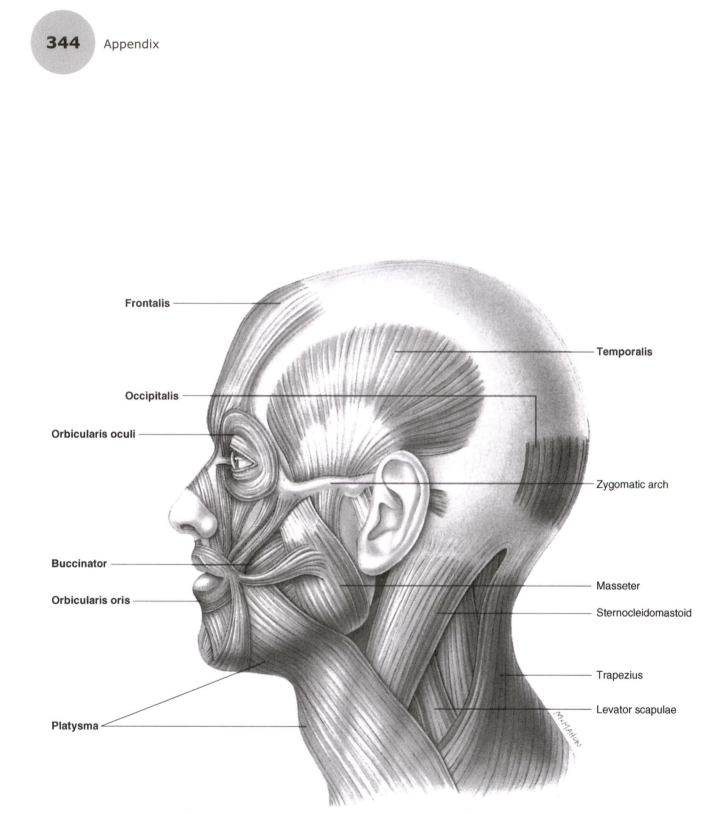

Figure A3. Some muscles of the head and neck (lateral view).

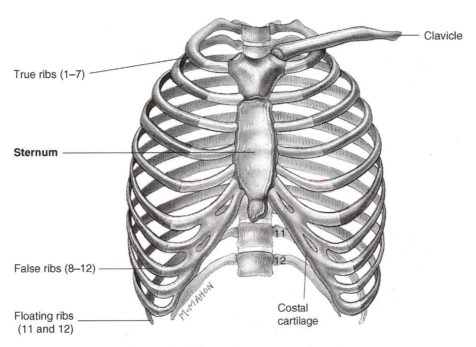

Clavicle

True ribs (1–7)

Sternum

11

12

False ribs (8–12)

Costal
cartilage

Floating ribs
(11 and 12)

Figure A4. Thoracic cage, anterior view.

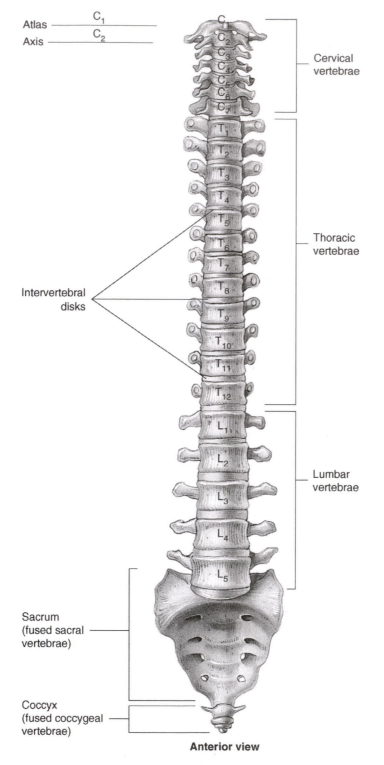

Atlas —— C_1

Axis —— C_2

C_3
C_4
C_5
C_6
C_7

Cervical
vertebrae

T_1
T_2
T_3
T_4
T_5
T_6
T_7
T_8
T_9
T_{10}
T_{11}
T_{12}

Thoracic
vertebrae

Intervertebral
disks

L_1
L_2
L_3
L_4
L_5

Lumbar
vertebrae

Sacrum
(fused sacral
vertebrae)

Coccyx
(fused coccygeal
vertebrae)

Anterior view

Figure A5. The vertebral column.

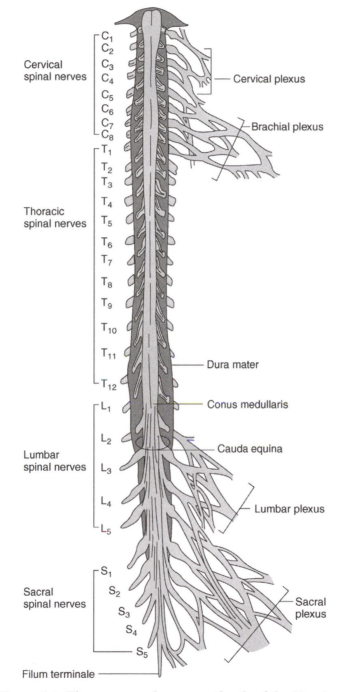

Figure A6. The names and emergent levels of the 31 spinal nerves.

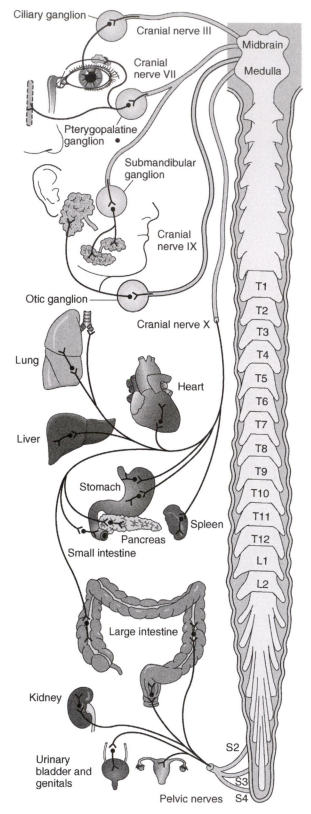

Figure A7. The nerve pathways of the parasympathetic division of the autonomic nervous system.

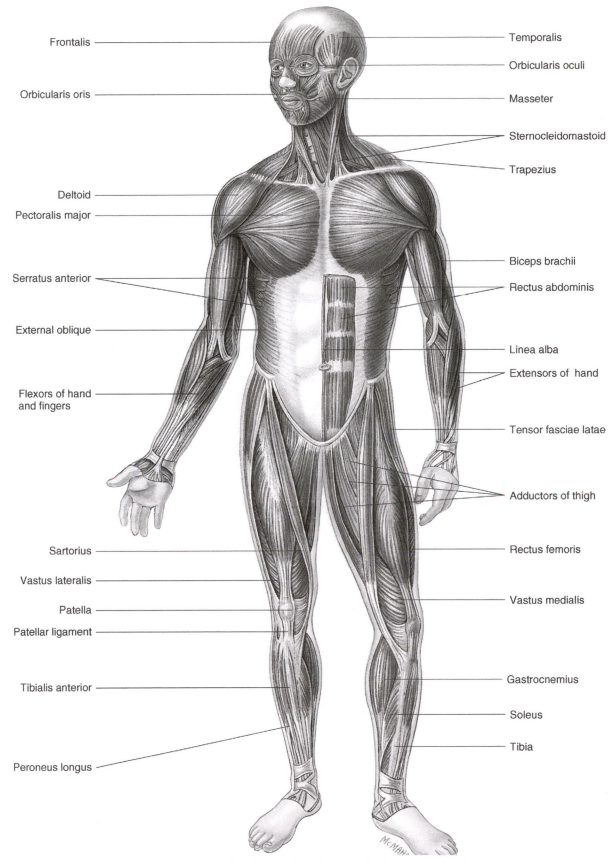

Frontalis

Orbicularis oris

Deltoid

Pectoralis major

Serratus anterior

External oblique

Flexors of hand
and fingers

Sartorius

Vastus lateralis

Patella

Patellar ligament

Tibialis anterior

Peroneus longus

Temporalis

Orbicularis oculi

Masseter

Sternocleidomastoid

Trapezius

Biceps brachii

Rectus abdominis

Linea alba

Extensors of hand

Tensor fasciae latae

Adductors of thigh

Rectus femoris

Vastus medialis

Gastrocnemius

Soleus

Tibia

Figure A8. The superficial muscles of the body (anterior view).

349

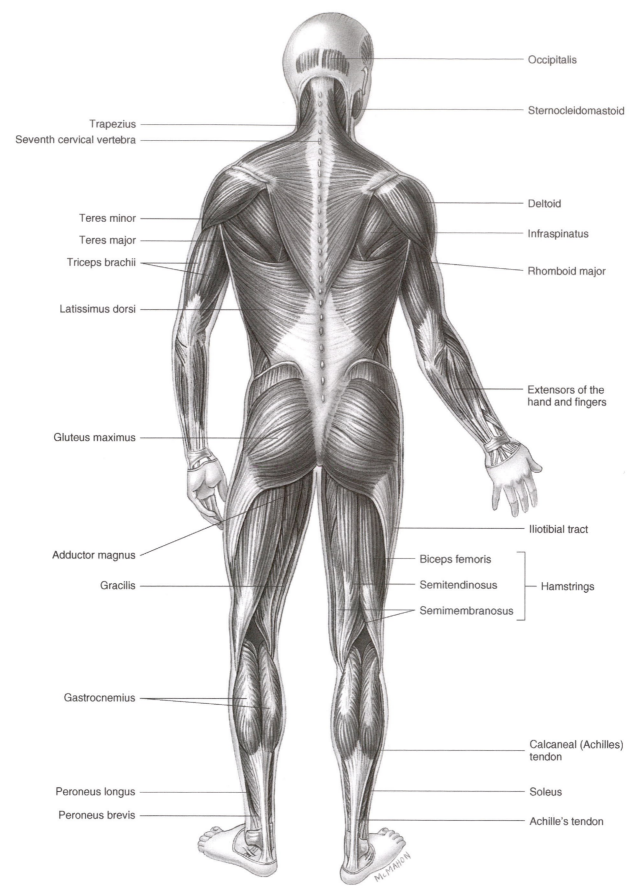

Figure A9. The superficial muscles of the body (posterior view).

Occipitalis

Sternocleidomastoid

Trapezius

Seventh cervical vertebra

Deltoid

Infraspinatus

Teres minor

Rhomboid major

Teres major

Triceps brachii

Latissimus dorsi

Extensors of the
hand and fingers

Gluteus maximus

Iliotibial tract

Adductor magnus

Biceps femoris

Gracilis

Semitendinosus

Hamstrings

Semimembranosus

Gastrocnemius

Calcaneal (Achilles)
tendon

Peroneus longus

Soleus

Peroneus brevis

Achille's tendon

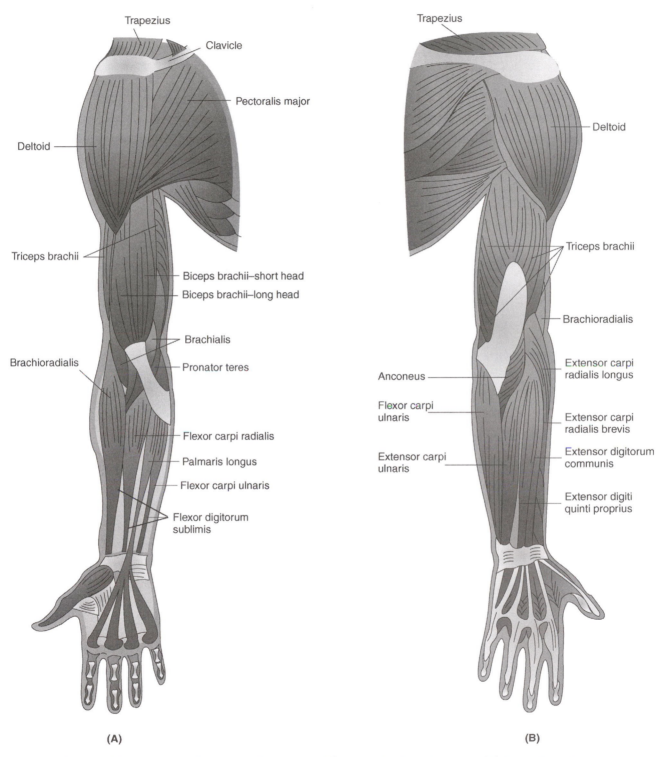

Figure A10. Muscles that move the arm and fingers (A) Anterior view (B) Posterior view.

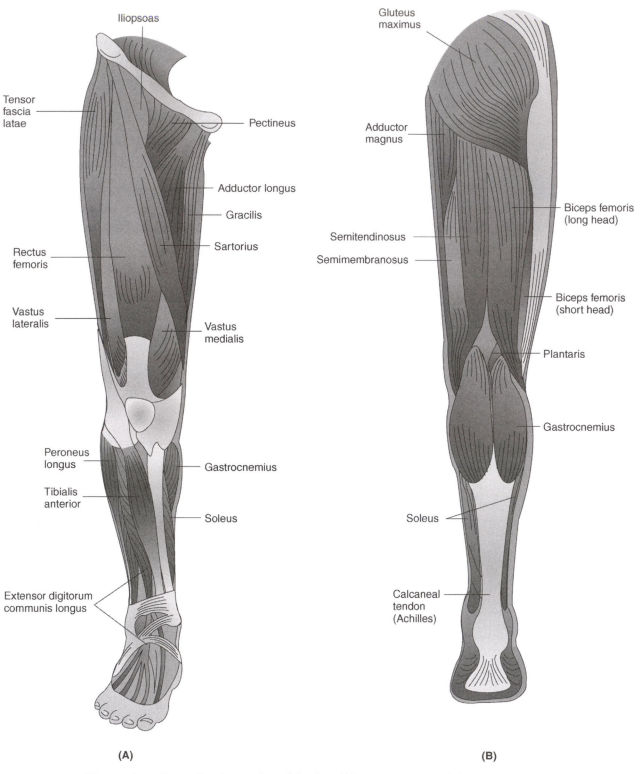

(A)

(B)

Figure A11. Superficial muscles of the leg (A) Anterior view (B) Posterior view.

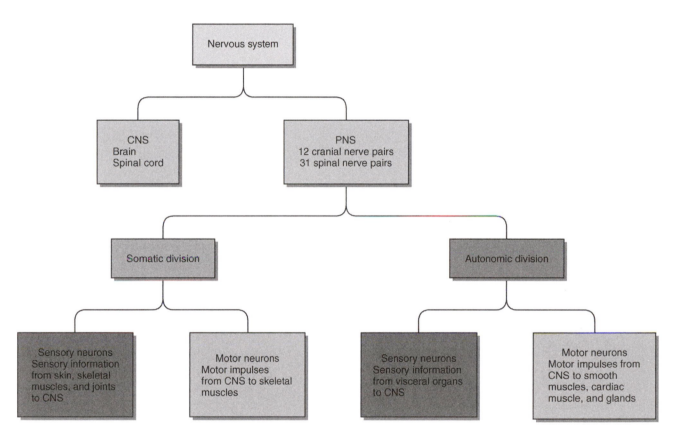

Figure A12. Divisions of the nervous system.

Suggested Readings

(1999). *A Normative Model of Physical Therapist Assistant Education: Version 99.* Alexandria, VA: American Physical Therapy Association.

Andrade, C., & Clifford, P. (2001). *Outcome-Based Massage.* Philadelphia: Lippincott Williams & Wilkins.

Anemaet, W., et al. (2000). *Home rehabilitation: Guide to clinical practice* St. Louis: Mosby.

Bandy, W., & Sanders, B. (2001). *Therapeutic Exercise Techniques for Intervention.* Philadelphia: Lippincott Williams & Wilkins.

Bates, A., & Hanson, N. (1996). *Aquatic physical therapy.* Philadelphia: WB Saunders.

Behrens, B., & Michlovitz, S. (1996). *Physical agents: Theory and practice for the physical therapist assistant.* Philadelphia: FA Davis.

Bennett, S., & Karnes, J. (1998). *Neurological disabilities: Assessment and treatment.* Philadelphia: Lippincott Williams & Wilkins.

Berryman-Reese, N. (1999). *Muscle and sensory testing.* Philadelphia: WB Saunders.

Bobath, B. (1990). *Adult hemiplegia: Evaluation and treatment* (3rd ed.). Oxford: Butterworth-Heinemann.

Bottomley, J. (2000). *Quick reference dictionary for physical therapy.* Thorofare, NJ: Slack Inc.

Cameron, M. (1999). *Physical agents in rehabilitation: From research to practice.* Philadelphia: WB Saunders.

Campbell, M. (2000). *Rehabilitation for traumatic brain injury: Physical therapy practice in context.* Philadelphia: Churchill Livingstone.

Campbell, S., et al. (2000). *Physical therapy for children* (2nd ed.). Philadelphia: WB Saunders.

Carr, J., & Shepherd, R. (2000). *Movement science: Foundations for physical therapy in rehabilitation* (2nd ed.). Maryland: Aspen.

Chabner, D. (2003). *Medical terminology: A short course* (3rd ed.). Philadelphia: WB Saunders.

Cipriano, J. (2003). *Photographic manual of regional orthopedic and neurologic tests* (4th ed.). Philadelphia: Lippincott Williams & Wilkins.

Davis, C. (1998). *Patient practitioner Interaction: An Experiential Manual for Developing the Art of Health Care* (3rd ed.). Thorofare, NJ: Slack Inc.

Domenico, G., & Wood, E. (1997). *Beard's massage* (4th ed.). Philadelphia: WB Saunders.

Dvir, Z. (2000). *Clinical biomechanics.* New York: Churchill Livingstone.

Edge, R., & Groves, J. (1999). *Ethics of health care: A guide for clinical practice* (2nd ed.). Albany: Delmar.

(1987). *Emergency care and transportation of the sick and injured* (4th ed.). Park Ridge, IL: American Association of Orthopedic Surgeons.

Evans, R. (2001). *Illustrated orthopedic physical assessment* (2nd ed.). St. Louis: Mosby.

Frazier, M., et al. (2000). *Essentials of human disease and conditions* (2nd ed.). Philadelphia: WB Saunders.

Goodman, C., & Snyder, T. (2000). *Differential diagnosis in physical therapy* (3rd ed.). Philadelphia: WB Saunders.

Goodman, C., et al. (2003). *Pathology implications for the physical therapist* (2nd ed.). Philadelphia: WB Saunders.

Guccione, A. (2000). *Geriatric physical therapy* (2nd ed.). St. Louis: Mosby.

Guide to Physical Therapist Practice (2nd ed.). (2001, January). *Physical Therapy Journal of the American Physical Therapy Association 81* (1).

Hall, S. (2003). *Basic Biomechanics* (4th ed.). Boston: McGraw-Hill.

Hamilton, N., & Luttgens, K. (2002). *Kinesiology: Scientific basis of human motion.* Boston: McGraw-Hill.

Hanna, M., & Gibson, J. (1987). *Public speaking for personal success* Dubuque, IA: William C. Brown Publishers.

Hayes, K. (2000). *Manual for physical agents* (5th ed.). New Jersey: Prentice Hall.

Herdman, S. (1994). *Vestibular rehabilitation.* Philadelphia: FA Davis.

Hillegass, E., & Sadowsky, H. (2001). *Essentials of cardiopulmonary physical therapy* (2nd ed.). Philadelphia: WB Saunders.

Hislop, H., & Montgomery, J. (2002). *Daniels and Worthingham's muscle Testing Techniques of Manual Examination* (7th ed.). Philadelphia: WB Saunders.

Hoppenfeld, S. (1976). *Physical examination of the spine and extremities.* Norwalk, CT: Appleton & Lange.

Kelly, D. (2002). *A Primer on lymphedema.* New Jersey: Prentice Hall.

Kendall, F., et al. (1993). *Muscles: Testing and function* (4th ed.). Baltimore: Williams & Wilkins.

Kettenbach, G. (1995). *Writing SOAP notes* (2nd ed.). Philadelphia: FA Davis.

Kisner, C., & Colby, L. (2002). *Therapeutic exercise: Foundations and techniques* (4th ed.). Philadelphia: FA Davis.

Lesh, S. (2000). *Clinical orthopedics for the physical therapist assistant.* Philadelphia: FA Davis.

Lieber, R. (2002). *Skeletal muscle structure, function & plasticity* (2nd ed.). Philadelphia: Lippincott Williams & Wilkins.

Lippert, L. (2000). *Clinical kinesiology for physical therapist assistants.* (3rd ed.). Philadelphia: FA Davis.

Long, T., & Cintas, H. (1995). *Handbook of pediatric physical therapy.* Philadelphia: Williams & Wilkins.

Loving, J. (1999). *Massage therapy theory and practice.* Stamford, CT: Appleton & Lange.

Low, J., & Reed, A. (1994). *Electrotherapy explained* (2nd ed.). Oxford: Butterworth-Heinemann.

Luckman, J. (2000). *Transcultural communication in health care.* Albany: Delmar.

Lukan, M. (2001). *Documentation for physical therapist assistants* (2nd ed.). Philadelphia: FA Davis.

Magee, D. J. (2002). *Orthopedic physical assessment* (4th ed.). Philadelphia: WB Saunders.

Martin, S., & Kessler, M. (2000). *Neurologic intervention for physical therapist assistants.* Philadelphia: WB Saunders.

Maxey, L., & Magnusson, J. (2001). *Rehabilitation for the postsurgical orthopedic patient.* St. Louis: Mosby.

Micholovitz, S. (1990). *Thermal agents in rehabilitation* (2nd ed.). Philadelphia: FA Davis.

Minor, M., & Minor, S. (1999). *Patient care skills* (4th ed.). Norwalk, CT: Appleton & Lange.

Myers, B. (2004). *Wound management, principles and practice.* Upper Saddle River, NJ: Prentice Hall.

Navarra, T., et al. (1990). *Therapeutic communication, a guide to effective interpersonal skills for health care professionals.* Thorofare, NJ: Slack.

Neumann, D. A. (2002). *Kinesiology of the musculoskeletal system, foundations for physical rehabilitation*. St. Louis: Mosby.

Nixon, V., & Schneider, F. (1985). *Spinal cord injury: A guide to functional outcomes in physical therapy management*. Maryland: Aspen.

Nordin, M., & Frankel, V. (2001). *Basic biomechanics of the musculoskeletal system* (3rd ed.). Philadelphia: Lippincott Williams & Wilkins.

Norkin, C., & Levangie, P. (1992). *Joint structure and function: A comprehensive analysis* (2nd ed.). Philadelphia: FA Davis.

Norkin, C., & White, D. (1995). *Measurement of joint motion: A guide to goniometry* (2nd ed.). Philadelphia: FA Davis.

Nosse, L., et al. (1999). *Managerial and supervisory principles for physical therapists*. Baltimore: Williams & Wilkins.

O'Sullivan, S., & Schmitz, T. (2001). *Physical rehabilitation assessment and treatment* (4th ed.). Philadelphia: FA Davis.

Pagliarulo, M. (2001). *Introduction to physical therapy* (2nd ed.). St. Louis: Mosby.

Payton, O. (1994). *Research: The validation of clinical practice* (3rd ed.). Philadelphia: FA Davis.

Perry, J. (1992). *Gait analysis: Normal and pathological function*. Thorofare, NJ: Slack.

(2000). *Physical therapist's clinical companion*. Springhouse, PA: Springhouse Corporation.

Pierson, F. (2002). *Principles and techniques of patient care* (3rd ed.). Philadelphia: WB Saunders.

Placzek, J., & Boyce, D. (2001). *Orthopedic physical therapy secrets*. Philadelphia: Hanley & Belfus, Inc.

Prentice, W. (2002). *Therapeutic modalities for physical therapists* (2nd ed.). New York: McGraw-Hill.

Prentice, W., & Voight, M. (2001). *Techniques in musculoskeletal rehabilitation*. New York: McGraw-Hill.

Prentice, W. (1998). *Rehabilitation techniques in sports medicine* (2nd ed.). St. Louis: Mosby.

Purtillo, R. (1999). *Ethical dimensions in the health professions* (3rd ed.). Philadelphia: WB Saunders.

Purtillo, R., & Haddad, A. (2002). *Health professional and patient interaction* (6th ed.). Philadelphia: WB Saunders.

Ramsden, E. (1999). *The person as patient, psychosocial perspectives for the health care professional*. Philadelphia: WB Saunders.

Rothstein, J., et al. (1998). *The rehabilitation specialist's handbook* (2nd ed.). Philadelphia: FA Davis.

Sahrmann, S. (2002). *Diagnosis and treatment of movement impairment syndromes*. St. Louis: Mosby.

Saidoff, D., & McDonough, A. (2002). *Critical pathways in therapeutic intervention, extremities and spine*. St. Louis: Mosby.

Salimbene, S. (2000). *What language does your patient hurt in? A practical guide to culturally competent patient care*. St. Paul, MN: EMC Paradigm.

Sawner, K., & LaVigne, J. (1992). *Brunnstrom's movement therapy in hemiplegia: A neurophysiological approach* (2nd ed.). Philadelphia: Lippincott.

Scott, R. (2002). *Foundations of physical therapy, a 21st century-focused view of the profession*. New York: McGraw-Hill.

Scott, R. (1999). *Health care malpractice, a primer on legal issues for professionals* (2nd ed.). New York: McGraw-Hill.

Scott, R. (1994). *Legal aspects of documenting patient care* (2nd ed.). Maryland: Aspen.

Scott, R. (1999). *Professional ethics: A guide for rehabilitation professionals.* St. Louis: Mosby.

Scott, R. (1997). *Promoting legal awareness in physical and occupational therapy.* St. Louis: Mosby.

Seymour, R. (2002). *Prosthetics and orthotics: Lower limb and spinal.* Philadelphia: Lippincott Williams & Wilkins.

Shamus, E., & Shamus, J. (2001). *Sports injury prevention & rehabilitation.* New York: McGraw-Hill.

Shankman, G. (1997). *Fundamental orthopedic management for the physical therapist assistant.* St. Louis: Mosby.

Sine, R., et al. (2000). *Basic rehabilitation techniques* (4th ed.). Maryland: Aspen.

Smith, L., et al. (1996). *Brunnstrom's clinical kinesiology* (5th ed.). Philadelphia: FA Davis.

Somers, M. (2001). *Spinal cord injury: Functional rehabilitation* (2nd ed.). New Jersey: Prentice Hall.

(1997). *Stedman's concise medical dictionary for the health professions* (3rd ed.). Baltimore: Williams & Wilkins.

(1997). *Taber's cyclopedic medical dictionary* (19th ed.). Philadelphia: FA Davis.

Tappan, F. (1988). *Healing massage techniques: Holistic, classic, and emerging methods* (2nd ed.). Norwalk, CT: Appleton & Lange.

Tecklin, J. (1999). *Pediatric physical therapy* (3rd ed.). Philadelphia: Lippincott.

Thibodeau, G., & Patton, K. (2002). *The human body in health and disease* (3rd ed.). St. Louis: Mosby.

Umphred, D. (2001). *Neurological rehabilitation* (4th ed.). St. Louis: Mosby.

Weiss, R. (1999). *Physical therapy aide: A worktext* (2nd ed.). Albany: Delmar.

www.hhs.gov

IMPORTANT! READ CAREFULLY: This End User License Agreement ("Agreement") sets forth the conditions by which Thomson Delmar Learning, a division of Thomson Learning Inc. ("Thomson") will make electronic access to the Thomson Delmar Learning-owned licensed content and associated media, software, documentation, printed materials, and electronic documentation contained in this package and/or made available to you via this product (the "Licensed Content"), available to you (the "End User"). BY CLICKING THE "I ACCEPT" BUTTON AND/OR OPENING THIS PACKAGE, YOU ACKNOWLEDGE THAT YOU HAVE READ ALL OF THE TERMS AND CONDITIONS, AND THAT YOU AGREE TO BE BOUND BY ITS TERMS, CONDITIONS, AND ALL APPLICABLE LAWS AND REGULATIONS GOVERNING THE USE OF THE LICENSED CONTENT.

1.0 SCOPE OF LICENSE

1.1 <u>Licensed Content</u>. The Licensed Content may contain portions of modifiable content ("Modifiable Content") and content which may not be modified or otherwise altered by the End User ("Non-Modifiable Content"). For purposes of this Agreement, Modifiable Content and Non-Modifiable Content may be collectively referred to herein as the "Licensed Content." All Licensed Content shall be considered Non-Modifiable Content, unless such Licensed Content is presented to the End User in a modifiable format and it is clearly indicated that modification of the Licensed Content is permitted.

1.2 Subject to the End User's compliance with the terms and conditions of this Agreement, Thomson Delmar Learning hereby grants the End User, a nontransferable, nonexclusive, limited right to access and view a single copy of the Licensed Content on a single personal computer system for noncommercial, internal, personal use only. The End User shall not (i) reproduce, copy, modify (except in the case of Modifiable Content), distribute, display, transfer, sublicense, prepare derivative work(s) based on, sell, exchange, barter or transfer, rent, lease, loan, resell, or in any other manner exploit the Licensed Content; (ii) remove, obscure, or alter any notice of Thomson Delmar Learning's intellectual property rights present on or in the Licensed Content, including, but not limited to, copyright, trademark, and/or patent notices; or (iii) disassemble, decompile, translate, reverse engineer, or otherwise reduce the Licensed Content.

2.0 TERMINATION

2.1 Thomson Delmar Learning may at any time (without prejudice to its other rights or remedies) immediately terminate this Agreement and/or suspend access to some or all of the Licensed Content, in the event that the End User does not comply with any of the terms and conditions of this Agreement. In the event of such termination by Thomson Delmar Learning, the End User shall immediately return any and all copies of the Licensed Content to Thomson Delmar Learning.

3.0 PROPRIETARY RIGHTS

3.1 The End User acknowledges that Thomson Delmar Learning owns all rights, title and interest, including, but not limited to all copyright rights therein, in and to the Licensed Content, and that the End User shall not take any action inconsistent with such ownership. The Licensed Content is protected by U.S., Canadian and other applicable copyright laws and by international treaties, including the Berne Convention and the Universal Copyright Convention. Nothing contained in this Agreement shall be construed as granting the End User any ownership rights in or to the Licensed Content.

3.2 Thomson Delmar Learning reserves the right at any time to withdraw from the Licensed Content any item or part of an item for which it no longer retains the right to publish, or which it has reasonable grounds to believe infringes copyright or is defamatory, unlawful, or otherwise objectionable.

4.0 PROTECTION AND SECURITY

4.1 The End User shall use its best efforts and take all reasonable steps to safeguard its copy of the Licensed Content to ensure that no unauthorized reproduction, publication, disclosure, modification, or distribution of the Licensed Content, in whole or in part, is made. To the extent that the End User becomes aware of any such unauthorized use of the Licensed Content, the End User shall immediately notify Thomson Delmar Learning. Notification of such violations may be made by sending an e-mail to delmarhelp@thomson.com.

5.0 MISUSE OF THE LICENSED PRODUCT

5.1 In the event that the End User uses the Licensed Content in violation of this Agreement, Thomson Delmar Learning shall have the option of electing liquidated damages, which shall include all profits generated by the End User's use of the Licensed Content plus interest computed at the maximum rate permitted by law and all legal fees and other expenses incurred by Thomson Delmar Learning in enforcing its rights, plus penalties.

6.0 FEDERAL GOVERNMENT CLIENTS

6.1 Except as expressly authorized by Thomson Delmar Learning, Federal Government clients obtain only the rights specified in this Agreement and no other rights. The Government acknowledges that (i) all software and related documentation incorporated in the Licensed Content is existing commercial computer software within the meaning of FAR 27.405(b)(2); and (2) all other data delivered in whatever form, is limited rights data within the meaning of FAR 27.401. The restrictions in this section are acceptable as consistent with the Government's need for software and other data under this Agreement.

7.0 DISCLAIMER OF WARRANTIES AND LIABILITIES

7.1 Although Thomson Delmar Learning believes the Licensed Content to be reliable, Thomson Delmar Learning does not guarantee or warrant (i) any information or materials contained in or produced by the Licensed Content, (ii) the accuracy, completeness or reliability of the Licensed Content, or (iii) that the Licensed Content is free from errors or other material defects. THE LICENSED PRODUCT IS PROVIDED "AS IS," WITHOUT ANY WARRANTY OF ANY KIND AND THOMSON DELMAR LEARNING DISCLAIMS ANY AND ALL WARRANTIES, EXPRESSED OR IMPLIED, INCLUDING, WITHOUT LIMITATION, WARRANTIES OF MERCHANTABILITY OR FITNESS OR A PARTICULAR PURPOSE. IN NO EVENT SHALL THOMSON DELMAR LEARNING BE LIABLE FOR: INDIRECT, SPECIAL, PUNITIVE OR CONSEQUENTIAL DAMAGES INCLUDING FOR LOST PROFITS, LOST DATA, OR OTHERWISE. IN NO EVENT SHALL THOMSON DELMAR LEARNING'S AGGREGATE LIABILITY HEREUNDER, WHETHER ARISING IN CONTRACT, TORT, STRICT LIABILITY OR OTHERWISE, EXCEED THE AMOUNT OF FEES PAID BY THE END USER HEREUNDER FOR THE LICENSE OF THE LICENSED CONTENT.

8.0 GENERAL

8.1 <u>Entire Agreement</u>. This Agreement shall constitute the entire Agreement between the Parties and supercedes all prior Agreements and understandings oral or written relating to the subject matter hereof.

8.2 <u>Enhancements/Modifications of Licensed Content</u>. From time to time, and in Thomson Delmar Learning's sole discretion, Thomson Delmar Learning may advise the End User of updates, upgrades, enhancements and/or improvements to the Licensed Content, and may permit the End User to access and use, subject to the terms and conditions of this Agreement, such modifications, upon payment of prices as may be established by Thomson Delmar Learning.

8.3 <u>No Export</u>. The End User shall use the Licensed Content solely in the United States and shall not transfer or export, directly or indirectly, the Licensed Content outside the United States.

8.4 <u>Severability</u>. If any provision of this Agreement is invalid, illegal, or unenforceable under any applicable statute or rule of law, the provision shall be deemed omitted to the extent that it is invalid, illegal, or unenforceable. In such a case, the remainder of the Agreement shall be construed in a manner as to give greatest effect to the original intention of the parties hereto.

8.5 <u>Waiver</u>. The waiver of any right or failure of either party to exercise in any respect any right provided in this Agreement in any instance shall not be deemed to be a waiver of such right in the future or a waiver of any other right under this Agreement.

8.6 <u>Choice of Law/Venue</u>. This Agreement shall be interpreted, construed, and governed by and in accordance with the laws of the State of New York, applicable to contracts executed and to be wholly preformed therein, without regard to its principles governing conflicts of law. Each party agrees that any proceeding arising out of or relating to this Agreement or the breach or threatened breach of this Agreement may be commenced and prosecuted in a court in the State and County of New York. Each party consents and submits to the nonexclusive personal jurisdiction of any court in the State and County of New York in respect of any such proceeding.

8.7 <u>Acknowledgment</u>. By opening this package and/or by accessing the Licensed Content on this Web site, THE END USER ACKNOWLEDGES THAT IT HAS READ THIS AGREEMENT, UNDERSTANDS IT, AND AGREES TO BE BOUND BY ITS TERMS AND CONDITIONS. IF YOU DO NOT ACCEPT THESE TERMS AND CONDITIONS, YOU MUST NOT ACCESS THE LICENSED CONTENT AND RETURN THE LICENSED PRODUCT TO DELMAR LEARNING (WITHIN 30 CALENDAR DAYS OF THE END USER'S PURCHASE) WITH PROOF OF PAYMENT ACCEPTABLE TO THOMSON DELMAR LEARNING, FOR A CREDIT OR A REFUND. Should the End User have any questions/comments regarding this Agreement, please contact Thomson Delmar Learning at delmarhelp@thomson.com.

System Requirements:
Operating System: Microsoft®Windows® 98 or XP
Processor: Pentium or faster
Memory: 54 MB of RAM
Hard Disk Space: 20 MB or more
CD-ROM drive: 2x or faster

Setup Instructions:
Physical Therapy Assistant Exam Review should automatically open to a welcome and instructions for a Setup when disk is inserted into the CD-ROM. If the program does not open to a Welcome Screen please:

1. From the Start Menu, choose *RUN*
2. In the *Open* text box, enter **d:setup.exe,** then click *OK* (substitute the letter of your CD-ROM drive for d:
3. A Welcome screen and installation instructions will prompt you for setup.

8191ⴷ

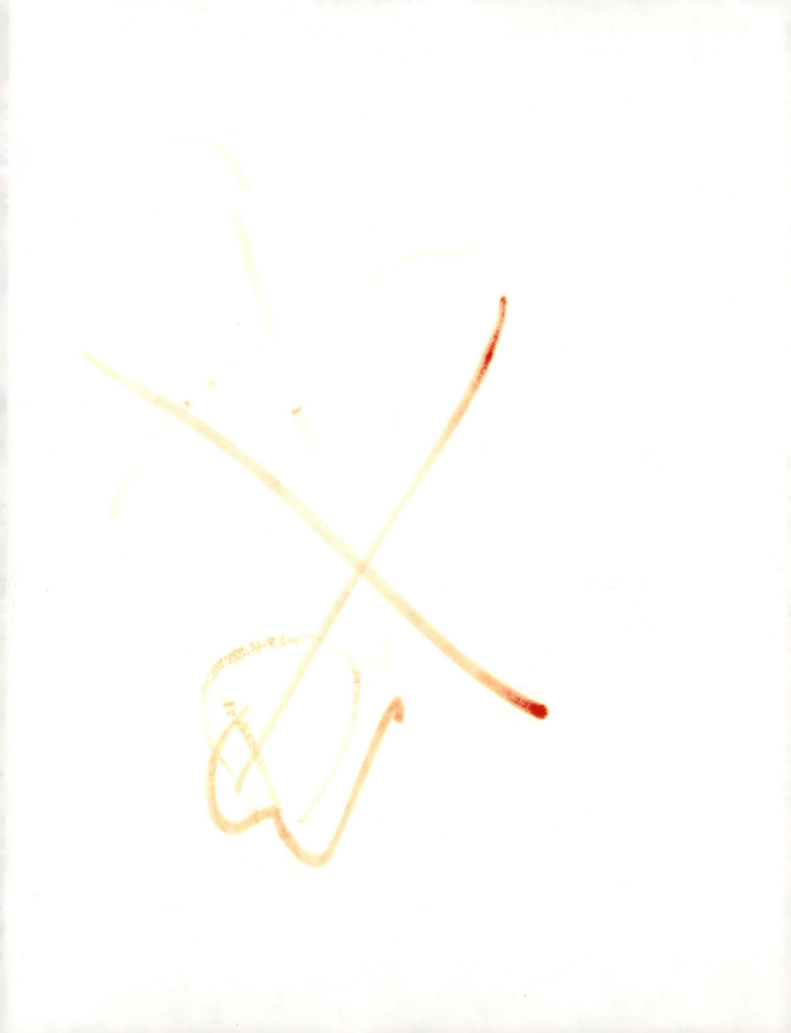

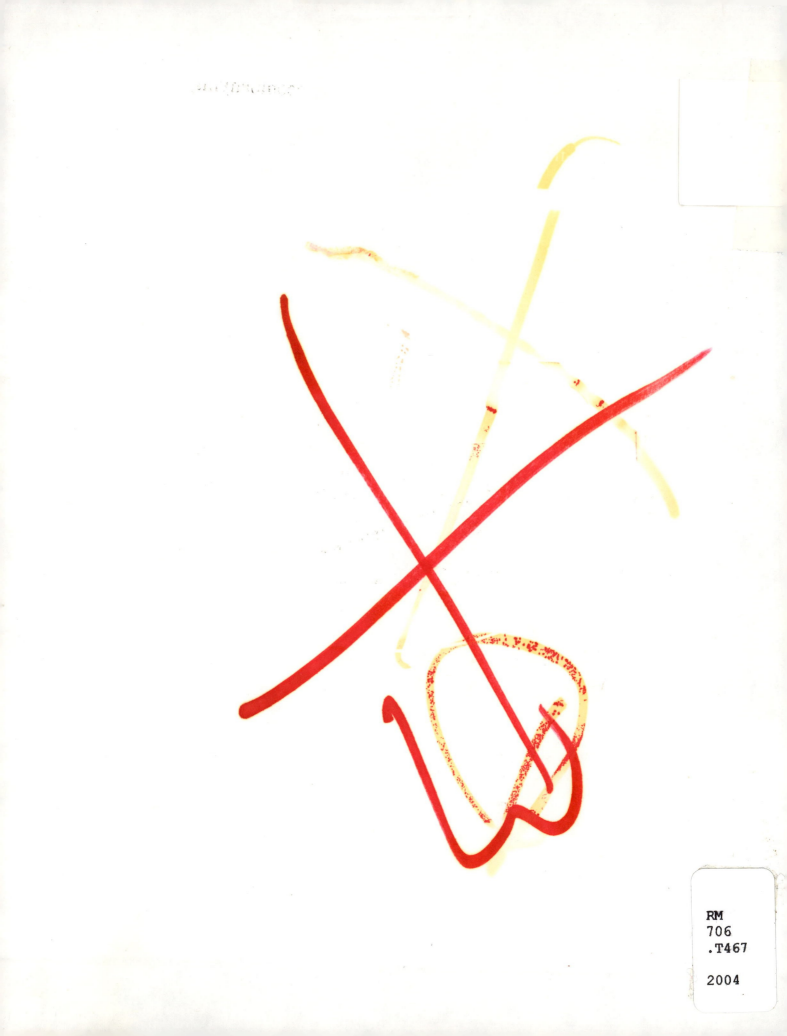

RM
706
.T467

2004